THE SUN SIGN DIET

THE
SUN SIGN
DIET

Gayle Black

Foreword by Ivan G. Black, M.D.

MACMILLAN PUBLISHING COMPANY
New York

COLLIER MACMILLAN PUBLISHERS
London

Macmillan Publishing Company
866 Third Avenue, New York, N.Y. 10022
Collier Macmillan Canada, Inc.

Library of Congress Cataloging-in-Publication Data
Black, Gayle.
    The sun sign diet.
    Bibliography: p. 447.
    Includes index.
    1. Reducing diets.   2. Nutrition.   3. Astrology and diet.   I. Title.
RM222.2.M5826   1986   613.2'5   85-23741
ISBN 0-02-511110-8

Macmillan books are available at special
discounts for bulk purchases for sales
promotions, premiums, fund-raising, or
educational use.

For details, contact:

Special Sales Director
Macmillan Publishing Company
866 Third Avenue
New York, N.Y. 10022

10 9 8 7 6 5 4 3 2 1

Designed by Nancy Sugihara

Printed in the United States of America

*To Margot and Shelly . . .
the brightest stars in my universe . . .
whose love and encouragement kept me going.*

CONTENTS

GEMINI 83

CANCER 119

LEO 157

VIRGO 193

LIBRA 231

SCORPIO 267

SAGITTARIUS 305

CAPRICORN 341

AQUARIUS 377

PISCES 411

FOREWORD

by Ivan G. Black, M.D.
(Dr. Black is no relation to the author.)

Gayle Black, the author of *The Sun Sign Diet,* has a fresh and simple answer to the question that is both the dieter's and the physician's major dilemma: If dieters are able to shed at least some unwanted pounds on a good diet, then why can't they manage to stay on the diet until they've lost the entire amount?

During my many years as a medical nutritionist, I have treated more than two thousand patients for the problem of obesity. It has been proven to me that there are many good diets, and that practically all of them have a chance of working if followed consistently. But for some heretofore mysterious reason, patients simply cannot hold to a diet for the time necessary to lose all the excess pounds.

Ms. Black gives us the reason. Diets designed with purely caloric or metabolic considerations in mind overlook several crucial elements: the dieter's particular temperament and particular personality traits—elements that have been part of the dieter's life from birth onward. A diet designed for all people, or for an "average" person, is doomed to failure from the start.

Like most doctors, I am familiar with the typical patterns of dieters. For the first few weeks they faithfully come to the office for their weekly visits. Usually there is an encouraging weight loss. Then, two or three weeks may pass without a visit. When the patients finally do return, they sheepishly tell of feeling too guilty and embarrassed to come in for the checkup and weigh-in because they broke the diet and regained some or all of the initial weight lost.

I have seen how various patients respond differently to my advice. Some patients demand that I yell at them like a drill sergeant when they do not achieve a good weight loss. It helps them do better the next week. Other patients want me to treat them as a kind and gentle grandfather would treat a beloved grandchild. This, I must state, is really asking a doctor to play God. How does one figure out how individual dieters prefer to be handled? Gayle Black eloquently and comprehensively communicates the diversity in individuals and delivers the proper approach for each dieter.

My experience in private practice has convinced me that some people do much better on simple repetitive diets, while others fail if they do not have variety in their prescribed dieting plan. Because *The Sun Sign Diet* addresses the needs peculiar to the individual, and allows for those occasional "bad days," the reducing diets presented here work. And they work without the dieter feeling deprived or frustrated . . . or guilty.

Besides being a nutritional doctor, I am also a sports medicine physician and have treated countless athletes for a myriad of injuries. Often, an athlete who is in superb condition will set a record one week, while the following week, under identical circumstances and for no apparent reason, he will perform way below the previous week's level.

Similarly, I have patients who lose five pounds one week, then eat the exact same food the following week and lose no weight at all. I have also noticed weeks when none of my patients has a good loss, as well as other weeks when everyone seems to be losing. In addition, I have found that there are certain days when many of my patients show an almost uniform twenty-point rise above their normal blood pressure, while on other days there may be a twenty-point drop.

With no clinical or pathological reasons to account for these phenomena, it was at this point that I acknowledged that there seemed to be a definite relationship between atmospheric conditions and the functioning of the human body. And I have seen many illnesses, from rheumatism to allergies, react to climate and season changes. Certainly, in my professional practice, I have noticed how the healing process is affected by changes in climatic conditions. And I have also noticed that at particular times of the year I hear from old patients who desire to start a diet again. Once again, supposedly inexplicable patterns emerge.

In addition to offering explanations for these atmospheric and climatic phenomena, *The Sun Sign Diet* offers detailed individual personality profiles and guidelines on individual eating habits. These can be a valuable aid to both patient and doctor.

Diets work, and they will work for a lifetime, if they take into consideration every aspect of a person's life-style. Rather than focusing merely on the effects of overeating, Gayle Black concentrates on the physical and emotional needs of individual dieters. I heartily applaud her for considering the whole person and whole life-style in her approach and in the preparation of these diets. *The Sun Sign Diet* provides nutritionally balanced foods with a high percentage of essential vitamins, minerals, carbohydrates, proteins, fats, and fiber.

I was delighted to support Gayle Black and to allow her to work with my patients, who filled out lengthy questionnaires as part of the documentation for her exhaustive research. I heartily recommend that dieters use the valuable information contained in *The Sun Sign Diet* to assist them in achieving successful weight reduction and in finding a lifetime maintenance program.

IVAN G. BLACK, M.D.

New York City
February 1986

AUTHOR'S PREFACE

Astrology is all about balance—balance on a cosmic scale. The astrologer attempts to bring you into balance with the changing universe. Astrology is, perhaps, the most natural of the sciences. It holds that nature, in spite of its excesses and mysteries, is, ultimately, order. The nature of the changing universe affects our lives. What happens up there has something to do with what happens down here.

It's all about cause and effect.

I was lucky. I was born under a star that guaranteed that I would find my way to astrology and health care. "Lucky," in this case, is a relative term.

In 1958, I almost died.

It was just after my sixteenth birthday when I came down with Guillain-Barré syndrome. You probably have never heard of it, and I pray you never get this vicious virus. It attacks the nervous system, the musculature, and the reflexes. In my case, it affected my eyes, and I could not see for months. After spending nine months in the hospital, the prognosis was still grim. My doctors did not believe I could ever regain control over my weak body.

They were wrong.

Fortunately more than one valid medical system has been created under the sun.

In the East, astrology is often an integral part of the diagnostic and healing process. Although our Western medical technology can help raise the standard of living and improve health care in the East, we should not discard ancient truths, truths that have survived and, indeed, flourished up until this day. We have a lot to learn from each other.

Balance.

When you come as close to the edge as I did, lying in that hospital bed, profound thoughts run through your mind. Modern medicine was doing as much as it could for me. But I knew there just had to be something else.

Yoga.

The year was 1959, and the yoga center my family brought me to was on the top floor of a seedy office building in some obscure section of New

York City. The setting was bleak. There was a candle and a mat on the floor. But there was also the illuminating aura of a beautiful swami. He claimed that even though this horrible Guillain-Barré syndrome had worked over my body pretty thoroughly, he could restore my health.

He was right.

But it wasn't easy. I threw myself into this ancient system and worked harder than I ever imagined I could. The stakes were high, but I had motivation: I was trying to regain control over my body, over my life.

And six months later I did.

An illness led me to yoga, and yoga would eventually lead me to astrology. It was a perfectly natural progression.

Cause and effect.

I became a yoga zealot. I had a mission. I wanted to tell the world about it; I wanted to repay this ancient system for giving me back my life. So I studied. I studied intensively for ten years, asked questions, and studied even more, until I became a certified yoga instructor.

My mind was transforming as well. So, while I continued my spiritual studies, I also worked toward a degree in psychology at Adelphi University. Armed with my credentials, I thought I had a lot of the answers.

But I still had a lot to learn.

I met another swami, who told me that if I was really serious about yoga and healing, I had to fill a void in my spiritual education: I had to learn astrology. And if I was ever to become a truly effective health-care provider, I had to move to an even higher level and study medical astrology.

From the moment we are born, our bodies and personalities are affected by the position of the sun. This influence will continue throughout our lifetimes. It may all be quite simple, but I have to admit that I'm still amazed by it, especially when I find myself accurately determining the life-style of a person just by referring to his or her natal chart.

When I was invited by the British government to share notes with some of their health-care professionals at the prestigious St. Thomas's Hospital in London, I rubbed elbows with doctors from every corner of the globe. I met doctors from India who not only had studied yoga, philosophy, and Eastern culture, but who also had trained at the finest medical schools in India. A great number of them, in fact many of the people I met there, were extremely knowledgeable about astrology. Many spoke of its great potential for unlocking medical mysteries.

My spiritual awareness paralleled my academic development. Not only was I in an environment that gave astrology its due, but, in my capacity as observer, I was able to see firsthand how powerful the stars really are. There are no accidents.

I spent a good deal of time with the patients at St. Thomas's. Examining their charts, the first thing I did was carefully note each patient's date of birth. Then, based on the patient's sun sign and transiting planets, I found that in most cases I could pick out obvious maladies or medical problems before even seeing them.

The hospital was my laboratory, and I became a researcher. I probed, I prodded, I questioned everyone and everything. I couldn't have been in a better place, with access to patients' histories and all the medical minds around me.

It all began to make sense. I kept clear and concise notes.

Why do we have periodic bouts with illness? Why do we have cyclical episodes at seven- and/or fourteen-year intervals?

Surgical patients provided revelation after revelation. I noted that if surgery was performed during a Mercury retrograde, the patient usually had to go back for more repair and further surgery. Years later, when I told a dear friend to delay stomach surgery for three weeks, she asked me why. When I told her that Mercury was in retrograde, she did what any rational person would do: She told me that I was crazy and that the surgeon, rather than the stars, had set the date for the operation. That was one time when I hated to be right, but three months later she again had surgery.

In medical astrology, the sun has rulership over different parts of the body. And I observed that Jupiter's position affected blood chemistry, usually showing up as diabetes and/or low blood sugar.

I also discovered the role the seasons played. Summer claimed higher birth weights, with June and July the top months. The preponderance of births occurred in June; the mortality rate was always higher in winter.

And, I wondered, was it a coincidence that many patients died at almost the same hour of the day that they were born?

Balance?

England also introduced me to the practice of homeopathy. The use of herbs and cell salts to treat certain diseases and conditions is an ancient and revered science in Europe. Thousands of years ago, the ancients discovered that there was a correlation between the herbs and cell salts, the disease, and the position of those planets whose course a doctor could follow.

Losing weight had always been a constant problem for me. Like so many people, I had spent years getting acquainted with diet doctors, clinics, and amphetamines. Struggling. Gaining, losing, succeeding—but ultimately failing. I lived for next week's diet encounter group. I tried everything.

Then something quite profound occurred to me.

I reasoned that if sun signs had so much power over health and well-being, why couldn't that power be harnessed to help one lose weight? And maintain weight?

So I decided to design my own diet. A diet based on the vitamins, minerals, nutrients, cell salts, and all the properties governed by my sun sign. A diet that would balance my system, that would, by the very foods I consumed, eliminate my constant battle of the bulge.

And it worked.

For the past several years I have been using the sun sign diet for my private clients, and, due to the success I've had with hundreds of people, I've gained a reputation as a weight-loss guru. But I'm not a magician, nor do I possess any supernatural powers. I can claim only a small part of the credit for my clients' success. After all, the stars impel—they do not compel. I have succeeded because I talk directly to people and address their special needs.

When I tell my Aries clients that they eat on the run, grabbing food on the way out the door, they are amazed at how much I know about them. When I tell Cancers that I understand their insatiable craving for sweets, and that it is not in their heads, they know that I am talking directly to them. And when I sympathize with the Virgos' picky eating habits and dislike of food additives, they are relieved to be talking to someone who really knows them.

Everybody is different. We each have to travel our own path to transformation. With this insight, a healthy, trimmer body is within everyone's reach.

Listen to your body. It not only knows what it wants, but it naturally wants what it needs.

Balance.

ACKNOWLEDGMENTS

I want to express my thanks to my creative Libra agent, Mel Berger of the William Morris Agency, whose enthusiasm, encouragement, and energy made the publication of this book possible.

To Hillel Black, a dynamic, positive Aries, and Arlene Friedman, a progressive, insightful Taurus, of the Macmillan Publishing Company, who first recognized the value of this work and its potential for helping individuals finally win the personal weight battle.

To my very special Gemini friend, Jill Cooper, whose extraordinary help, love, and talent guided me, and whose friendship sustained me.

To Marian Cohn, another creative, talented, Libra whose professional expertise assisted me in the preparation of this book.

To Robert Schaefer, who got me off "to a flying start," and to Barney Smith, Rachel Rothschild, Gill Ziff, Betty Rothbardt, Eileen Kurtis-Kleinman, Seymour Feig, Jane Dakin, Joel Black, Michael Cole, Diane Powers, Jackie Seplow, Florine Dorfmann, Dorothy and Morton Pavane, and Dr. Constance Buxer, who were always there when I needed them. And to my parents, Sylvia and Nathan Black.

To Joyce and Nick Monte, Keepers of the International Health and Beauty Spa at Gurney's Inn, Montauk, New York, who supported me in my research and allowed me to conduct hundreds of interviews with their approving guests. And similarly, to Frieda Eisenkraft, director and owner of the lovely Deerfield Manor, East Stroudsburg, Pennsylvania, who graciously opened her spa to my research.

To all of my friends, who understood my commitment to this project and who left me alone. To my clients, who waited so patiently for their appointments and who accepted the many cancellations. And to the thousands of wonderful people from continent to continent, who took the time and had the patience to fill out my lengthy questionnaires.

My heartfelt gratitude and appreciation to you all.

INTRODUCTION

If you want to lose 3 to 5 pounds a week, eat many of the foods you crave, binge on sinful foods four times a month, and dine in the most elegant gourmet restaurants, this diet is for you. The Sun Sign Diet has worked for thousands of people and is a revolutionary approach to dieting. The Sun Sign Diet helps you explore and understand how your own sexuality relates to overeating. It helps you recognize and change self-sabotaging habits. You will learn which food combinations best meet your personal weight loss goals. Whether at home, on the job, or dining with friends or business associates, the Sun Sign Diet helps you achieve your ideal weight without ever feeling hungry. You will learn the secrets to lifetime thinness.

Medical science has ascertained that everyone's chemical, mineral, and vitamin needs are different—and yet diets are prepared for the masses. But you and your body chemistry are not general; you're unique. For a diet to work, you must take into consideration your own specific needs. One of the wonder diets may work for you . . . another may not. If a diet does not meet your individual needs, it's ultimately destined to fail.

We each have our own astrological blueprint, a stamp of our special identity. A natal horoscope indicates to all individuals the weakest and strongest parts of their bodies. Certain health problems are peculiar to each zodiac sign. Have you ever noticed how some months you are more irritable or depressed, or totally incapable of following a diet? This can be attributed in part to the fact that we are all influenced by the rotation of the planets.

The sun is the most powerful force in the heavens; the controller of human vitality. Scientists who have studied its light report that all elements on earth are represented in solar radiation. It should come as no surprise, then that the sun signs are extremely significant in astrology; 75 percent of the time the sun sign will reign supreme over all the other planets in one's birth chart.

Over the years I have found that, invariably, people's behavior, desire, motivations, and eating habits fall into the twelve zodiac signs: Aries, Taurus,

Gemini, and so on. Each sign bestows upon you mental and emotional characteristics, even an individual body type and structure and specific psychological proclivities.

Human bodies basically come in twelve different shapes, represented by the twelve signs. Research has indicated that people of the same zodiac sign have a basic genetic form and a tendency to develop fat in the same localized areas. By recognizing the conscious and unconscious components of your psyche, you will be able to avoid the dieting pitfalls that have plagued you up to now. By studying those conscious and unconscious factors and understanding their importance in the dieting process, you can gain control of your eating for the first time. You will no longer be ruled by impulsive or compulsive eating. You will be in control.

Obviously, you have never found the ideal weight loss program. Most diets are not programmed for individual likes, dislikes, cravings, and pre-determined fondness for food.

With this diet you never have to fail again.

By combining a nutritionally sound approach to dieting, taking into consideration ancient therapies and modern medicine, I have designed a program that incorporates behavioral characteristics, personality traits, libidinal tendencies, and chemical and metabolic makeup. Now anyone, at any age, can maintain a healthy body weight and can expect to add years to their life, in addition to finally conquering their overweight.

Under your special sun sign, I describe your personality profile and eating habits, along with inherent behavior patterns that often spell success or failure in the dieting process. You will readily recognize yourself. (If you are on the "cusp," read the cusp section *in addition to your sun sign.*)

The reducing diets are designed to produce an average weight loss of 3 to 5 pounds per week. Included in each reducing diet is a list of supplemental vitamins and minerals which are vital to your well-being. Some of the reducing diets offer you choices in the foods you consume; others do not allow for any substitutions. You will note that each sun sign diet has carefully planned, specifically tailored reducing diets, some programmed for more than two weeks and some for as little as three days. Each diet is followed by special diet notes. A diet is only successful when the motivations, behavioral patterns and nutritional demands of each individual are considered, and these diets have been designed for your life-style and temperament and should not be interchanged with diets of other signs.

There are no transgressions when you follow the Sun Sign Diet. It is biochemically created to replenish your body with necessary cell salts, nutrients and fuel for optimum daily functioning.

Forget what you've experienced on all other diets: On the Sun Sign Diet, you will lose weight and feel more alive than you ever have before in your life. The Sun Sign Diet takes the total person approach and considers your total life-style.

I have included a lifetime maintenance food list, from which you will have the option to choose your own menus. To get started, included are two sample maintenance menus and instructions on handling maintenance planning, special-occasion dining, restaurant eating, and food shopping.

In fact, you don't even have to think of it as a diet. Instead, consider it a way of life. You will not have to subject yourself to any guilt for the inevitable cheating that can occur. Last, but not least, your diet takes into consideration the fact that you are human. And being human you have certain sensory cravings. On this diet, you will be allowed to eat many of the foods you crave. I have even included a binge day for each of you, allowing for the foods that give you that ultimate sense of satisfaction—the foods you crave.

How do I know what foods you crave?

It's written in the stars. Now get ready for that "heavenly body" you always dreamed about.

YOUR SUN SIGN

The stars determine the way you eat.

Aries	March 21–April 20	the hit-and-run eater
Taurus	April 21–May 21	the gourmet eater
Gemini	May 22–June 21	the erratic eater
Cancer	June 22–July 23	the emotional eater
Leo	July 24–August 23	the restaurant eater
Virgo	August 24–September 23	the analytical eater
Libra	September 24–October 23	the balanced eater
Scorpio	October 24–November 22	the sensuous eater
Sagittarius	November 23–December 21	the optimistic eater
Capricorn	December 22–January 20	the disciplined eater
Aquarius	January 21–February 19	the experimental eater
Pisces	February 20–March 20	the ambivalent eater

General Diet
and Maintenance
Guidelines for
All Sun Signs

The Importance of Drinking Water

To lose weight, you must drink eight glasses of water each day.

What Function Does Water Play in Your Body?

- Aids in chemical changes that take place in the body.
- Carries food to and wastes away from the body's cells.
- As urine, flushes away wastes of metabolism. Wastes increase during weight reduction, since fat is being broken down for energy.
- Used in digestion as saliva (about one gallon per day) and in digestive enzymes (about one-half gallon per day).
- Regulates your temperature by insulation or evaporation of perspiration.
- Maintains muscle tone. If you do not consume enough water, your muscles will eventually become soft and flabby.

How Can You Fight Fluid Retention?

The most important way is by drinking more water. This will produce more sodium excretion. *Drinking more water will actually prevent the body from storing it,* which the body does when insufficient amounts are taken in. This is a survival reaction of the body, since every necessary chemical reaction must occur in body fluid.

How Does Inadequate Water Intake Contribute to Obesity?

Your kidneys need water to filter the toxic wastes of normal metabolism. Without an adequate amount of water, the body produces less urine. For further self-preservation, the body then uses the liver to detoxify the blood. However, then one of the other functions of the liver—fat and carbohydrate metabolism—is neglected. This causes fat to be dumped into storage areas instead of being used for energy, and obviously results in further obesity.

Why Is Water Stressed in Preference to Other Fluids?

- Water, especially bottled water, has very few impurities.
- Most soda has sodium as a preservative, which, we know, is a cause of fluid retention.

- Soda gets us hooked on sweet drinks, and we then start craving other sweets.
- Coffee and tea are not as good as water due to their caffeine content, which stimulates the appetite.

Remember: All sun signs must follow water advice,
all signs need water,
so start drinking it now.

Daily Reminders

- You may healthfully repeat this diet until your desired weight is achieved.
- Drink no-sodium diet soda to insure better weight loss.
- Many times you will not find a beverage indicated after a meal in your own reducing diet. If not specifically listed, you may choose from the beverage list, noted in your "General Guidelines."
- You will note that I often do not include coffee with milk. Do not add milk to your coffee if not indicated; it will upset the enzyme action and you will not lose weight. Try to get used to drinking your coffee black, or switch to tea. Occasionally, when there is no fruit in your reducing diet meal, you may, if you absolutely must, have 2 oz. of milk in your coffee. Just remember, it will slow down your weight loss.
- Remember, *you must drink 8 glasses of water each day,* regardless of any other liquid you consume.
- Choose your condiments from the seasonings list.
- Consider the most likely times during the month that you are under stress emotionally or physically; plan for the "binge days" with that in mind. Women should consider their unique cravings during and before their menstrual cycle.
- Read all the notes, and your diet regimen before going to sleep each night, for education, motivation, and information.
- Awake with a positive approach, knowing that you are on your way to a heavenly body.
- At the conclusion of your individual Sun Sign Diet, carefully read "Maintaining Your Ideal Weight" for lifelong success and fitness.

Shopping List of Seasonings, Extracts, and Diet Aids

BEVERAGES

Black coffee (regular and decaffeinated)
Tea
Herbal teas
Iced tea sweetened with Nutrasweet
Club soda (no-sodium brand)
Diet soda (no-sodium brand) 3 cans per day

Evian	Perrier (no-sodium brand)
Mineral water	Seltzer (no-sodium brand)

Remember: All carbonated sodas contain additives that make for the carbonation. It is far better and will ensure better weight loss if you drink just plain water.

CONDIMENTS

Apple-cider vinegar	Horseradish*
Bouillon cubes*	Lemon juice (concentrate or fresh)
Diet jelly*	Lipton Trim soups (2 per day)
Diet margarine*	Pritikin 2-calorie no-oil salad dressing
D-Zerta diet gelatin	Sugar substitute (Sweet 'n Low)
Herb-Ox low-sodium soups	

*Note: These items are allowed only when indicated on your diet.

HERBS AND SPICES

Basil	Kelp
Cayenne pepper	Marjoram
Chervil	Oregano
Chives	Parsley
Cinnamon	Pepper
Curry powder	Peppercorns
Dill	Peppermint
Garlic	Sage
Ginger	Thyme

DIET AIDS

Glucomannan—2 capsules a half hour before meals, total six capsules daily. Please refer to your individual Sun Sign chapter for important information about Glucomannan, a dietary fiber that you may choose to use as a supplement to your reducing diet. And remember: 8 glasses of water a day.

When reading about the behavior patterns of your unique sun sign, there may be statements with which you disagree. Please keep in mind the following: Often, many of our true (subconscious) feelings never surface. Allow yourself to be free and open, and understand that not all desires and tendencies are—for many individual reasons—manifested on a conscious level.

Maintenance Eating Hints

Being fat is not an accident; it is a life-style. To lose weight permanently and to keep it off, a diet must fit your life-style, make you feel good, give you energy, and allow you to exist on this planet without feeling deprived.

You will note in your individual sun sign chapter that I have listed special maintenance foods. These foods are governed by your sun sign, and I suggest that you choose as many foods as possible from that list. I also include a 2,000-calorie sample maintenance diet for your individual sun sign, and I suggest that you use your own creativity to design your own maintenance menus. But first you will need to determine the number of calories per day needed for maintenance, based on the following, generally accepted equations for measuring the calorie-to-weight ratio. Multiply your *ideal* weight by:

13, if sedentary
15, if moderately active
20, if vigorously strenuous

Example:
Ideal weight 120 pounds, sedentary = 1,560 calories/day

Purchase a good calorie book. For those of you who will be counting carbohydrates, you will have to test out your maintenance carbo level, which is usually about 100 grams.

After you have reached your goal weight, weigh yourself every three or four days. If you have gained 3 pounds, resume your diet regimen with any day of your Sun Sign reducing diet. If you have gained more than 5 pounds, begin again with Day One of your Sun Sign reducing diet.

How can you allow for bingeing while on maintenance eating? If you allow yourself a daily calorie count of 1,500 calories, program it for the week (i.e., 1,500 calories × 7 = 10,500 calories per week). If you know that you want to splurge for a certain meal, be sure to deduct the calorie count of that meal from the total weekly calorie allowance. In this way you can adjust your eating over the entire week and you will not have that starved feeling. NOTE: Never plan less than 1,000 maintenance calories per day.

Is it harder for some people to lose weight than it is for others? Yes. There are many differences in metabolism, often influenced by an individual's sun sign. That is why, for the very first time, you will succeed on this diet where other diets have failed. Each reducing diet is designed to address the chemical makeup and uniqueness of your sun sign.

Restaurant Eating Tips

Your boss asks you to entertain a client at one of the finer Italian restaurants in town, or your girlfriends plan a baby shower at a quaint French restaurant. For many dieters, eating out is their downfall on an otherwise successful diet. Observe the following guidelines and you will not have to worry about enjoying the pleasures of a good restaurant meal.

General Restaurant Eating Guidelines

- Always order water the moment you sit down. Order a pitcher of water and start drinking. Have at least two glasses.
- If you wish to order wine, you may. If you choose not to, order coffee or tea when others order their alcoholic beverages. Don't worry, they will not think you are strange. Many people do this, and the caffeine in the tea or coffee will give you a lift. If you wish to limit your caffeine intake, order club soda. NOTE: This is all done to keep you away from the rolls or garlic bread.
- Ask that dressing not be added to your salad. You may always use lemon and/or vinegar.
- Request whatever you want prepared the way you want it. Don't accept fried when broiled or steamed is your desire. Don't be embarrassed. You are there to be served.
- Remember, the smaller the portion, the more you'll lose.

Your individual sun sign chapter includes restaurant eating menus that reflect the foods you like. Follow the suggestions in "Restaurant Eating" in your chapter, as well as those that appear below, and you will enjoy dining out without jeopardizing your successful dieting and maintenance eating.

Do's and Don'ts

CHINESE RESTAURANTS

- Do not allow the chef to use MSG (monosodium glutamate) in your food.
- Do not order anything prepared with cornstarch.
- Do not order anything fried in batter.
- Do order anything poached, steamed, stir-fried, or simmered in natural juices.
- Do drink lots of tea.
- Do order white rice.

ITALIAN RESTAURANTS

- Do not order heavy cheese sauces or dishes.
- Do not order anything swimming in oil or butter.
- Do not order fried food.
- Do order food in a light tomato sauce, or prepared with garlic and/or wine.
- Do eat a small portion of pasta.
  NOTE: When ordering pasta, order only linguine, capellini, or fettucine.

AMERICAN RESTAURANTS

- Do not order casseroles (they are filled with all sorts of no-no's).
- Do not order food breaded and fried.
- Do not order food prepared with mayonnaise.

JAPANESE RESTAURANTS

- Do not order anything fried.

All About "Cusp Periods"

If your birthday falls during one of the cusp periods listed below, you will have planetary influences from two signs, or as we say in astrology, you are "on the cusp" of two signs.

Aries and Taurus	Libra and Scorpio
April 19–22	October 22–25

Taurus and Gemini May 20–24	Scorpio and Sagittarius November 20–24
Gemini and Cancer June 20–23	Sagittarius and Capricorn December 19–23
Cancer and Leo July 22–25	Capricorn and Aquarius January 19–22
Leo and Virgo August 22–26	Aquarius and Pisces February 18–22
Virgo and Libra September 21–25	Pisces and Aries March 18–22

Since your eating behavior will be influenced by the influence of the cusp period, you will want to read about this special period *in addition* to reading your sun sign chapter. Most people are familiar with their zodiac sun sign, but even those people born on the cusp are often unacquainted with what that means. According to traditional astrology, the cusp is the twenty-four-hour period in which the planets in the solar system move into a new position in the zodiac; thus you are receiving influences from the new ruling sun sign as well as some influences from the old. For example, on April 21 the zodiac sun sign moves from Aries to Taurus. That day is called the "cusp of Aries–Taurus," and while anyone born on that day is a Taurus, many Aries traits will be evident in personality and eating habits.

Many astrologers, myself included, believe that cusp influences are evident not only in individuals born on the exact day of the cusp, but also in anyone born during the few days of the *cusp period.* My observations of the food personalities of these people indicate that the cusp period actually seems to begin about two to three days before the end of one sun sign and to extend two days into the beginning of the next.

What does this mean to you, practically speaking? If you were born during the first two days of one sun sign *or* the last two or three days of the next, your personality will display a blend of traits from both signs on your cusp, and I would suggest that you read the personality profiles for both sun signs in this book to get a complete picture of your own food personality.

However, although your birthday falls in the "cusp period," *you only have claim to one sun sign,* as shown in "Your Sun Sign" at the beginning of the book. The sun is by far the largest member of the solar system— about 740 times more massive than its nine major planets combined, and ten times wider than the largest planet, Jupiter. The sun's rays are the strongest in the solar system, and therefore your sun sign (as determined by the position of the sun in relation to the earth on the day you were born) *always* rules about 80 percent of your health, behavior, and nutritional and chemical makeup. It is for this reason that you must follow the diet and nutrition plans designed specifically for your sun sign.

Aries-Taurus

You are not as impulsive as your Aries friends, but when it comes to eating you will dive into the unknown. You often eat with quick Arien fervor, downing a traditional meat-and-potatoes bill of fare.

You do not consider yourself an epicure, but do know that when you are hungry, you want to eat. Right then and there! And it better be hearty food. No delicate little tidbits for you. Remind yourself to pace your eating . . . a little slower, please.

Taurus–Gemini

You have much less of a weight problem than your Taurus friends. Thank your lucky stars that your Gemini influence keeps you juggling three or four projects at once, running from place to place, while simultaneously speaking on the phone, and writing poetry or prose. Your quick mind is always in high gear, which acts to motivate your body to do the same. Fortunately, all this physical and mental activity keeps the calories burning.

Gemini–Cancer

Somehow you wonder how come all your Gemini friends are so thin and you are not. Well, my friend, while blessed with the sensitivity, compassion, and nurturing traits of your Cancer mates, you also share their desire for ice cream, sweets, and alcohol. The Gemini part of you just likes to pick at food here and there, so you prefer to snack your way through life. However, as you already know, all this snacking usually adds up to many, many pounds. You are usually the one that says, "But I hardly ever eat a decent meal."

Cancer–Leo

You love to look great, my Leo friend, but somehow you find every time you have an emotional problem to solve, it is usually over some wonderfully reassuring goody. You waiver between titillating your taste buds Cancer-style, and your desire for thinness, Leo-style. You often are heavier one month, then thinner the next. Looking spectacular is important to you, and so you have often solved the problem at the outset by stocking your closet with outfits in two or three different sizes. Take heart, my cusp friend: Leo wants center stage, so diet you will.

Leo–Virgo

You have much more control than your social, partying Leo friends. Your desire to have a perfect body (Virgo) and your feeling that you can "never be too rich or too thin" (Leo) keeps you on the straight and narrow path of forever dieting. However, because you are a social butterfly and feel that eating is a very warm, wonderful experience to be shared with friends, you can easily give yourself the excuse to digress from your diet. You wonder how you could have deviated from your diet when you had such good intentions. But never fear, with this cusp influence you can get yourself back in line with your Virgo whip.

Virgo–Libra

You seek food that is nutritious, wholesome, and natural. No additives or preservatives for my September friends. But your Libra influence also demands that it be served in the most attractive, delicate manner. Unlike the typical Virgo, your Libra influence has presented you with a sweet tooth, often sabotaging your good diet intentions. Fortunately, however, Virgo puts you back on track before too much damage has been done. The demands of Virgo perfection coupled with the Libra demand for beauty adds up to one cusp personality that will always make dieting a priority.

Libra–Scorpio

The Libra side of you has confidence that if you cheat today you will make up for it tomorrow. You can also count on the fact that Scorpio will not tolerate your losing control for too long. "Fat today, thin tomorrow" is a slogan you know well, for both Libra and Scorpio love to indulge themselves. Luckily, the more evenly balanced Libra eating pattern will act to modify the sometimes extreme Scorpio influence. For this reason you can usually count on being a winner at the losing game.

Scorpio–Sagittarius

You are not as controlled as your Scorpio friends, but neither are you as extreme. However, carefree, fun-loving Sagittarius is not the best influence on your dieting habits. If you have been telling yourself that you will start your diet tomorrow, blame Sagittarius. But you can always count on that Scorpio control and determination to surface when you need it. That time is now, with your Sun Sign Diet.

Sagittarius–Capricorn

You have more control over your diet than your Sagittarian friends seem to have, so consider yourself fortunate at having been born on this cusp. The carefree attitude of Sagittarius has been tempered by the ever-driving, goal-oriented Capricorn tenacity, and you will feel guilty when you cheat. That's Capricorn telling you that you will never walk the path to success that way. So you are caught between hoping your diet problem will take care of itself, and really knowing that nothing will change if you are not the master of your eating destiny. With regard to dieting, you often take a "light view of a weighty subject."

Capricorn–Aquarius

This can be a most beneficial cusp. The Capricorn part of you is "determined" to lose weight and will persevere, and the Aquarius part of you is often too involved with work and projects to think about food. In addition, you are one cusp that is usually "nutritionally savvy" and can accomplish anything you set your mind to do (even if it means eating with chopsticks).

Aquarius–Pisces

Even though your eating habits change from day to day and seem a bit unusual to most people, you are still able to keep your weight under control. However, there is no one more vulnerable than you to putting on the pounds when you have been wounded in love. Your appetite as well as your figure is often symbolic of cupid's bow.

Pisces–Aries

It does not take you as long to program yourself to diet as some of your Piscean colleagues, and when your mind is made up, you actively put your energy into a positive direction. You want a diet that is easy to follow, very portable, and quick to yield good results. You are not likely to allow outside influences to sabotage your diet regimen, and have been known to enlist the support of others. You are aggressive in your pursuit of a "heavenly body."

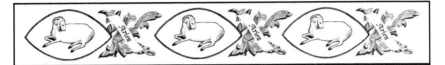

ARIES

March 21–April 20

The Aries
Personality

"I'm hungry—now."

You are the first sign of the zodiac, Aries, and like your sign, want to be first in everything. You are one of the most energetic, ambitious people around, a natural leader and a born competitor. You are adventurous and courageous, and you love a challenge more than anything. You confidently throw yourself into whatever it is you are doing at the moment the way a fearless child jumps into the deep end of a pool, shouting, "Last one in is a rotten egg!" You are a marvelous PR person and can sell the Brooklyn Bridge to your best friend twice over in one week.

Well, I can count on you, spontaneous, self-starting Aries, to be the first to try a new diet, too. In fact, with typical enthusiasm, you will fire up your friends to do the same. The difference is, they will probably finish the diet while you somehow will get lost along the way. But not this time: You know when you have something good.

Impetuous and impulsive, you are great at new beginnings, but fall short on follow-through. The eternal, cosmic infant, you want what you want when you want it, and you want it *now.* Instant gratification. Indeed, one of the main reasons you put on weight so easily is that you tend to grab the first thing you see to satisfy your hunger. Furthermore, you eat so quickly that your brain does not have time to signal when you are full. And while you eat—and act—in haste, you repent at leisure. You lose interest in most diets quickly because of their duration. Like the great humorist Mark Twain, who remarked how easy it is to stop smoking (he said that he himself stopped a thousand times), you can start a new diet every day of your life.

Sticking with it seems to be the only thing you are capable of putting off until tomorrow.

Your eating habits—or lack of them—contribute to your weight problems, immoderate Aries. There is no particular set pattern to the time of day or night you eat. You eat when you are happy and you eat when you are sad. You go through phases when you eat only peanut butter and cucumber sandwiches every day for three weeks, or follow semistarvation diets, such as eating only grapes one day and drinking only packaged liquid diets the next. You rarely just sit down to eat a meal, however. Driven and constantly on the go, you cannot seem to do one thing at a time. When you are eating, you are usually busy doing something else—watching television, talking on the phone, reading, working, or even walking. In fact, most of your food is consumed on the run—in your car, at your desk, or simply standing up—probably right in front of the refrigerator door. Depending on just how busy you are, you may nibble on one of your all-time favorites —cheese and fruit washed down with some wine. Of course, when you have a good spurt of energy going, dynamic Aries, you are not exactly what I would call a gentle picker, anyway. Wolfing food is more your style. It is so much more gratifying. One Aries friend of mine, watching me eat pizza with a knife and fork, finally lost what little patience he had, told me to put down those damn utensils, and proceeded to give me a lesson in eating pizza he-man-style—the only style the macho male Aries knows. (Even you female Aries have an inborn sense of how to succeed in a man's world.) He rolled up his wedge-shaped slice by cracking it lengthwise in the middle, and with the sides all curled up, he stuffed practically the entire slice into his mouth. Four or five bites later it was all gone.

You give new meaning to the term fast food, Aries. You love takeout foods because you can get to them quickly. But shopping malls and street fairs are your true delight. Designed for the eat-and-run Arien mentality, they offer the genuine moveable feast. To your heart's content, restless one, you can travel from one stand to the next, indiscriminately sampling all the foods you love to eat. A couple of chili dogs, anything Chinese, pita bread filled with falafel and hot sauce—the more spicy the better to titillate your taste buds, fiery Aries. You are crazy for pasta regardless of its shape (you will even finish off a bowl of spaghetti *after* it gets cold). In fact, all starchy products gratify your appetite; potato chips and pretzels in a plastic bag you can tear open with your teeth are an Arien specialty. There is something fantastic about those Aries teeth: You can even open beer bottles with them.

You also do not like to be caught without food. First of all, it seems your stomach gives you little advance notice that it is getting empty. All of a sudden the electrical impulses in your brain sound the alarm: I am starving.

I must eat. *Now.* So you have learned to be prepared wherever you are. You carry immersion heaters when you travel and store little CARE packages in your pockets and handbags. (One Aries friend of mine traveling south of the border was forced to turn over a half-eaten bag of cookies, two tins of sardines, and three flip-top cans of mushrooms to customs.) Taking such precautions eliminates the need for room service (you cannot stand to wait for the order to be sent up) and the need to hang around the dining room until it opens at seven in the morning. And if you wake up hungry in the middle of the night, you know you will not starve to death.

Amazing as it seems, I have seen you forget to eat, hardworking one. You are the classic workaholic and will sacrifice sleep as well as sustenance in the name of your ambitions. With your me-first attitude, you love to conquer, and you love to play the game of life called change. Nothing is so frustrating to you as boredom, which plays havoc with any Aries diet. You like to be in high gear, always doing something, always finding some new avenue to explore.

Please learn to slow down just a little, Aries. Even walking, you look like a charging ram, with your head leading your feet by about six inches. Many times you have gone to the refrigerator to refuel yourself, when in fact what you have needed was a good night's sleep. Give in, exuberant one. Food cannot recharge your ever-running battery when you are suffering from exhaustion. Sometimes you just have to let that motor of yours rest. Try to slow the pace of your life just a bit—especially at mealtimes. Try to make your meal last at least twenty minutes. I know that is a monumental task for you, Aries. Take it as a challenge. Realize you are not going to starve to death. Your need for immediate satisfaction and your natural impulse to live for the moment makes you eat sometimes as though there were no tomorrow. Well, there is. And you will live to see it, impatient Aries, even if your stomach rumbles now and again.

You like to be in control—so take control of your eating habits, and you will be well on your way to physical fitness. I know you have tried out the herbal wraps, the saunas, the stretchers, the ointments, the waist trimmers —all those gimmicks that promise to take off ten pounds by yesterday. And you have already discovered they don't work. You need to spend some of that pent-up, restless energy of yours exercising daily. It is natural and even soothing for you to be physically active, Aries. Indeed, your sign is the number-one health-spa-goer. Aerobics and weight training are excellent outlets for your low-tolerance irritability, anger, and frustration. Do whatever you need to do to release energy—play a competitive game of sports, start a new hobby, make love. Or just close your door and yell and scream if you have to. It is less costly in calories than raiding the refrigerator.

When you have gained too much weight, Aries, I know you will get right in there and find a solution. You are a special breed. A born winner. Strong-willed and positive-thinking, you know how to make your dreams come true. You generate your own good luck and never have to say "give me a break." You have the phoenix-like ability to come back from defeat. No sooner have you broken one diet than you start once again on another. And I am pretty sure of the reason you never see one through to the end: It is difficult for you to relinquish control and submit to a given regimen.

Well, independent one, we are going to harness some of that indefatigable will of yours to break the old patterns. The Sun Sign Diet I have prepared for your success leaves no room for your control, Aries, but it will give you the control over your body that you have always wanted. And it will not take long. You will have the most instant results possible—if you follow the routine.

The challenge is to stay with the diet with the same enthusiasm, concentration, and focus until the end. You will have to be willing to give up one form of control for another. You will, in fact, become a leader in this manner. Remember, my forceful friend, I do know you and your biochemical needs as well as you might know yourself. This is a revolutionary approach to successful dieting, and I expect you to be the pioneer who proves it.

Sexual Appetite

Passionate Aries, so much of your overeating is done out of anger, impatience, or sheer physical frustration. Bursting with fire, you have enormous energy and certainly a need to express it physically, whether in the bedroom or the gymnasium. When you fail to find a physical outlet for your urges, you often wind up looking into the empty bottom of an ice cream container. Well, it is one way to cool off—but very fattening.

You need a mate who can take the heat, not one who tries to handle your fiery sexual nature by dampening it. Hot-blooded Aries, you demand adventure and romantic excitement at all times in a relationship. You expect to hear bombshells, or fireworks at least, every time you kiss and embrace. You need a partner who understands your strong sexual drives and who can match your physical strength and endurance, as well as your lusty imagination. You also want a lover who knows how to fan the flames of passion and who will understand that your sudden rages and outbursts are not to be taken seriously. You just need to blow off smoke once in a while and to maintain a bit of high drama in your life. Life is so boring without it, and boredom drives you directly to the icebox.

To be really comfortable in a relationship, you do need to feel you are in control, headstrong one. Pick lovers who will allow you this freedom. Just let them know upfront who you are, and let them decide for themselves if they like you the way you are or if they don't. Come on, Aries, I know you are never shy about your personal projection.

For all your swagger and bluster, you can be as ingenuous as a child, and you need affection like one as well. Without it, you feel starved and look for (oral) gratification where you can find it. As large as your ego appears to be already, narcissistic Aries, it nevertheless demands constant feeding. Your mate will need to have the patience and understanding of a saint to survive your sometimes self-centered, self-absorbed ways, and still have love left over to give you the emotional nourishment you require.

Open, honest, earnest, and direct as you are, Aries, let's face it: You are not an easy person to live with. Sometimes you can come on like a ten-ton truck of bricks. You are flirtatious and often like the chase more than the catch. You need to feel wanted, but are not always so demonstrative with your own affections. You expect total trust and freedom from your mate but won't grant your partner the same rights. The slightest digression on his or her part, and you will be out the door. You often hurt people with your tactless way of speaking. You are hot-tempered and easily and quickly agitated and irritated. You demand complete allegiance from your partner, whom you expect to share your loves and hates with equal conviction and vehemence. And you absolutely, positively must be in control. Sexually and otherwise, you can be very dominating, even domineering. Unassertiveness is not one of your native afflictions, pushy Aries.

Why do we put up with you? Well, you do have this childlike charm, which is rather irresistible at times. You may easily fly off the handle, but you are quick to forgive and forget. You don't hold many grudges for long, and no one can accuse you of talking behind another's back. Your motto is, "What you see is what you get," and your straightforward, blunt manner can be a totally refreshing experience. You can also be very entertaining. Your desire for adventure, your spontaneous, exuberant nature make life with you exciting and unpredictable. And that kind of life has its definite appeal in an otherwise humdrum, workaday world.

To make relationships work for you, Aries, keep communications open in that forthright manner you have mastered so well. Frequent trips to the cupboard are a sure sign that you are keeping things bottled up, whether your sexual desires or your anger. If you don't already know this about yourself, recognize that you are a very physical person; then speak out your needs. Don't expect your lover to read your mind. Communicate about the fact that you appreciate a partner who is as uninhibited as you are, someone ready for thrills. As for your anger, recognize it to be an outlet for mental health. But learn to practice laughter afterward. Your anger and impatience stem from your inability to control every situation. Recognize that your need to command puts your entire physiology into a constant state of flight. When you let go a bit, you will discover you are calmer and steadier emotionally—and just as important and powerful, even though you have relinquished some hold. Also, try to broaden your outlook, to be less self-absorbed. Try giving a bit more. Your creative energy is an inspiration for us all.

And take the time to learn what really makes your lover tick. You tend to look at a cover over and over and think you have read the book. Learn how to peruse the inside pages. You may be happy to discover the gratification for your efforts to be quite instantaneous.

One final note about gratification, desirous Aries. Let your lovers know that a lot of foreplay is not your cup of tea. Eager Ariens like to get right down to serious business when it comes to lovemaking. I believe what actually works best in bed for you is pleasing yourself, Aries. Make an agreement with your partner that you will each occasionally be responsible for your own orgasms and pleasure, taking turns. That way you can be sure to find your fulfillment in the bedroom, and not in the kitchen.

If no lover is around, don't worry, Aries. Just take up some new challenge and revel in the natural high you get from initiating action. It's your own special kind of orgasm, and very low in calories.

Eating/Entertaining at Home

Aries, you are a showman. You love to entertain because you do it so well. You can pull off a big bash with great panache, though Lord knows how you do it, inattentive to small details as you are. The night before a dinner party will usually find you in a frenzy of last-minute shopping, cooking, and cleaning. Anyone else would be bushed, but you go on cooking up a storm. You will set your table with equal flair, rolling napkins and displaying food in enterprising ways. Whatever you cannot accomplish in the night, you will finish at the crack of dawn. Thank goodness for pressure cookers and microwave ovens, speedy cooking devices you couldn't live without.

You are a vivacious host and love companionship at your table. You tend to invite lots of guests at a time because you hate to think someone is left out. And as long as company lets you talk, garrulous Aries, there will be no shortage of lively conversation at your dinner party.

Neither will there ever be a shortage of food. Heaven forbid your guests should go home starving. Cheese platters and fruit trays and dips, dips, dips will abound. *Two* entrées, Aries? I guess it is your enthusiasm to please everyone's palate. What saves *you* from overeating on these occasions is that you are too busy attending to your company to give much attention to your own needs.

You do enjoy making others happy, but you alays set up your entertaining so that you are a winner. One Aries acquaintance of mine prepares quiche quite well, and knows it. Whenever she has company coming, she calls them ahead of time and says, "I am making quiche Saturday night and would like to know how you would like it, with mushrooms, spinach, anchovies, or broccoli?" In this way, she typically retains "control," making what she does best but allowing her guests to feel the choice was theirs.

And when it comes to cooking, you do have chutzpah, Aries. You like to serve foods you are sure no one else has in quite the same combination. Prosciutto with garlic toast or chocolate-dipped orange slices, for instance. You will scurry about and chatter so quickly, your guests will just assume they didn't catch your words correctly, and the tasty dish won't give your cooking secrets away.

Food Shopping

Nothing would make an Arien happier in a supermarket than to roller-skate down the aisles, buying food on impulse. Any other way you regard as a waste of time. Put you in front of a slow checkout counter, and we can watch your hair catch fire.

You rarely scrutinize your pantry before leaving home, nor do you shop with a list. You tend to overbuy because you have no idea what foods you really need and you select according to whim. Convenience foods are a priority, of course, and a nice-looking package that will stack or store with ease is a winner for fast-paced Aries. And if it is a type of food that will travel well—in the car, on a bicycle, or walking down the street—it is a natural to find its way into your shopping cart.

You are a fool for a good sale, Aries. Your body charges with electricity at the word, and you are out the door in minutes. When you're preparing for special company, however, the sky is the limit.

Your shopping choices are often motivated by the latest television ads you have seen. An advertised item may catch your eye, and you quickly snatch it from the shelf. "Are you hungry?" you ask yourself. Of course you are. You are hungry from the moment you wake up.

Due to your erratic purchasing style, there are some weeks when you come home to find six jars of ketchup in the pantry. That's okay, you rationalize: It won't spoil, and someday you will use it up. But you are not big on preparing leftovers, Aries, and the perishables you overbuy often go to waste. For the sake of your diet, Aries, shop for food only after eating a full meal. It can save you money as well as pounds.

While we are on the subject of shopping, let me pass on a helpful hint. Aries women are convinced that clothes shopping is the best way to eliminate the need for a shrink...and it is cheaper in the long run. I would suggest that when those pent-up angers, energies, and frustrations just get too much for your body, Aries, grab your credit cards and say, "Charge!" It is cheaper in calories, too.

Social Dining

When dining out, Aries will choose a restaurant for its quality, portion size, and exotic fare. You love ethnic foods, and the spicier the better. You also appreciate offbeat diners with a great short-order cook. Ambiance is important but not primary.

You would also never return to a restaurant where the service had been bad. When you are hungry, you want to eat—pronto. You will not wait on line even for the best restaurant in town, and you like something served to you the moment you are seated. A waiter who rushes over with fresh breadsticks, crudities, and water can expect a lavish tip from Aries. But if the food is not brought in a reasonable amount of time, you will not tip at all. It is black or white and no in-betweens for you, Aries. You get irritable and impatient waiting long periods between courses, especially since you have probably finished all the food on your plate in record time, long before everyone else, so the waiting seems longer.

Above all, hungry Aries, you must avoid buffet-style or smorgasbord restaurants. They are the downfall of any Aries diet. When you see the cornucopia of food on display, no matter how hard you try, you will wind up gorging on the delectables. Yes, even if the foods you take are allowed on your diet, you cannot be trusted to stop at one helping. While everyone else is enjoying their first, you will be on to seconds and thirds. Face it, Aries, your excitement, fast-paced eating habits, and hearty appetite are no match for the temptations of a restaurant buffet.

Special-Occasion Dining

Always seeking new adventure, you like to take unique vacations. Strolling through the markets of Marrakesh, your senses are captivated by the strange new smells of local foods. You just *must* try that concoction of halvah, honey, almonds, and coconut topped with bittersweet chocolate. Or sailing on a Venetian canal, vendors everywhere you turn whet your appetite with their fabulous ice cream sandwiches, called *biscotti.* Well, how can you leave Italy without trying one?

I don't expect you to curb your social life or your taste for adventure, Aries. Just try to learn some self-control on these outings. You will enjoy not only the occasion but the self-satisfaction of staying with your diet.

Your Health

Your vitality and enthusiasm, Aries, keep you from being plagued by pro-longed illness. However, your active life-style can be overtaxing at times. This coupled with your aversion to doctors (you never give in and admit that a visit to the doctor's office is necessary) can periodically weaken you, making you quite susceptible to illness. It is important not to overestimate the strength of your body—no matter how much work you have to do. Also, Aries, learn to have patience with your body's recuperative abilities. You're too restless to let any ailment keep you in bed longer than a day. Your desire for overnight recovery may send you back to the sickbed a week later, if not controlled. Finally, you must ensure that you get proper sleep each night. No engine can perform to maximum efficiency without rest—not even yours, busy Aries.

Aries rules the cranium and the facial bones, arteries of the head and brain, blood vessels of the brain, cerebral nervous system, the face, ears, eyes, mouth, teeth and upper jaw, and eyes. Aries are subject to:

Accidents	High blood pressure
Dental problems	Insomnia
Ear infections	Migraines
Eye infections	Neuralgia
Fevers	Nose infections
Flu	Strokes
Headaches	Ulcers
Head colds	Vertigo

The Aries diet must be rich in foods containing sufficient amounts of protein, vitamins C, B-12, essential fatty acids (EFA), folic acid, iron, phos-phorus, and chlorine. Vitamin C helps prevent the head colds to which you are prone, EFA are effective in alleviating some of the cold symptoms, and iron replenishes energy spent by your hectic life-style. Also, be sure to incorporate the B-vitamin category foods into your daily diet; absorption from food is far superior to that in capsule form.

Aries, you are also accident-prone due to your impatient, reckless nature. To keep your joints and tendons supple and elastic, thus minimizing any harm done by accident, your diet should include foods rich in the mineral chlorine.

Potassium phosphate is the Aries cell salt. Cell salts are naturally occur-ring minerals that are normal constituents of the body cells. They are found in trace amounts in foods, and plants, animals, and human beings require these compounds for proper nutrition. And, like vitamins, cell salts get used up. Potassium phosphate is the "brain cell building block" or "nerve nutrient" cell salt. It combines with albumen and oxygen to create the gray matter of the brain. Without potassium phosphate, this gray matter cannot be manufactured, and without gray matter the brain and nerves cannot function. Potassium phosphate is also needed for the growth and reproduction of nerve and brain cells; because of this property, it is used for the treatment of insomnia, mental fatigue, depression, headaches, and migraines. The nervous headaches and migraines that Aries commonly suffer are often due to a lack of potassium phosphate. The cell salt also has antiseptic properties and is thus effective in alleviating certain skin disorders; it can help in the general maintenance of healthy, clean pores. Aries should include foods rich in potassium phosphate in their diet as often as possible.

FOODS RICH IN POTASSIUM PHOSPHATE

Apples	Mustard
Cabbage	Olives
Cauliflower	Onions
Celery	Potatoes
Cucumbers	Radishes
Dates	Spinach
Lemons	Walnuts
Lettuce	Watercress
Lima beans	

Aries, you often eat poorly because of the hectic pace you keep. When you realize you have not eaten since breakfast, you grab something quickly and wolf it down. Or many times you eat only one meal a day in an attempt to control your diet. In the long haul this is not a good approach to dieting, and I would like to suggest that you try to space your meals more evenly. It will help temper the pace at which you eat and allow you to feel as though you have really eaten. Try to cut down on the amount of coffee you drink—it only serves to make you more hyper.

Make sure that you do have enough quality protein in your diet and try to eliminate refined white sugar.

You have a lot to accomplish in your life, and while you do have a basically healthy constitution, why not try to do everything to keep it that way.

Aries Daily Nutritional Supplements

- One general multivitamin with minerals
- Time-release B-complex (B-100s)
- 2,000 mg vitamin C with bioflavonoids
- 400 mg vitamin E

Remember, Aries...

The following diet is uniquely prepared to address your sun sign and *should not be interchanged with any other Sun Sign Diet.* It is important that you follow the diet exactly as it appears, for optimum weight loss and assimilation. Before starting your Aries diet, carefully read "General Diet and Maintenance Guidelines for All Sun Signs," found at the beginning of this book. Remember, drink 8 glasses of water daily.

I know, Aries, that you have always tried the latest diet that will give you quick results. Patience is not one of your virtues. This diet has been designed to give you quick results without jeopardizing your nutritional well-being. It is short enough for you to stay with it without getting bored.

Good luck, and *go for it.*

The Aries
Seven-Day
Reducing Diet

Your Aries Seven-Day Reducing Diet has been designed to address your life-style. Either too busy and on the go to stop to eat, or too involved at work to go out to eat, you need some foods you can eat on the run and others you can eat at your desk. Well, your Sun Sign Diet includes menus that address both needs. And since you must eat *toute de suite* when hunger strikes, your diet foods are easily accessible for instant gratification.

Of course, the Aries diet includes a two-day crash program, too, so that you can have instantaneous results. Options are included so that you may choose the one most suited to your tastes. The complete diet is only seven days, and you may repeat it as often as necessary until you achieve your goal. You will be encouraged to continue week after week because you will shed the pounds quickly.

If you are not in a super hurry, you may exclude the crash days. Simply start with Day Three and repeat after five days. *Under no circumstances are you to do the crash diet more than once a week.*

To tantalize your tongue, I have included some of the hot and spicy foods that are your passion. The Aries diet is also prepared for your own chemical and nutritional needs. High-performance protein foods, such as anchovies, herring, caviar, and sardines, are included to meet your high-energy life-style. Foods rich in vitamins B-12 and C, folic acid, iron, chlorine, and phosphorus are incorporated into your menus.

Underneath that superhero style of yours, Aries, you really are a mere mortal soul like the rest of us. Understanding that, I have included an Aries

Total Binge Day for you, too. Whenever you feel you just cannot go on any longer without pulling out your hair, use your Total Binge Day, but no more than four times a month.

Well, Aries, with all your needs comfortably met, you will have no excuse not to succeed—as long as you make one commitment to yourself: For one week, you will give up control and follow the diet *exactly as designed.* There are sound nutritional reasons for each and every menu combination, and unless substitutions are indicated, you may not do so. You may repeat your favorite day over and over again, or you may switch lunch and dinner on any given day, but you may not switch meals from one day to the next. If you are not hungry, you do not have to eat.

In addition, I have included a menu based on your workaholic personality and your needed protein requirement, "Eating at Your Desk Day."

At the end of your Aries Seven-Day Reducing Diet you will find itemized information in the "Notes for Aries Seven-Day Reducing Diet," which explains the reasons for inclusion of certain foods. These foods are noted with an asterisk (*) in the diet menus.

To further speed up your weight loss and suppress your appetite, you may choose to try a diet aid known in the United States as Glucomannan. It is extracted from the Japanese konjac root, a tuber that is very high in fiber. A final monograph on its effectiveness has not yet been established by the FDA, as it has no history of use in the United States before 1958; however, the konjac root has been cultivated and eaten in Asia for over a thousand years.

Glucomannan contributes to a decrease in cholesterol and triglyceride levels, and aids in maintaining low-density lipoprotein levels. It acts as a dietary fiber to increase viscosity and moisture content of food as it is digested, so that it forms a smooth, soft mass that moves easily through the intestinal tract. Digestion is slowed, so normal blood sugar levels are maintained after a meal. Two capsules taken three times a day may cut your appetite in half!

Furthermore, to help tame your robust appetite for starchy bread products, I suggest the use of 2 teaspoons of apple-cider vinegar in an 8-ounce glass of water with any of your meals. The potassium/phosphorus balance will help you digest your meals and will provide essential minerals you need. You may also drink this anytime you need a quick pick-me-up during the day.

Good luck, Aries, with your new challenge. Warrior that you are, I know you will win "the battle of the bulge" with the latest diet technology.

ARIES DAY ONE AND DAY TWO

You may choose between the two-day buttermilk crash or the two-day fruit crash.

BUTTERMILK CRASH—DAY ONE

Drink 2 qts. no-sodium buttermilk.

Buttermilk has powerful enzymes as a result of the fermentation process. (The word enzyme comes from the Greek *enzymos,* which means ferment.) The buttermilk will cleanse your intestinal tract and stop your craving for sugar, starch, and salt. It is thick and creamy and you will find it to be most satiating.

BUTTERMILK CRASH—DAY TWO

Drink 2 qts. no-sodium buttermilk.

You may have regular tea (no lemon), herbal tea of your choice, or decaffeinated black coffee. (If absolutely necessary, you may have 1 cup regular black coffee per day.)

The above buttermilk enzyme crash produces dramatic weight loss: 3 to 4 pounds in two days!

FRUIT CRASH—DAY ONE—THE PINEAPPLE DAY

Eat 2 large fresh pineapples for the day.

Pineapple is extremely rich in bromelin. Bromelin has a high enzyme content which actually helps to burn fat. Because of its high chlorine content (needed by Aries), pineapple purges the body of waste and is a fine diuretic.

You may cut up the fresh pineapple and put in the blender with 3 ice cubes and a little water and a sugar substitute to make a thick juice.

Pack pineapple into a container and take it to the office. The weight loss will be worth the energy.

Remember, drink 8 glasses of water every day.

FRUIT CRASH—DAY TWO—THE APPLE DAY

Eat 3 lbs. of juicy apples *or* 2½ lbs. of apples and 2 hard-boiled eggs.

You may have water, tea—red zinger, country apple, or herbal—or decaffeinated black coffee. You may use a sugar substitute, in moderation. Absolutely no other beverages are permitted.

Apples are body cleansers; they purify the blood. They are high in potassium, magnesium, sodium, vitamins B and C, and fiber. Additionally, the phosphoric acid in the apples stabilizes the blood sugar level and stops hunger urges.

Up to a 3-pound weight loss is to be expected on the Fruit Crash.

Remember, drink 8 glasses of water every day.

DAY THREE

By now you are feeling so very light and have lost quickly. Get set for the next five days.

BREAKFAST
>1 large apple*
>
>1 oz. Monterey Jack, Swiss, cheddar, or Gruyère cheese

MIDMORNING SNACK
>6 oz. unsweetened grapefruit juice in glass of club soda

LUNCH
>2-egg* mushroom, broccoli, or spinach omelette (use very, very little butter), topped with 2 Tbsp. caviar

MIDAFTERNOON SNACK
>6 oz. tomato juice with 1 heaping tsp. horseradish*

DINNER
>4 oz. glass dry red wine (optional)
>
>1–2 lb. lobster, boiled or broiled (no butter)
>
>>*or*
>
>6 oz. broiled brook trout,* halibut,* or scallops in wine or lemon juice
>
>Large salad of endive, spinach, Chinese cabbage, celery, watercress,* and parsley,* sprinkled with lemon juice or 2 Tbsp. Pritikin no-oil dressing

EVENING SNACK

>**D-Zerta Diet Gelatin Candy**
>Stir in 2 cups water to 2 packages D-Zerta diet gelatin. When hardened, cut into bite-sized pieces. Have all you want.
>
>*Remember, drink 8 glasses of water every day.*

DAY FOUR

BREAKFAST

    1 cup assorted honeydew and cantaloupe balls

    1 oz. sunflower seeds*

MIDMORNING SNACK

    6 oz. unsweetened grapefruit juice* mixed with 1 glass no-sodium club soda

LUNCH

    3½ oz. canned chinook salmon* with 2 tsp. horseradish

    ½ can artichokes canned in water, or ½ box frozen artichokes

    no-sodium seltzer with lime

MIDAFTERNOON SNACK

    1 cup Lipton Trim Soup

DINNER

    ¼–½ baked or broiled chicken* prepared in Mexican salsa* (available in health food store) or tomato juice.

    1 cup fresh, frozen, or canned asparagus*

    1 cup sliced cucumber sprinkled with basil and dill with 2 Tbsp. Pritikin no-oil salad dressing

    no-sodium Perrier with a twist of lime

EVENING SNACK

    D-Zerta diet gelatin—all you want

    Yoo-Hoo diet chocolate drink with 1 Tbsp. powdered milk

    Remember, drink 8 glasses of water every day.

DAY FIVE

BREAKFAST
4–5 kiwi fruit,* or 1½ papayas, or 1 cup strawberries*

black coffee or tea (no milk)

MIDMORNING SNACK
1 oz. sunflower seeds*

LUNCH
3½ oz. kippered herring with horseradish*

sliced cucumber with dill

or

1 large raw green pepper* stuffed with 3½ oz. tomato herring* and 3 small canned pimientos*

or

1 large raw green pepper stuffed with 3½ oz. water-pack tuna and 3 small canned pimientos, and 2 Tbsp. salsa (optional)

no-sodium diet soda, iced tea, or coffee

MIDAFTERNOON SNACK
6 oz. can tomato juice (mixed with 1 tsp. horseradish optional)

DINNER
1 large baked potato* seasoned with tarragon, chives, and basil, topped with cayenne pepper

as much fresh or frozen asparagus* as you wish; season with 2 Tbsp. Parmesan cheese

1 cup sliced lettuce and cucumber seasoned with lemon juice

EVENING SNACK
1 cup air-blown popcorn

1 can Yoo-Hoo diet chocolate drink with 1 Tbsp. powdered milk

Remember, drink 8 glasses of water every day.

DAY SIX

BREAKFAST

¼–½ fresh pineapple *

tea, black coffee, or water (no milk)

MIDMORNING SNACK

2 cups herbal tea

LUNCH

Tuna * and Artichoke Salad

Drain a can of water-pack artichokes and mix with 3½ oz. water-pack tuna. Serve on endive, garnished with 4 black or green olives. Use cayenne pepper * or 2 Tbsp. horseradish for seasoning.

(An excellent lunch for you, Aries, that can be kept on hand. Easy to carry to the office.)

or

Almond * Turkey Salad

4 oz. sliced turkey breast with 4 whole almonds, alfalfa sprouts, carrots, celery, and a few raisins. Season with Pritikin no-oil salad dressing or lemon juice.

MIDAFTERNOON SNACK

6 oz. unsweetened grapefruit juice mixed with 1 glass no-sodium seltzer or club soda

DINNER

6 oz. veal * scallopine with 6 broccoli spears (Sauté veal in white wine or Marsala wine and lightly steam broccoli; season spears with lemon juice, garlic, and pepper.)

as much salad of watercress, parsley, lettuce, green peppers, and scallions as you desire, with 1 Tbsp. Pritikin no-oil dressing

D-Zerta diet gelatin—as much as you want

Remember, drink 8 glasses of water every day.

DAY SEVEN

BREAKFAST

1 whole pure bran muffin* with 1 tsp. diet margarine and jam

or

8 oz. vanilla or coffee yogurt*

MIDMORNING SNACK

6 oz. grapefruit juice in 1 glass no-sodium club soda

LUNCH

½ avocado* (may substitute ½ cantaloupe) stuffed with ¼ cup cottage cheese with grated nutmeg and cinnamon; top with 10 pistachio nuts*

MIDAFTERNOON SNACK

1 tangerine

1 can Yoo-Hoo diet chocolate drink

DINNER

1 cup Broccoli Watercress Soup*

8 oz. frozen Celantano Lasagne (any supermarket)

or

8 oz. vegetable or durum wheat pasta* sprinkled with 2 Tbsp. Parmesan cheeese and 2 Tbsp. ricotta cheese, garlic, pepper

1 cup fresh strawberries

EVENING SNACK

1 can Yoo-Hoo diet chocolate drink

Remember, drink 8 glasses of water every day.

EATING AT
YOUR DESK DAY

BREAKFAST
>1 apple and 1 oz. cheddar, Swiss, or Gruyère cheese
>
>*or*
>
>8 oz. container vanilla, lemon, or coffee yogurt
>
>1 oz. sunflower seeds

MIDMORNING SNACK
>orange pekoe tea with sugar substitute (2 cups)

LUNCH
>¼ lb. cold roast beef (purchase at deli)
>
>1 large sliced tomato
>
>no-sodium diet soda, iced tea, black coffee, or Yoo-Hoo diet chocolate drink

MIDAFTERNOON SNACK
>2 cups orange pekoe tea with sugar substitute

DINNER
>4 oz. cold roast beef, turkey, chopped liver, or pickled herring in wine sauce
>
>1 tomato
>
>¼ cup mixed salad (drain any oil off)
>
>1 can Yoo-Hoo diet chocolate drink
>
>*Nothing else today.*
>
>*Remember, drink 8 glasses of water every day.*

Notes for Aries Seven-Day Reducing Diet

Aries Diet Notes—Day Three

After your two Crash Days, you are ready for a high-protein day filled with all the necessary foods for your body. If you look in the list of your maintenance foods you will note that your entire reducing regimen is resplendent with your particular vitamin and mineral requirements. This is absolutely essential to keep your energy level high and to keep you feeling good.

* Apples are a good source of sodium, potassium, magnesium, and vitamins B and C. Apples purify and renew the blood.
* Horseradish is a great for Aries because it, too, is a blood cleanser.
* Eggs are rich in vitamins E, B-12, folic acid, phosphorus, and chlorine—all essential for Aries.
* Brook trout and halibut are rich in B-12.
* Watercress and parsley are included in all your salads because they are an excellent source of calcium; it is important that you include these as often as possible.

Aries Diet Notes—Day Four

A quality-protein day, low in calories.

* Sunflower seeds are an excellent source of vitamin E and calcium.
* Unsweetened grapefruit juice mixed with no-sodium club soda or seltzer is an excellent pick-me-up that goes right to the bloodstream and assuages hunger.
* Salmon is rich in vitamin B-6 and phosphorus, and an excellent source of low-cholesterol protein with staying power.
* Chicken is rich in so many vitamins and another good source of vitamin B-6. Salsa sauce can be purchased in any health food store. Make sure that it has no sugar. It is comprised of chilis, a pepper rich in vitamins A and C. It is good for the digestive and circulatory systems, and guaranteed to tantalize your taste buds.
* Asparagus is an excellent diuretic food. It also contains the enzyme asparagine, which helps to break up accumulated fats in the cells.

Aries Diet Notes—Day Five

* Kiwis and strawberries are rich in vitamin C and have excellent enzyme action that starts your metabolism working.
* Sunflower seeds have excellent laxative properties.
* Herring is rich in vitamin B-12, and the fermentation of the horseradish aids digestion.
* Pimientos and green peppers are rich in calcium and vitamin C.
* Potatoes are rich in potassium and will be most filling but will act as a fine diuretic to rid the body of excess water. When combined with asparagus it shows up as a good weight loss on the scale.

Aries Diet Notes—Day Six

* Pineapple is rich in chlorine, stimulates urination, and has excellent enzyme properties. It also has an invigorating effect upon the kidneys and liver. Important for you, Aries.
* Tuna is rich in all the B vitamins and an excellent low-calorie choice. (Use only water-pack tuna.)
* Cayenne pepper is the natural Aries spice; it revitalizes your body. Use it as often as you like.
* Almonds are rich in potassium, manganese, and phosphorus, and, when combined with vitamin B-rich turkey, are an excellent protein food.
* Veal is also rich in phosphorus, easily digested, and low in calories.

Aires Diet Notes—Day Seven

Another low-calorie vitamin-packed day.

* Bran muffin is a good source of fiber, and yogurt has vitamin B-12 and acts as an intestinal cleanser by neutralizing putrefying bacteria.
* Avocado is rich in vitamins E, B-12, and folic acid, and provides fiber in the diet.
* Pistachio nuts are rich in vitamin E.
* Broccoli is rich in all the vitamins in your diet, especially calcium, and when combined with watercress is a powerful internal cleanser and energy booster. You may prepare this soup once a week and freeze the rest.

Broccoli Watercress Soup

1½ cups instant chicken broth (Campbell's is especially good.)
2 cups water
3 cups frozen chopped broccoli
2 bunches watercress (Should equal about 1 cup.)
1 tsp. lemon juice

Cook broccoli just until tender. Combine water and chicken broth, cooked broccoli, and watercress in blender (you will probably have to do this in two separate batches). Heat soup. Serve with chopped chives. Makes about 4 cups.

* Pasta is a source of B vitamins and a complex carbohydrate that excites most Aries. It has excellent staying power for eliminating any hunger pangs. Remember to purchase only whole wheat pasta or durum wheat pasta, because of their low calorie content.

Aries Diet Notes—Eating at Your Desk

This menu is guaranteed to give you quality nutrition while working. It is high in protein and low in carbohydrate, so as to modify any slack periods during the day. After a hard day's work you will be happy when you step on the scale tomorrow morning. May be used as often as your schedule requires.

Aries Total Binge Day

Aries, with all the extremes in your life, you sometimes need to let go. I have given you that option with a binge day. Now remember, Aries, you have a tendency to go overboard, so be careful.

Before You Binge
1. Drink water.
2. Drink water.
3. Drink water.
4. Rest.
5. Brush your teeth and rinse with your favorite mouthwash.
6. Chew sugarless gum for 20 minutes.

You may find that the desire to binge has passed. However, if you are still suffering from intense food frustration, follow these basic binge rules:

Rule One
Under no circumstances should you ever binge before completing Day Five of your reducing diet. This will ensure a maximum weight loss with a minimum of food frustration.

Rule Two
If, for example, you binge on the sixth day of your diet, resume your diet the following day (Day Seven) with the menu for Day Six. If you binge for just one meal, such as lunch on Day Six, resume your reducing diet with dinner on Day Six of your reducing diet.

Rule Three
Bingeing is for when you get that creepy, anxious feeling, when you feel like pulling out your hair—strand by strand—and you cannot endure dieting for even one more moment. Before you climb the walls, give yourself a binge day. It's hoped that this will not be necessary more than four times a month, however.

Rule Four
After you have lost your first 10 pounds, you may vary your binge day with the binge day of the sun sign opposite yours, which is Libra.

Remember, an occasional binge day—when necessary—will still allow you to lose weight (without guilt). Here, Aries, is your binge day menu.

Binge Day Menu

BREAKFAST

> 1 large pumpernickel bagel with 1 Tbsp. cream cheese and 2 oz. lox
>
> coffee or tea with ½ cup milk
>
> > *or*
>
> 1 glass skim milk
>
> 1 Hostess chocolate cupcake
>
> > *or*
>
> 1 Sara Lee caramel pecan roll or 1 slice cheesecake

LUNCH

> 4 oz. white wine or dry sherry (optional)
>
> 2-inch slice Italian or French bread with 2 oz. any hard cheese or 2 oz. Brie
>
> > *or*
>
> 1 slice pizza with mushrooms
>
> 1 no-sodium diet soda or light beer
>
> ½ cup ice cream, Tofutti, or chocolate fudgesicle

DINNER

> 1 oz. liquor or 4 oz. dry red wine (optional)
>
> large platter of steamers dipped in lemon juice
>
> 1–2 lb. lobster (no butter) or 6 oz. any broiled or baked fish (no butter) of your choice
>
> 1 cup mixed salad with 1 Tbsp. dressing
>
> tea or espresso with lime

Maintaining Your Ideal Weight

Aries Maintenance Foods for Optimum Health

W hen you have achieved your desired weight goal, you should follow a maintenance diet rich in the specific nutrients that you, Aries, need each and every day.

Vitamin C

Vitamin C serves many crucial functions in the body. One of its more important tasks is aiding in the formation of collagen. Collagen is a substance that constitutes about 35 to 40 percent of the body's protein. It fortifies cells, keeping them in their natural formations and enabling them to resist infection. Vitamin C is also extremely important in the production of white blood cells, which protect the body from invading bacteria. Proper intake of vitamin C helps to maintain a healthy production of collagen and white blood cells, and thus increases the body's immunities to bacteria and infections such as head colds, which often afflict Aries.

FOODS RICH IN VITAMIN C

Alfalfa	Beets
Almonds	Blueberries
Apples	Broccoli
Asparagus	Brussels sprouts
Bananas	Cantaloupe

41

Carrots
Celery
Chicken
Cranberries
Currants
Grapefruit
Green peppers
Lemons
Oranges

Orange juice
Paprika
Parsley
Pineapple (fresh only)
Skim milk
Strawberries
Tomatoes
Watercress

Vitamin E

Vitamin E is considered the sex and anti-aging vitamin. It increases sexual potency and virility, and acts as an antioxidant; it has the ability to unite with oxygen and prevent it from being converted into toxic peroxides. This leaves the red blood cells filled with a greater supply of oxygen, which the blood carries to all organs of the body. Vitamin E also supports the proper functioning of the pituitary and adrenal glands, sensitive areas for Aries.

FOODS RICH IN VITAMIN E

Apples
Asparagus
Avocados
Broccoli
Cabbage
Carrots
Cheese
Chicken
Eggs
Halibut
Liver
Milk

Mushrooms
Parsley
Peanut butter
Salmon
Sardines
Shrimp
Spinach
Sunflower seeds
Sweet potatoes
Turkey
Wheat germ

Vitamin B-12 and Folic Acid

Vitamin B-12 is essential for healthy metabolism of proteins, fats, and carbohydrates, and is important for the maintenance of nerve tissue and a healthy nervous system. Vitamin B-12 is also valuable in preventing insomnia, a problem common to Aries. Folic acid is a member of the B-complex vitamins, and is more effective when taken with vitamin B-12. Vitamin B-12 and folic acid work together to help manufacture choline. Another of folic acid's functions is to carry carbon necessary for the production of red blood cells. A deficiency of folic acid can cause anemia, a typical Arien illness. Folic acid is also important for proper functioning of the adrenal gland.

FOODS RICH IN VITAMIN B-12

Alfalfa sprouts	Milk
American cheese	Muscle meats
Beef	Pickled foods
Bran	Prunes
Chicken	Sardines
Chicken liver	Shellfish
Cottage cheese	Skim milk
Dairy products	Soy bean products
Eggs	Swiss cheese
Green peas	Trout
Herring	Yogurt
Liver	

FOODS RICH IN FOLIC ACID

Asparagus	Kidney
Avocado	Lamb
Beet greens	Lima beans
Broccoli	Liver
Brown rice	Peanuts
Chard	Potatoes
Cottage cheese	Smoked ham
Endive	Spinach
Green leafy vegetables	Turnips
Kale	Wheat bran

Essential Fatty Acids (EFA)

Essential fatty acids (EFA) help maintain the overall coagulation rate of the blood. They also break up cholesterol deposits in the arteries, thereby preventing arteriosclerosis, to which Aries is prone. EFA have also proven very effective in reducing both the number and severity of head colds.

FOODS RICH IN EFA

Avocado	Sardines
Chicken	Soy bean products
Eggs	Sunflower seeds
Mayonnaise	Tuna
Peanuts	Walnuts
Pecans	Wheat germ

Iron

Iron is one of the more important minerals in the body. It works in the red blood cells uniting copper with protein to produce hemoglobin. Iron also assists in the production of globulin, which transports oxygen to the muscles, giving them the ability to contract. Lack of iron leads to anemia, but a daily diet sufficient in iron will ensure proper oxygenation and a good supply of energy, so necessary for Aries to maintain your hectic schedule —especially when you miss meals.

FOODS RICH IN IRON

Alfalfa sprouts	Green beans
Almonds	Kidney
Avocados	Lamb
Beef	Liver
Beets	Mushrooms
Broccoli	Olives
Chicken	Onions
Dried beans	Red wines
Egg yolk	

Phosphorus and Chlorine

The level of phosphorus is the second highest of any mineral in the body. It is necessary for proper skeletal and tooth development, as well as proper functioning of the kidneys. It should be included in the Arien diet to avoid the dental problems and the bladder and kidney infections to which you are susceptible.

Together with chlorine, phosphorus also aids in the proper maintenance of your body's acid-alkaline balance. The chlorine also keeps joints and tendons supple and elastic, which can be quite beneficial to accident-prone Aries.

FOODS RICH IN PHOSPHORUS

Almonds
Apples
Avocados
Beef
Beef liver
Beets
Cherries
Chicken
Corn
Egg yolk
Grapefruit
Halibut
Lima beans

Liver
Milk
Mushrooms
Nuts
Parsley
Pumpkin seeds
Rice
Salmon
Scallops
Spinach
Tuna
Veal

FOODS RICH IN CHLORINE

Asparagus
Beets
Cabbage
Carrots
Cheese
Eggs
Fish

Meat (in general)
Milk
Onion
Parsnips
Pineapple
Watercress

Aries Sample Maintenance Menu

When you reach your desired goal, please follow the maintenance eating hints found in "General Diet and Maintenance Guidelines for All Sun Signs" at the beginning of this book for proper calculations of caloric intake.

I am including a sample maintenance menu based on your sun sign for optimal Aries maintenance. When creating your own menus for yourself, try to choose many of the foods you eat from your Aries Maintenance Foods lists.

2,000 CALORIES PER DAY

BREAKFAST	CALORIES
½ grapefruit	35
1 bran muffin	112
with 2 Tbsp. cream cheese	99
8 oz. skim milk	80
cup of black coffee	0
	326

LUNCH	
Super tuna melt:	
1 English muffin	145
½ cup tuna salad	170
2 slices tomato	10
1 oz. Swiss cheese melted on top	106
½ cup coleslaw	90
no-sodium diet soda	0
	521

MIDAFTERNOON SNACK	
1 banana with 2 Tbsp. peanut butter	282

DINNER	
6 oz. veal scallopini	298
4 oz. spaghetti with tomato sauce	85
1 cup spinach	42
1 light beer	98
½ cup chocolate ice cream	133
with 2 heaping Tbsp. Cool Whip dessert topping	30
	686

EVENING SNACK	
4 Triscuit crackers with 1 oz. Muenster cheese	188
TOTAL DAILY CALORIES	2,003

Remember, drink 8 glasses of water every day.

Restaurant Eating the Aries Way

Perhaps you have seen the following dishes on restaurant menus. Both the dishes and the types of restaurants chosen will appeal to the Aries palate and satisfy your nutritional needs. Aries, you like everything hot: Cayenne pepper is your middle name. If it doesn't excite your taste buds and start a fire on your tongue . . . it's hardly a dinner worth eating. Your meal ticket is ethnic and exotic—Chinese hot and sour soup or Mexican dishes made with jalapeño peppers that let you know you are alive.

Most of the recommended dishes contain the nutrients specified in your Aries Maintenance Foods lists. For example, on your Mexican guide the first chicken entrée is rich in iron, vitamins C and B-12, and EFA.

Mexican Restaurant

APPETIZERS

Green salad with hot Mexican dressing

Chicken salad made with fresh vegetables and a spicy sauce

ENTRÉES

Layer of tortilla with shredded chicken and cheese in a spicy to-mato sauce

Fresh shrimp in a green parsley, wine, and garlic sauce
Chicken in hot mole sauce

Rolled tacos (ask waiter to have tacos baked, *not* fried) topped with guacamole sauce

Chinese Restaurant

APPETIZERS

Assorted vegetables with bean shoots, served in a hot, spicy sauce

Shrimp balls with curry sauce

ENTRÉES

Diced chicken and peanuts in a hot pepper sauce

Scallops in garlic sauce

Beef in chili sauce

Eggplant in garlic sauce

Indian Restaurant

APPETIZERS

Rice with Sambhar curry

Wheat crepes with onions

ENTRÉES

Jumbo prawns, marinated and roasted with tomatoes, onions, and cucumber; served in lemon and mint sauce

Chicken marinated in yogurt, garlic, and ginger

Bombay fish curry, cooked in spiced gravy

Barbecued lamb cooked in piquant sauce with tomatoes and onions

Italian Restaurant

APPETIZERS

Calamari and mussel salad, seasoned with garlic and lemon

Baked clams (if very lightly breaded)

ENTRÉES

Chicken sautéed with mushrooms and artichokes

Veal with tomato, pepper, and mushrooms

Broiled striped bass

Sliced filet mignon with peppers and spicy tomato sauce

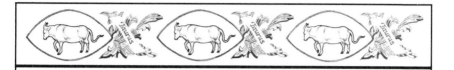

TAURUS

April 21–May 21

The Taurus
Personality

"I'm a creature of comfort."

Determined, deliberate, patient, tenacious, stable, steady. And stubborn, stubborn, *stubborn*. Taurus, you have all the necessary traits to be a successful dieter—if and when you decide you *want* to lose weight.

You are not very fond of change. Rigid Taurus, symbolized by the bull, pretty much likes things status quo. Your motto: "Look before you leap." When you get set in your ways, you are immovable. Remember, Taurus, your patterns of eating are so fixed, you probably never change brands of food.

And how you love to eat. Food is a major part of life's enjoyment for sensuous Taurus. Not just any food. Only the best—and plenty of it—for your refined taste buds. You know how to order from the menus of the finest gourmet restaurants. However, you actually prefer hearty home cooking just about anytime. Meat and potatoes are right up your alley (make that filet mignon, of course). And you simply lose your head over cakes, pies, and other baked goods. You are an excellent cook, and might bake these goodies yourself.

Taurus is an earth sign. Like Mother Earth herself, the Taurean nourishes life and is a producer. In any kind of work you do, you want to point to practical, tangible results. Nothing equals the pleasure you derive from watching guests eat food you have prepared, except, of course, the pleasure you get from eating it yourself.

You consider yourself to be a connoisseur of wine as well as food. You are up on the newest and best Chardonnay and Beaujolais; you're especially

51

fond of Cabernet Sauvignon and know all the vineyards and specialties of each region. You're proud of your wine cabinet and talk in vocabularies of aroma, intensity, hint of flavor, and good body.

All that fancy talk aside, Taurus, the plain truth is you just love the warm feeling that wine has on the lips. All your senses are very keen, but taste and touch are especially vital to you. You want to "feel" what you serve and eat. You crave substance. Tactility. Foods you can really get your hands on and teeth into—a juicy hamburger on a bun, an overstuffed sandwich, a succulent whole lobster you can take apart limb by limb—are Taurean delights. But only in private. Ever conscious of how you look to the world, you are not inclined to exhibit in public the primal sides of your nature.

Oh, yes, Taurus knows how to create the "right" impression. You are very conscious of your surroundings and your outward appearance. You value your reputation and social status. You know who you are, however. Ruled by the planet Venus (named after the mythological goddess of beauty), Taurus radiates grace, poise, and self-confidence.

When it comes to your dress, you spare no expense. I know a number of svelte Taureans whose sole motivation to keep weight off is the price tag of their size-8 wardrobe. Words like *savvy* and *classic* describe your sartorial style. If you wear a watch, it is a Cartier or Rolex. Your clothes are custom-made in the finest fabrics. You are particularly fond of beautiful leathers and suedes, but you also love denim—fine-tailored denim. If you are the female of the species, you luxuriate in silk lingerie. Those rich textures feel so good to the touch.

In all matters of the senses, the Taurean is . . . well, epicurean. You are a lover of great art and music. Probably, you paint, sculpt, play an instrument, or sing. At the very least, you buy season tickets to the opera or ballet, collect records, have a fine-art museum membership, or collect one-of-a-kind artifacts with which you decorate your home.

You like to feel like royalty for a day when you spend your money, and you do it with elegance and style. *Never* ostentatiously. Generally speaking, however, you are considered by some to be conservative in financial matters. You are familiar with the latest tax differential savings plans, high-yield, tax-free municipal bonds, and the best growth plans for now and the future. You are conscious of selecting safe ways to keep your savings increasing. In protecting your capital, you feel it is better to err on the side of conservatism. Playing the commodities futures market is not your game.

Nevertheless, for a night on the town, you will treat your date to *haute cuisine* at an elegant eatery, first-row-center seats to the hottest new musical, and after-theater drinks and dessert at the Hilton, where violins serenade in the background. But after the first date, you will henceforth prefer to spend a quiet evening *à deux,* eating home-cooked meals in front of your TV.

Face it, Taurus, you are just not the jet-set type. It's not that you don't appreciate the finer things in life. You *do*. But you would rather enjoy them at home more than anyplace else in the world.

Earth is your element. Your feet are planted in terra firma, and you derive greatest enjoyment from having a little corner of it to call your own. Property is the ultimate possession to materialistic Taurus. It represents security, especially property that can be changed into cash. A cozy summer home is important to you, preferably one in the mountains and probably with a fireplace you can cuddle up to, along with a good book and some David's cookies.

Eating again, Taurus? I know, taking away your goodies is like taking away a part of yourself. Simply put, you are a creature of comfort, Taurus. And Mother Nature's great pacifier is food. The heartier and more plentiful the fare, the cozier and more comfortable the Bull.

Herein lies your problem, Taurus. You just cannot seem to get enough of those wonderful oral sensations. You are first to the dinner table and last to leave. As long as food is abundant and wine is flowing, you will savor and sip until every last morsel and drop is gone—long after everyone else is finished. If food remains on the table when you are finally full, tomorrow you will feast on leftovers. ("Waste not, want not," says ever-thrifty Taurus.) You are really not concerned with the history of food, its origins or ingredients, but with the pure, simple, sensuous pleasure of eating it.

While you exercise balance and restraint in other areas of your life, when it comes to food, you sometimes overdo it. And speaking of exercise, a call for "Tennis, anyone?" would not get a rousing response from lazy Taurus.

Headstrong as you are, you will probably prolong attempting to start a diet longer than any other sign in the zodiac, Taurus. It is hard for you to change your mind about something, even when you know the attitudes you hold are no longer correct. When you do make up your mind to diet, you will forge ahead with that same bullish streak, allowing no one to sabotage your plans, until you reach your goal. Not even your legendary appetite, Taurus, is a match for your indomitable will and perseverance.

Sexual Appetite

Taurus, your need for physical contact is primal. Better than anyone, you realize that touch affirms our place in the world and that of the people around us. Just a simple touch of the hand is a universal gesture of reassurance and comfort, and I know how important that is to tactile Taurus. Your need to touch, snuggle, cuddle, hug, and kiss is essential to your well-being, and certainly to keeping your appetite under control.

I remember a friend of mine once dated a very dashing Italian. He confirmed everything I had ever heard about Italian men. He was passionate, volatile, and loved to laugh. And how he adored touching. His hands were always grabbing her hands. She lost weight while she was seeing him because he hardly ever freed her long enough to eat. Anyhow, her need for comfort was quite satisfied.

I personally believe that all Taureans are Italian lovers in disguise, or need to have Italian lovers.

Let me add that I do not mean the Casanova type, either. That is not your style at all, loyal Taurus. You are definitely monogamous. In your deepest core, you are searching for a secure and lasting relationship. You hate to be toyed with and like to know where you stand in matters of the heart, because you have deep-seated security needs. If your spouse is not in tune with this, or if he or she is flirtatious, your marriage will suffer. By the same token, it takes a lot of conflict to drive you out of a marriage. You consider your spouse your possession and are quite stubborn about this.

You are so strong and dependable, Taurus, that your partner often feels he or she can lean on you. That is no problem for you as long as you feel emotionally nourished. However, you may have to learn to *take* more in marriage to establish a happy balance. Earthy, emotional, and pragmatic as you are, you are usually very busy giving in relationships. The truth is, you are highly vulnerable and fear rejection, both emotionally and sexually, although you may never let anyone know this.

Only your sexual drive rivals your need for security, affectionate Taurus. Sometimes your physical needs are, to put it in a word, consuming. You are a tender, gentle, and protective lover. And very sexy. Regardless of gender, Taurus has an air of sophistication, strength, grace, and power that is very alluring. You appreciate the sexual appeal of power. Wealth is a turn-on, and that is one reason you like to accumulate power and cash.

Male Taurus, you do not need to prove yourself as many men do. Your confidence in your sexuality is always apparent, never overt, and always vital. Your primitive approach is earthy, reassuring, and stimulating. And Taurean female, you may look fragile and helpless, but you are quite headstrong and persistent, especially when it comes to making sure your romantic interludes have just the proper ambiance. You need an outlet for your affections, and you are not likely to look outside your marriage for it. Cook up a storm for your mate as only a Taurus woman knows how, and if he's Taurean, too, you can surely recapture his heart with a great home-cooked meal.

And you know how to create an evening of romance, Taurus—male or female. A roaring fireplace, soft music, shimmering candlelight, tinkling crystal, and lots of champagne and laughter. And food. This is the time and place (in private) to bring out that hands-on fare you so relish—foods you can tear, hold, nibble, suck, gnaw, and lick. (You alone, Taurus, can make eating frozen ice cream on a cone look deliciously hot!)

When the repast is over, you may want to suggest to your mate how lovely it would be to give each other massages. (Often someone will discourage touching because he or she does not feel like making love and assumes touching will lead to sex. Communicate to your partner that you simply love to cuddle, Taurus.) You especially love to be stroked, and delight in long neck rubs.

Remember, lusty Taurus, good sex can be as satisfying as good food to pacify your urge for sensory gratification. A word of caution: Sometimes your stubbornness, your need to always be right, your need to constantly be in control, to possess and to change others to suit you gets in the way of a healthy sexual relationship. This can turn a good relationship into a frustrating one. Work on moderating these characteristics, Taurus, and you will not find yourself at the refrigerator door.

Eating/Entertaining at Home

Taurus, I will always know your home when I enter it. Your innate talents for architecture and interior design will be evident everywhere. Your furniture will be custom-made in the finest polished hardwoods and brass, and it will have richly textured upholstery. Copies of *Gourmet* magazine, *The Connoisseur, Travel & Leisure, National Geographic,* and some European publications will sit on the rack or a shelf, all lined up very neatly, of course.

An aroma of fresh-baked bread or pie might waft from your kitchen. There, cookbooks will line at least one counter, and outside your window, I will probably find a well-kept vegetable garden, planted and tended by your earth-loving hands.

A peek into your pantry will find it stockpiled with food and every staple imaginable. Acquisitive Taurus, you like to keep a reserve (in the bank, too), just in case a snowstorm, hurricane, or avalanche happens suddenly to strike.

By nature, you are a homebody. You are likely to be found in the evenings in front of the TV set, satisfying a chronic sweet tooth with a bowl of sugared cereal. It is also likely that you like to snack late at night, a dieter's catastrophe.

When it comes to company, however, activity in the Taurus household will center around the dining room table. You, domestic Taurus, love family gatherings, and if guests bring gourmet foods they have prepared, you will certainly ask for recipes.

Home entertaining, Taurus-style, is elevated to an art. Despite your penchant for hearty home cooking, you are a gourmet host and love to create a pleasant, elegant ambiance for dinner guests. You would never dream of eating off paper plates. Ugh-ugh. Only the finest china, crystal, and linen will be set on your table. Even a Taurean's pet doesn't eat from a can. You serve yours the same freshly cooked cuisine you serve yourself and company.

You invariably make ten times more food than necessary and are simply rejected to the core if guests do not try everything you so carefully prepared. Have some compassion for your dieting friends, Taurus—remember not every sign in the zodiac is blessed with your tenacity, determination, and will to resist so gracious and tempting an onslaught.

In any event, your guests should be prepared to enjoy hours of leisurely eating and conversation at your table, Taurus. Your only problem is, when you are ready to retire, your house guests may not want to leave. The Taurus brand of pampering is not just nice, it is habit-forming.

Food Shopping

When you shop for food, Taurus, you demand honesty, promptness, and courtesy. When it comes to brand names and purchases, you are very staid and conventional. You like to stick to the tried-and-true.

Aesthetic Taurus, you are attracted to lovely looking things, but the shape and packaging of food items will not convince you to buy. Neither will gimmicks like cents-off coupons, contests, or gifts packaged inside. It is not the price on the outside of the package that will motivate Taurus to buy, although you are conscious of getting your money's worth.

Supermarkets do take advantage of the lackadaisical Taurean, stacking the most expensive brands on the middle shelves. Along you come, Taurus. Oh, it really does take so much effort and exertion to bend down or reach up. So, you give into comfort and take what is nearest on the middle shelf. Well, you are inclined to look for the best quality, anyway. Steak is steak, but filet mignon is eating!

You always look for freshness when purchasing food. It is the bakery section—the fresh bread, rolls, cake, and cookies—where you inevitably meet your Waterloo, Taurus. Even if you successfully maneuver your cart up the aisle past these tempting goodies, you will continually hear them call out to you as you shop. "Taurus, here I am," they say. "On the shelf—a freshly baked brown bread with raisins. I am soft and delicious." Oh, if you could just make it to the checkout . . . then suddenly that silly little package of whole wheat bread catches your eye. Is food shopping really worth this torture? Well, I have faith in you, resolute Taurus; even these seductive sirens will not lure you off the path once you have taken the decisive step to lose weight.

Social Dining

The restaurants of your choice, Taurus, tend to be elegant and comfortable, preferably with big upholstered chairs or booths. As for ambiance, you eschew the cold look of high-tech and feel quite at home amid rustic charm or old-world grace. Applied to you, the term gourmet does not have the connotation of "food snob," but simply denotes a lover of good food and wine. Dinner will start with a bottle of fine wine and linger over cognac or a liqueur. You, Taurus, understand deep in your heart that the dining table is the proper place to share sentiments.

Hard as it may be, you should get used to asking for the à la carte menu. In the long run it will save you pounds *and* dollars. You are concerned about getting your money's worth at a restaurant. One look at the prices on a menu and your mind begins to calculate value. However, once your taste buds are titillated and your belly filled, you will forget about how much the meal depleted your life's savings. I do not mean to imply you are stingy, Taurus. It is not the big things that rouse your conservatism, but the smaller ones, such as ordering up room service at a hotel. It costs more than dining in the restaurant. However, after the champagne arrives and the tray is placed on the dresser with a single red rose in a vase, you will say to yourself, in true form, "You know, I really deserve this."

You do love the good life, Taurus. But remember, you also have very great willpower and strength of convictions. If you have made up your mind to diet, the next time you are dining out, you will stick to it.

Special-Occasion Dining

Vacation time and travel are occasions when you tend to indulge your eating habits, Taurus. Your favorite kind of trip is when you eat your way through a country, testing local culinary specialties. If it rains, of course, there is nothing else to do but eat. Well, that means paying the piper sometime, Taurus. So you might as well just decide before you begin your travels to call up those deep reserves of inner resolve and pull back the reins on those stampeding senses of yours—or find some other means than food to keep them gratified.

Excursions by train or plane will present a special problem for you only if you are not prepared. When you are hungry, even airplane food can look pretty tempting when the stewardess sets a tray down in front of you. Call ahead and order a fresh fruit plate or have your nearest catering shop prepare a lunchbox of fresh tomatoes, sliced chicken, and salad. Treat yourself to a glass of wine on board, and you have a nourishing meal minus the calories.

A friend of mine who travels often is a confirmed "brown bagger." She is also a Taurus. She purchased a lovely piece of jewelry at Tiffany's and promptly asked the salesperson whether she could have a dozen of those "little bags" and a dozen of the larger ones. You've got it, savvy Taurus: the small ones for the short trips, the large ones for the long. Always a class act, you are.

Your Health

Taureans have a great deal of natural good health and endurance. So blessed are you, Taurus, with a strong constitution that you would be considered the healthiest sign in the zodiac were it not for your fondness for fattening foods and the consequent tendency toward obesity. Whether male or female, Taureans also tend to have a beautiful visage, even when the excess pounds accumulate.

Your notorious stubbornness, bull-headed Taurus, is a reflection of your strong physical resistance. You are also fortunate to have inner fortitude and willpower unequaled by any other sign. These qualities ultimately will enable you to conquer your passion for sweet and starchy foods.

Taurus rules the neck and throat, base of the brain, pharynx, larynx, thyroid gland, vocal cords, carotid arteries, jugular vein, chin, jaw, and lower teeth.

Every sun sign has a proclivity to have some diseases more than others. Possible problems for Taurus are:

Asthma and sinusitis	Problems of carbohydrate and
Bronchitis	sugar metabolism and others
Diseases involving the neck,	due to overindulgence in rich
larynx, and ears	foods
Goiter	Throat infections
	Thyroid glands
	Vocal cords

The throat and neck are particularly sensitive areas for you, Taurus. Stroking either of these areas is a sure way to calm down an agitated bull— the human variety, that is. Lemon juice is useful to help your throat, and you can reduce your chances of strained vocal cords by wearing scarves and covering your neck in cold and damp weather.

Taurus, your ruling cell salt is sodium sulfate, which controls the amount of bile secreted into the duodenum to break down foods, and aids and regulates the elimination of unwanted water in the body. Cell salts are naturally occurring minerals that are normal constituents of body cells. They are found in trace amounts in foods and are required by all plants, animals, and people for proper nutrition. And, like vitamins, cell salts get used up. Sodium sulfate is an important constituent and is found only intercellularly in the fluids.

FOODS RICH IN SODIUM SULFATE

Beets	Pumpkin
Cabbage	Radishes
Cucumber	Spinach
Horseradish	Swiss chard
Onions	

Your diet also should be rich in nutritious foods, short on fat and starchy food products. You should include a lot of seafood and iodine-rich foods as well as those foods rich in niacin and vitamins E and A. You retain fluids and have to keep your metabolic fires burning in order to lose calories.

But have faith. You are about to find the way. Certain food combinations do decrease the appetite naturally and also decrease the craving for starches and sweets. Don't worry, Taurus, I will not deprive you forever of your goodies. After all, what's life without them? Once you reach your maintenance goal, they will be introduced again into your diet. In the meantime, you will never have the need for so many sweets, Taurus, once you start your very own Sun Sign Diet.

Taurus Daily Nutritional Supplements

- One general multivitamin with minerals
- 400 mg vitamin E
- 2,000 mg vitamin C

Remember, Taurus...

The following diet is uniquely prepared to address your sun sign and *should not be interchanged with any other Sun Sign Diet.* It is important that you follow the diet exactly as it appears, for optimum weight loss and assimilation. Before starting your Taurus diet, carefully read "General Diet and Maintenance Guidelines for all Sun Signs," found at the beginning of this book. Remember, drink 8 glasses of water daily.

You will not feel totally deprived dear Taurus, because this diet has been prepared to meet your biological, chemical, nutritional, and behavioral needs.

Good luck, and *go for it.*

The Taurus
Seven-Day
Reducing Diet

This diet has been specifically designed for the Taurus constitution; to counteract sugar and carbohydrate cravings, to eliminate water, and to speed up your metabolism, while still achieving the maximum amount of weight loss with the minimum amount of discomfort.

Although I am opposed to crash dieting per se, I have included an optional one-day buttermilk crash day for those of you who need quick results to gain inspiration and motivation. It will also act as an enzyme booster to your system and an internal cleanser. If you do not like buttermilk, do not fret. Just eliminate this day and start with Day One.

Please take note of the items marked with an asterisk (*) in your daily diet plan. In the section "Notes for Taurus Seven-Day Reducing Diet," you will find a detailed explanation as to why you must have these foods for your successful weight loss, and further explanation as to the vitamins, minerals, and nutritional value to you, Taurus.

To further speed up your weight loss and suppress your appetite, you may choose to try a diet aid known in the United States as Glucomannan. It is extracted from the Japanese konjac root, a tuber that is very high in fiber. A final monograph on its effectiveness has not yet been established by the FDA, as it has no history of use in the United States before 1958; however, the konjac root has been cultivated and eaten in Asia for over a thousand years.

Glucomannan contributes to a decrease in cholesterol and triglyceride levels, and aids in maintaining low-density lipoprotein levels. It acts as a dietary fiber to increase viscosity and moisture content of food as it is digested, so that it forms a smooth, soft mass that moves easily through the intestinal tract. Digestion is slowed, so normal blood sugar levels are maintained after a meal. Two capsules taken three times a day may cut your appetite in half!

Furthermore, to help tame your robust appetite for starchy bread products, I suggest the use of 2 teaspoons of apple-cider vinegar in an 8-ounce glass of water with your meals. The potassium/phosphorus balance will help digest your meals and will provide essential minerals; it also helps you to speed weight loss and to assimilate food more quickly.

Even the most self-disciplined souls will run out of willpower at some point. When you feel you are about to go absolutely stir crazy and can go on no longer, I suggest you use a binge day. It will satisfy all those sinful cravings, and if followed exactly will not have you putting on an ounce. Do not permit yourself more than four a month. You will find all the instructions in the binge section following the Diet Notes.

With your indefatigable perseverance and your Taurus Seven-Day Reducing Diet in hand, you're a sure bet for success.

ONE-DAY ENZYME*
POWER BOOSTER DIET

MENU

2 qts. of cultured no-sodium buttermilk* for the entire day

(You may combine with ice cubes and Sweet 'n Low and beat to a frothy drink in the blender.)

You may drink tea, herbal tea, or water. No coffee allowed (it will stop the enzyme action). *Absolutely no other beverages.*

Space your buttermilk throughout the day. You will not be hungry. Buttermilk is very satiating, filling, and soothing. The high calcium content will make you feel relaxed. You will lose more weight than if you fasted all day.

---

* Paavo O. Airola, N.D., in his book *Health Secrets from Europe,* states that the word "enzyme" comes from the Greek *enzymos,* which means *ferment.* Man fermented bread and made it rise with the help of enzymes. He preserved vegetables by the enzymatic process of "pickling" them, or making sauerkraut or sour pickles. All of these foods are storehouses of enzymes. And primitive man was healthy.

DAY ONE—THE FIVE-P DAY

(Potatoes, Pineapple, Papaya, Parsley, Peppers)

BREAKFAST

as much fresh pineapple* as you want
(Pineapple contains bromelin so very important for enzyme digestion.)

or

as much fresh papaya* as you want
(Papaya is loaded with digestive enzymes that work on fat and get
metabolism going.)

or

up to 10 oz. of any unsweetened fruit juice

or

2 juicy apples*

black coffee, tea, or herbal tea (absolutely no milk allowed today.)

LUNCH

1 large baked potato, with ½ bunch parsley and 1 chopped red or
green pepper seasoned with dill and chives

black coffee, tea, herbal tea, or no-sodium diet soda

This potato will satisfy your Taurus carbohydrate craving. The parsley and peppers have extraordinary enzyme power and will easily
digest the potato and will supply you with a healthy fix of phosphorus and vitamin C. This is extremely important in the first days of
dieting, both for your nerves and toxic elimination.

You must get the sugar out of your system and learn how vital
you can feel with these foods. Can I count on you, Taurus, not to
be stubborn about this?

MIDAFTERNOON SNACK

water, water, water

10 unsalted almonds
(The almonds are an excellent source of protein and will help you
get over the midafternoon slump. Go to a health food store and get

the freshest ones you can find. You do not have to have all 10 if you do not wish.)

DINNER

¼ broiled chicken,* or

8 oz. of white meat turkey,* or

4 oz. of water-pack tuna

watercress, mushrooms, and/or fresh or frozen spinach

D-Zerta diet gelatin—as much as you wish

no-sodium Perrier or seltzer, coffee, or tea

Remember, drink 8 glasses of water every day.

In between meals for the first dieting day you might take the amino acid tryptophan, which the body is able to convert to niacin (60 mg tryptophan = 1 mg niacin). Tryptophan is a natural amino acid produced by the body and it sends messages to the brain that control the sugar craving and is often a help during the dieting process. Take a 250–500 mg supplement three times a day between meals with water, but not within two hours of consuming protein.

You may also find that herbal teas are most comforting for you and may be drunk throughout the day.

DAY TWO

A protein day to get your metabolism burning and rid of excess water weight and sugar.

BREAKFAST

    1 apple and 1 glass of water (have at same sitting so absorption is quicker)

    black coffee, tea, or herbal tea

LUNCH

    ½ broiled or baked chicken (without the skin)

    tossed house salad seasoned with apple-cider vinegar* and/or lemon juice

    coffee, tea, no-sodium diet soda

MIDAFTERNOON SNACK

    water, water, water

    8 oz. tomato juice

DINNER

    4 oz. white wine (optional)

    ½ broiled or baked chicken (without the skin)

    1 large serving of freshly steamed asparagus (as much as you want) seasoned with lemon juice
    (Asparagus has an enzyme known as asparagine, which helps to break up accumulated fats in the cells and to alert the metabolism to flush excess water out of the system. It is nature's diuretic food.)

    coffee, tea, 2 tsp. apple-cider vinegar in 8 oz. water, no-sodium seltzer with lime, or no-sodium diet soda

    1 plain graham cracker

Remember, drink 8 glasses of water every day.

DAY THREE

A low-calorie, enzyme-balanced day for good weight loss.

BREAKFAST

1 cup fresh blueberries *

(If not in season, use ½ cup defrosted frozen unsweetened blueberries, take out night before, and put in refrigerator. Blueberries have specific enzymes for activating digestive juices.)

1 hard-boiled egg

black coffee, tea, or herbal tea

LUNCH

1 all-beef frankfurter (no roll)
1 cup sauerkraut *
mustard if desired
(It is important that you have the sauerkraut with the frankfurter. The fermenting process has a specific catalytic reaction on the protein of the frankfurter.)

large head of lettuce and sliced tomato

no-sodium diet soda, black coffee, or tea

MIDAFTERNOON SNACK

water, water, water

8 oz. tomato juice

DINNER

6 oz. broiled, baked, or steamed shrimp, salmon, or flounder *

large serving of freshly steamed asparagus*—as much as you wish

sliced whole tomato

glass of water with apple-cider vinegar

no-sodium diet soda, coffee, or tea

1 plain graham cracker

Remember, drink 8 glasses of water every day.

DAY FOUR

Another high-protein day to fortify your energy in preparation for a cleansing day tomorrow.

BREAKFAST

> 1 cup fresh strawberries, or ½ fresh pineapple, or 1 apple, or 1 whole papaya

LUNCH

> 4 oz. sliced cold lean roast beef, or
> 4 oz. turkey, or
> 4 oz. chicken, or
> 4 oz. pickled herring in wine sauce, or
> 4 oz. broiled liver
>
> 1 whole tomato or 2 kiwi fruits
>
> no-sodium diet soda, black coffee, tea, or apple-cider vinegar cocktail

MIDAFTERNOON SNACK

> water, water, water
>
> 1 whole orange

DINNER

> same as lunch, plus:
> 1 large serving steamed broccoli
>
> D-Zerta diet gelatin—as much as you wish
>
> herbal tea
>
> *Remember, drink 8 glasses of water every day.*

DAY FIVE

Energy-packed day of vital, alive foods to bring a smile to your face.

BREAKFAST

> 1 oz. oatmeal, bran buds or grapenuts flakes*
>
> ½ cup skim milk
>
> ½ orange
>
> tea

LUNCH

> ½ avocado * with
>
> ½ cup skim-milk ricotta cheese or creamy cottage cheese, and 3 green or black olives
>
> 2 Wasa Crisp Bread or 2 breadsticks
>
> iced tea, coffee, or no-sodium diet soda

MIDAFTERNOON SNACK

> water, water, water
>
> 1 oz. pumpkin seeds
> (You can buy them in one ounce packages in the health food store. Excellent source of vitamin E; excellent staying power.)

DINNER

> 2 medium size baked potatoes*
> seasoned with ½ cup plain yogurt mixed with scallions and chives, and green peppers and watercress
>
> herbal tea, coffee, or apple-cider vinegar cocktail
>
> (You will feel so satisfied that you may not be able to finish the meal.)

Today's menu will meet your carbohydrate cravings. The high-potassium foods will be sure to give you a surge of energy. Wait until you step on the scale tomorrow.

Remember, drink 8 glasses of water every day.

DAY SIX

BREAKFAST

>1 big fat slice of pumpernickel bread* spread with diet margarine
>
>½ sliced orange
>
>coffee, tea

LUNCH

>up to 3 cups of fresh fruit salad
>(Make sure that only fresh fruits are used; enzymes are destroyed in the canning or cooking process.)
>
>tea or herbal tea

MIDAFTERNOON SNACK

>water, water, water
>
>20 luscious green grapes

DINNER

>1 cup whole wheat or durum wheat pasta,* seasoned with ¼ cup Aunt Millie's Spaghetti Sauce without sugar, and 1 whole green pepper
>
>salad of ½ head lettuce, watercress, parsley, raw mushrooms, and zucchini, seasoned with lemon garlic and pepper
>
>*or*
>
>8–10 oz. of baked, broiled, or poached filet of sole, haddock, halibut, or flounder (no butter)
>
>*and*
>
>1 cup fresh asparagus, or
>1 artichoke,* or
>1 cup broccoli*
>
>salad of lettuce and tomato seasoned with 1 tsp. oil and vinegar
>
>tea, herbal tea, no-sodium Perrier or seltzer with lime
>
>At this point the choice of carbohydrate or protein dinner is yours. I have given you this option so that you have a choice as to what you feel your body craves. Both will satisfy equally and create excellent weight losses. All your vitamins and nutrients have been met.
>
>*Remember, drink 8 glasses of water every day.*

DAY SEVEN

BRUNCH *

 2 scrambled eggs with 1 tsp. diet margarine with 2 Tbsp. black caviar

 coffee or tea

or

 2 eggs scrambled in 1 oz. diet margarine and 1 oz. melted Swiss cheese and ½ toasted bagel

 coffee or tea

or

 2 eggs scrambled with 2 oz. lox or 4 oz. pickled herring, ½ toasted bagel, and (optional) 6 oz. dry champagne, or Bloody Mary, or café brulé (black coffee with 1 orange or 1 lemon peel and 1 tsp. brandy flavoring)

MIDAFTERNOON SNACK

 water, water, water

 2 plain graham crackers

DINNER *

 4–6 oz. filet of sole (broiled without butter), sprinkled with chervil or chives and garlic pepper

 large portion of broccoli or spinach

 sliced lettuce and cucumbers

 1 sliced tomato

 no-sodium diet soda, coffee or tea, or no-sodium sparkling water with a twist of lime

 Remember, drink 8 glasses of water every day.

ALTERNATE BRUNCH DAY*

BREAKFAST

all the fresh fruit salad you want—oranges, apples, grapefruits, papayas, mangos, and pineapple—with ½ cup skim-milk ricotta cheese or ½ cup cottage cheese and ½ toasted bagel

DINNER

1 glass white wine (optional)

largest steamed lobster you can find (no butter sauce)
large green salad with lemon dressing

espresso, tea, or no-sodium sparkling water

or

1 lean hamburger or steak tartare, flavored with capers, basil, and mustard

You may choose to substitute and repeat another day's menu if you wish, but for best nutrition you should follow the diet as outlined. Go shopping at the beginning of the week and have all your food ready. Brown-bag whatever you need for lunch if it is not possible to obtain otherwise. It is a one-week diet that you may repeat over and over again until you achieve your best weight. If there is something on the menu that you do not like, don't eat it. Remember, this diet will keep you feeling fit and fine, and in good spirits. You have two options for a brunch and dinner meal at the end of the week. I have also enclosed some lunch options for substitution when necessary. If you find the Day One reducing diet too difficult to do each week, do it every other week. I am sure you are proud of your weight loss. Before you know it, you will have your desired trim body.

Notes for Taurus Seven-Day Reducing Diet

Enzyme Power Booster Notes

* It would be a most beneficial way for you to start your diet. If you wish you might even stay on it for two days, but that is all. I know that it is not easy to get a Taurus to stop *chewing*, so this might seem very martyr-like. However, get your determination and tenacity up, and do it. You will be happy at the results. Use only no-sodium buttermilk. (Many Taurus clients have lost up to 4 pounds on two days of buttermilk.)

Taurus Diet Notes—Day One

The enzyme action of the fresh fruit breaks down fat and acts to speed up your metabolism, giving it an extra boost for the day. All of the breakfast choices are high-quality enzyme fruits.

* Pineapple should be served ripe, so that the fructose is at its optimum and the enzymes are strong. It has natural diuretic qualities and an invigorating cleansing effect upon the kidneys and liver.

* Papaya contains the digestive juice "papain," which has a soothing effect upon the digestive system, especially the intestinal tract. Papaya is also rich in vitamins A, B, and C.

* Apples are rich in potassium and phosphorus, have a good deal of fibrous roughage, and are readily available. Your breakfast choice is simply up to you.

* Potatoes are a perfectly digested food leaving no waste in the intestine. One medium potato has 503 mg of potassium, which has a soothing effect on your nerves, Taurus. It is also high in protein, vitamins A and B, and alkaline salts. You should be sure to eat the skin.

* Do not eat the skin of the chicken or turkey. The white meat turkey has less cholesterol and calories than the dark meat, but you are by no means restricted. Both provide vitamin E, vitamin B-3, and folic acid.

Taurus Diet Notes—Day Two

This is an excellent low-calorie, high-protein day.

* Lunch: If you wish, you may have 2 Tbsp. no-oil Pritikin salad dressing.

* Dinner: If either for lunch or dinner you want less than ½ of a chicken, have only what you require.

Taurus Diet Notes—Day Three

* Blueberries have been included because of their good enzyme quality, vitamin C content, and high mineral count. Marvelous laxative properties.

* Sauerkraut, like buttermilk, is a fermented food. All fermented foods are high in enzymes. It is important to have with the frankfurter because it aids in digestion and breaks down the protein. Enjoy.

* Fish should be served without butter. Use lemon juice. You may season your asparagus with 2 Tbsp. of Parmesan cheese if you desire.

Taurus Diet Notes—Day Four

* Start your day out with just fruit so that your digestive system is ready for lunch. Remember no milk or milk products when you have fruit. The milk lactose will suppress the enzyme action of the fruit.

Lunch and Dinner: Both meals are high in protein and low in carbohydrates, designed to meet your mineral and vitamin requirements. Drink at least 8 glasses of water. The more you drink the more you will lose. If you have diet soda, make sure it is no-sodium diet soda.

Taurus Diet Notes—Day Five

* Oatmeal and bran buds or grapenuts flakes are complex carbohydrate foods. By now, Taurus, I know that you are screaming for this type of warm comforting breakfast.

* ½ medium avocado offers much nutritionally. It has 604 mg of potassium is high in fiber and vitamin E. It should not be considered "fattening" when incorporated in the manner of your reducing diet. It also has excellent satiating power.

* Potatoes have one of the highest nutrient content of all vegetables. They are rich in vitamins A and B, and protein. Potatoes also contain alkaline salts which aid in neutralizing acid waste and help cleanse the body by eliminating toxins, such as uric acid. Potatoes are very rich in potassium and will keep you energized as you continue your dieting process. You should feel very good by the end of the day and even better when you step on the scale tomorrow.

Well, you are probably feeling really good by now and I am sure that you are noticing your weight loss.

Taurus Diet Notes—Day Six

* Pumpernickel bread—can a Taurus really live without it?

* Spaghetti—make sure you buy durum wheat or vegetable spaghetti or macaroni. It is much lower in calories, and is more easily digested.

* Artichokes are the forgotten vegetable. You may use fresh, frozen, or water-pack in a can.

* Broccoli is high in vitamins A, B-2, potassium, and fiber.

Taurus Diet Notes—Day Seven

* Brunch and dinner are high in protein, low in carbohydrate, packed with all the essential nutrients to stop your sugar and starch cravings. By now, have you even thought about it?

* Alternate Brunch Day—this has been included for your variety and personal choice. However, you may not mix menus from either day to another. Now that you see your weight loss, wasn't it worth it?

TAURUS TOTAL BINGE DAY

Taurus, with all your set opinions as to why diets do not seem to work for you, the main one seems to be that you cannot live without an occasional sweet goody or binge. I have given you that option with a binge day. No more frustration for you.

Before You Binge

1. Drink water.
2. Drink water.
3. Drink water.
4. Rest.
5. Brush your teeth and rinse with your favorite mouthwash.
6. Chew sugarless gum for 20 minutes.

You may find that the desire to binge has passed. However, if you are still suffering from intense food frustration, follow these basic binge rules:

Rule One

Under no circumstances should you ever binge before completing Day Five of your Taurus Reducing Diet. This will ensure a maximum weight loss with a minimum of food frustration.

Rule Two

If, for example, you binge on the sixth day of your diet, resume your diet the following day (Day Seven) with the menu for Day Six. If you binge for just one meal, such as lunch on Day Six, resume your reducing diet with dinner of Day Six of your reducing diet.

Rule Three

Bingeing is for when you get that creepy, anxious feeling, when you feel like pulling out your hair—strand by strand—and you cannot endure dieting for even one more moment. Before you climb the walls, give yourself a binge day. It's hoped that this will not be necessary more than four times a month.

Rule Four

After you have lost your first 10 pounds, you may vary your binge day with the binge day of the sun sign opposite yours, which is Scorpio.

Remember, an occasional binge day—when necessary—will still allow you to lose weight (without guilt). Here, Taurus, is your binge day menu.

Binge Day Menu

BREAKFAST

1 frozen Aunt Jemima toaster waffle with 2 tablespoons low-calorie pancake syrup

6 oz. orange juice or 1 whole orange

coffee with ¼ cup regular milk

or

6 oz. orange juice or 1 whole orange

1 pumpernickel or whole wheat raisin bagel with 2 tsp. cream cheese, diet butter and/or jam (or ¼ cup cottage cheese substituted for cream cheese)

coffee with ¼ cup regular milk

MIDMORNING SNACK

2 cups unbuttered popcorn (throughout day if you do not have evening snack)

LUNCH

1 slice mushroom or spinach pizza

1 scoop vanilla, chocolate, coffee, or strawberry ice cream (can substitute Tofutti)
no-sodium diet soda

or

1 burrito or taco

1 scoop of vanilla, chocolate, coffee, or strawberry ice cream (can substitute Tofutti)
no-sodium diet soda

DINNER

2 glasses dry white wine (optional)

bouillabaisse (steamed fish stew), or
steamed shrimp and chinese vegetables, or 1½ lb. lobster

mixed green salad with 1 tsp. blue cheese dressing

black coffee

EVENING SNACK

¾ cup Special K cereal, with ½ cup skim milk, two packets Sweet 'n Low—sweet dreams

Maintaining Your Ideal Weight

Taurus Maintenance Foods for Optimum Health

When you have achieved your desired weight goal, you should follow a maintenance diet rich in the specific nutrients that you need each and every day.

Vitamin E

The most important duty of vitamin E, is that of antioxidation—or, in other words, to prevent oxygen from forming with toxic peroxide, thus keeping the blood pure. Vitamin E also helps prevent blood clots and decreases the possibility of stroke. In addition, vitamin E will help prevent wrinkling of the skin and maintain a youthful complexion. It is an important aid in maintaining the reproductive glands in good order.

FOODS RICH IN VITAMIN E

Apples	Eggs
Asparagus	Halibut
Avocados	Liver
Broccoli	Milk
Cabbage	Mushrooms
Carrots	Parsley
Cheeses	Peanut butter
Chicken	Salmon

Sardines	Sweet potatoes
Shrimp	Turkey
Spinach	Wheat germ
Sunflower seeds	

Iodine

Iodine is the essential trace element in the thyroid hormones. These hormones are responsible for regulating a variety of functions including growth and protein production. Iodine is necessary for the development and functioning of the thyroid gland which aids in the regulation of your metabolism and actually stimulates your metabolic rate and, thus, helps to burn excess fat. A lack of this element can result in lowered vitality, an inability to think clearly, low resistance to infection, and a tendency toward obesity. Iodine serves as an aid to the maintenance of healthy, supple arteries. Iodine is an important element in the Taurean diet. The Taurean lust for food and alcohol may at times strain the heart.

FOODS RICH IN IODINE

Apples	Iodized salt
Brussels sprouts	Kale
Cantaloupe	Lamb
Cheese	Liver
Clams	Salmon
Crab	Seaweed
Grapefruit	Shrimp
Green peppers	Spinach
Haddock	Turkey
Halibut	

Niacin (B-3)

Niacin is one of the B vitamins. Niacin aids in weight reduction by reducing the level of cholesterol in the blood and by stabilizing blood sugars. Thus niacin must be included in your maintenance foods.

FOODS RICH IN NIACIN

Alfalfa sprouts	Beef (lean)
Apricots	Brown rice
Avocados	Chicken

Corn   Mushrooms
Dried dates   Peanuts
Green peas   Peas
Halibut   Potatoes
Ham   Rice
Lentils   Salmon
Liver   Tuna

Rutin

The primary function of rutin is assisting the body in proper utilization of vitamin C. Taureans' most sensitive area is the throat region, making you susceptible to sore throats, swollen glands, and colds, so it is important that you include rutin in your daily menu. Rutin also acts as an anticoagulant, strengthening capillaries and reducing the possibility of bruising.

FOODS RICH IN RUTIN

Apricots   Lemons
Cabbage   Oranges
Cherries   Paprika
Grapefruit   Plums
Grapes   Prunes
Green peppers   Tangerines

Taurus Sample Maintenance Menu

When you reach your desired goal, please follow the maintenance eating hints found in "General Diet and Maintenance Guidelines for all Sun Signs" at the beginning of this book for proper calculations of caloric intake.

I'm including a sample maintenance menu based on your sun sign for optimal Taurus maintenance. When creating your own menus for yourself, try to choose many of the foods you eat from your Taurus Maintenance Foods lists.

2,000 CALORIES PER DAY

BREAKFAST	CALORIES
½ grapefruit	50
1 corn muffin	125
1 Tbsp. diet grape jelly	6
1 cup milk	100
	281

LUNCH	
4 oz. hamburger	246
1 hamburger bun	120
10 french fries	130
½ Tbsp. tomato catsup	145
no-sodium diet soda	0
	641

MIDAFTERNOON SNACK	
2 Tbsp. peanut butter	190
½ apple	40
	230

DINNER	
3½ oz. table wine (optional)	85
1 cup Manhattan clam chowder	80
6 oz. veal scallopine in lemon	300
salad of tomato, onions, and parsley in 1 Tbsp. olive oil	144
	609

EVENING SNACK	
1 cup ice milk	185
1 peach	40
	225

TOTAL DAILY CALORIES	1,986

Remember, drink 8 glasses of water every day.

Restaurant Eating the Taurus Way

Perhaps you have seen the following dishes on restaurant menus. Maybe you have ordered them, or maybe you have not, wondering if the calorie content was just too high. Note that all the recommended dishes here are chosen especially for your particular Taurean tastes and nutritive needs. All the foods listed within each restaurant category total no more than 600–700 calories per dish and contain the essential nutrients and vitamins necessary for your well-being. Note the high levels of niacin found in the beef entrées of both the American and French menus and also the inclusion of iodine found in the salmon and other fish fare. Hearty steak or filet mignon is included to satisfy your eating style, Taurus, and note that potatoes and sweets are listed to please your tastes.

American—Steakhouse

APPETIZERS

Marinated herring

Half grapefruit

Oxtail soup

ENTRÉES

Sirloin steak (4 oz.)

Broiled lamb chops

Filet of lemon sole, sauté meunière

Roast prime ribs of beef

Filet mignon and lobster tail (no butter)

French Restaurant

APPETIZERS

Bay scallops and oysters in champagne sauce

Filet of bass in herb sauce

Oysters baked in white wine and purée of mushrooms

ENTRÉES

Broiled sirloin with galette of potatoes

Veal chop in tarragon sauce

Sirloin steak with special red wine sauce

Sirloin steak with five different peppers

Roast baby chicken with white wine sauce and mushrooms

Rack of lamb with herbs

Italian Restaurant

APPETIZERS

Shrimp sautéed with herbs, lemon, and white wine

Thinly sliced filet mignon with green herb sauce

Tomato or clam juice

ENTRÉES

Pepper steak, flambé

Sirloin sautéed with red wine and mushrooms

Boneless chicken sautéed with fresh vegetables and white wine

Thin egg noodles with basil and garlic

Sliced filet mignon with peppers and tomato sauce

Chinese Restaurant

APPETIZERS

Hot and sour soup

Spiced cold beef

ENTRÉES

Sliced beef with watercress in hot garlic sauce

Curry beef

Sea cucumber with crabmeat

Lamb with spring onions

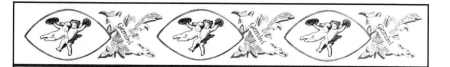

GEMINI

May 22–June 21

The Gemini
Personality

"I'm not hungry, I'll just pick."

If you have given into your Gemini nature, you have probably read the end of the chapter first. You always assume the best part of the book is at the end and read back to front, skimming the pages to get the "feel" of the message. Instead of skipping to the end this time, read the sections in order. You will find it has been well worth the wait.

Are you the Gemini who is so busy and nervous, juggling a dozen projects at once, that you forget to eat? Or are you the Gemini who, although forever moving, never forgets about food, and as you are finishing lunch, you are already planning dinner? Many-sided Gemini, the dual nature of your sign makes you as varied in your reactions individually as it does collectively.

Quick-witted, versatile, spontaneous, most Geminis are blessed with comparatively few weight problems, thriving less on food and more on the perpetual whirlwind of change and excitement they generate. Born under the fast-spinning little planet Mercury, they too trail-blaze a bright orbit that keeps them (and everyone around them) continually alert and alive. Mentally agile Gemini, you can become so enthralled working through your latest brainstorm that eating is the farthest thing from your mind. A new idea for a short story or article, an ingenious way to recess the track lighting in your living room, the kingpin answer to the computer game that has stumped you for weeks—all interest you much more than what you are putting in your mouth.

Gemini-Cancer cusp dwellers live on the frenetic energy that propels

June people through life, but they sustain themselves with a never ending supply of food to refuel and calm their high-strung nerves.

Whether you are too preoccupied with life's many changes and opportunities ever to think seriously about eating, or whether those very vicissitudes inspire you to dream even more longingly about the pleasures of food, you, Gemini, can never stop your mouth from pursuing one of your most enjoyable activities—talking. Overweight or slender, Geminis bring the art of conversation and repartee to new heights. Conversing with one friend or in the midst of several conversations hardly makes a difference to a Gemini. In fact the more variety and people to talk to the better. They communicate with such remarkable ease that friends and colleagues often find themselves standing back, marveling at the facile Gemini mind and scintillating humor.

You are especially adept at presenting your innovative, avant-garde ideas with a fun-spirited social charm. You love the creative sparks that fly when you are surrounded by others able to play off your mental leaps and turns. When working on a particularly inspiring project, you are even known to talk to the inanimate objects with which you are working. If you are cooking, you talk to the food you are preparing; if you are designing, you talk to the objects you are arranging; if you are writing, you definitely talk to your characters or talk through your ideas.

Open and inquisitive, you have a genuine curiosity about people. You love to add new friends and acquaintances to your already large collection. Socializing around a smorgasbord is a perfect way for Geminis to fulfill their gastronomical cravings while meeting their social needs. Snacks and hors d'oeuvres especially appeal to you because you are free to nibble a wide selection of tidbits, while talking to a great number of people. A sit-down dinner seems confining to a free-wheeling Gemini, who would much prefer to munch many different kinds of foods and mingle among a whole roomful of people.

If the buffet happens to feature delicacies from all over the world and the company also spans the international spectrum, Geminis feel truly in their element. The globe is simply an extension of your turf, and no place, person, food or fact is too remote for you to explore. You love to travel, and can make an adventure of a picnic in a nearby state park just as easily as you can a three-day trek in the Himalayas.

Sophisticated, you naturally refer to foreign foods by their proper names. When most of us had a crescent roll and coffee with steamed milk for breakfast, you were eating croissant and cappuccino; lunch was not noodles in green garlic sauce for you, it was tortellini with pesto. Were you to magically transport yourself to any country in the world, your marked linguistic ability would enable you to converse like a native within a few months, even if you never spoke a word of the language before you arrived.

Overcoming a language barrier and finding out about that mysterious new person who can only communicate in French or Italian or Swahili is just the kind of mental challenge Geminis love.

The phone is one of modern life's marvelous conveniences that makes it so much easier for you to talk with people. In your ideal world, every room in the house would contain two telephones as well as at least three cordless telephones, plus one in the car, for those moments when you just cannot wait to share a bit of juicy gossip or brilliant thought.

There is practically no activity you find impossible to do while talking on the phone. Your agile brain thrives on doing many things at once . . . talking, eating, watching television, and reading a magazine all at the same time. However, this dexterity can be a bit dangerous for dieting Geminis. Barely noticing how much you are eating, you can consume pounds of homemade chocolate chip cookies, spreading peanut butter evenly on top of each one. Your childhood love for sugar-coated breakfast cereals takes on new meaning as you go through each little box from the assortment packs, which you "improve" with butterscotch chips and bits of thin pretzel sticks. When bingeing, Gemini, your inventiveness knows no bounds, but wouldn't it be put to better use if you used it to reorganize the computer system at work or finish the advertising campaign presentation you wanted to show your client next week?

Instant foods appeal to you for the same reason—you never have to shift from high gear to make freeze-dried instant coffee, frozen spinach, or de-hydrated onions. Gemini you are equally fascinated by space-age eating. Tucked away in one corner of your kitchen cabinet are the nutritious powders and neatly packaged foods of the astronauts, which naturally you've tried.

Usually, you are less concerned with the nutritional value of food than you are with the taste.

But, ever difficult to pin down, Gemini, there are those of you who are very health-conscious, sprinkling bran flakes over your granola, sunflower seeds and alfalfa sprouts on your salads, wheat germ in your fresh fruit and yogurt. From time to time you may eat only vegetarian-style cooking—for variety and a cleansing of your system. Logical, scientific Gemini, you may even try a macrobiotic zen diet, fascinated by the principles of ying/yang that form the basis for this unique style of eating.

As long as you are talking or writing or redesigning, you are fine. But if you are also nibbling throughout your day, you are probably watching the scale climb higher each time you step on it. Clever Gemini, you are as ingenious and impatient when trying to lose weight as you are in all your endeavours, so it makes sense that you would be the one to try every battery-operated weight loss mechanism on the market.

Progressive Gemini, I'm sure you have also tried acupuncture and hypnotism to curb your appetite—with frustrating results, no doubt. Your excellent sense of fashion also helps you conceal your weight problem. You are an expert at disguising excess pounds with well-chosen, artistically arranged layered clothing that gives you an intriguingly offbeat bohemian/intellectual appearance. Why expend the effort to lose weight when people find you irresistible as you are, you rationalize. But you are always optimistic, and you are constantly looking for new ways to keep yourself trim and in shape.

Sexual Appetite

Perceptive Gemini, you understand the complexities and fluid nature of love. Your dual nature allows you to grasp the many sides of the human heart, and you realize that freedom to enjoy a wide variety of experiences is a prime ingredient for a relationship's growth and survival. Free-spirited Gemini, you could never find happiness in a love affair that followed rigid conventions. You know that diversity adds a sexy excitement to love, ensuring a continually renewed fire that will never become cold ash. It is just your passion for discovering the new and different that makes you such an imaginative lover and in pursuit of romance you can become inspired.

You especially love to give and receive an endless stream of little surprise gifts—one reason that loving a Gemini can be so much fun. Two hand-dipped chocolate-covered strawberries wrapped around a pale yellow rose, a record of avant-garde Japanese flute music, a book of short stories by a contemporary South American writer all find their way to your lover's doorstep, with a beautifully phrased note attached. Love can make you particularly eloquent, especially on paper. (There is even a side to the Gemini personality that can be a bit shy, which makes you even more charming.)

Flirting is one of your greatest joys in love. It is as scrumptious and as rich to you as a box full of assorted chocolate truffles but much more nourishing and completely calorie-free. You flirt with great style and humor, and you are well aware that it is hard for almost anyone to resist your captivating curiosity and well-chosen witty words. Quick-paced retorts, with a delicious undertone of sexual attraction, satisfy your interest in people. You are particularly intrigued by someone who lives an unusual life, such as an astronaut, skydiver, or trapeze artist. If on a given evening you manage to talk with a Peruvian poet, a Balinese dancer, *and* an anthropologist who recently sailed on a raft from the Ivory Coast to Brazil, how gratifying to your Gemini heart and mind, which crave a steady diet of the extraordinary.

In love, the Gemini head rules the Gemini heart, and it is through the head that the heart is won. Geminis will respond much more passionately to your declarations of love if you tell them that not only do they possess the most beautiful eyes you have ever seen in your life, but it is their brilliant and original mind that first attracted you.

Although, Gemini, you are known for a small gastronomical appetite, your sexual appetite is much heartier. You are a wonderfully innovative lover—as adventurous in lovemaking as you are in eating. You know when to add just a bit of spice or tenderness to keep romance always sparkling. You love variety—the Kama Sutra was probably written for you—and your ability to make fantasy a delightful part of sexual passion keeps your lover forever enthralled. Appeal to a Gemini's taste for spontaneity—and you have made a conquest.

Sometimes, however, you become so involved in a project at work that you temporarily forget about your love life and the person who may be waiting for you at home. You seem to have difficulty striking the right balance between work and love, devoting yourself to one at the exclusion of the other. You need both to create harmony in your twin-sided life, so try to respond to the gentle messages your slightly neglected lover may be sending. "Remember me, Gemini?" you might hear over the telephone at the office, 11 o'clock one late night. "Weren't we supposed to go out to dinner to your favorite Thai restaurant?" You may forgo dinner, but you are certainly game to make it up by going out dancing till dawn.

Just as you prefer to sample several delicacies at once, so do you enjoy entertaining a host of lovers. You quickly tire of or grow impatient with your lovers. Either they fall short of your expectations or they become too familiar and the relationship starts to feel too routine to you.

Until you feel you have found the perfect person who answers all your erotic and romantic dreams, you would much rather move on to a new lover than to spend the time working out a sexually unsatisfying relationship. However, when cupid's wily arrow strikes ever-mobile Gemini, your innate knowledge of love's eternal fluctuations helps you build a lifelong commitment. You, Gemini, embrace the ebb and flow of an evolving relationship. Forever altering and adopting your own views about life, you are quite comfortable with the fact that loving someone changes each day as feelings, desires, and expectations change.

But even your most enlightened insights and most determined resolves weaken when the shifting, restless Gemini wanderlust takes hold. Then, the urge to try something new may distract you, making you seem aloof or distant, and utterly confusing your partner. Instead of finding solace in the jar of peanut butter, talk with your lover about your feelings. Chances are, you will find the compassion you are seeking—your partner is just as bright as you are, otherwise you would never have been attracted in the first place. And since you could never tolerate a possessive lover, the itch to break free probably emanates from you—so both you and your mate will benefit from some honest communication. At times like these, you, who are so gifted with words, would rather resort to eating bowlfuls of tortilla chips and M&M's, while waiting impatiently for your lover to read your mind. Forget this method of communication and use more realistic ways of expressing your needs.

You may be surprised by what a little joint creative thinking and talking will yield. You may end up planning a vacation to Hawaii or Thailand. Nothing revives a relationship for a Gemini more effectively than an exotic vacation. You will be amazed how quickly your sexual and romantic juices begin to flow again.

Eating/Entertaining at Home

Full of whimsy and inventiveness, Gemini, you entertain with a true sense of fun and spontaneity. There is always a bit of surprise that greets your guests each time they visit. That is what makes your style so unusual—your ability to put together an eclectic assortment of elements, which you blend beautifully.

Never the traditionalist, you might decide to prepare a buffet for thirty, featuring finger food from countries and cities beginning with the letter *I* —Israel, India, Italy, Istanbul, Ireland—and maybe you will decide to start with dessert first. A genuinely gracious and adept host, you attend to your guests' every whim, deftly offering seconds, refilling glasses, bringing out yet another dish to try.

Another night, you may invite friends over for an evening of bridge. You especially love to socialize—talk, eat, flirt—while stimulating your mind with a challenging game. Beforehand, though, you usher everyone into the kitchen for assembly-line service from your streamlined, recessed stainless-steel counter space. On gray and black stoneware plates, you pile steaming homemade Italian pasta over generous chunks of French goat cheese. Complementing this may be a salad with feta cheese and olives imported from Greece. For dessert, you might treat your bridge partners to Swedish ginger cookies with Turkish coffee.

Perhaps you are the Gemini who does not cook; no matter, the takeout Chinese food you have ordered with beer imported from China and tea from the mainland Republic is every bit as enjoyable as if you were to prepare it all yourself. While your friends eat dumplings with hot sauce, you savor telling them how you happened to acquire the special tea.

Whether you serve a smorgasbord of hors d'oeuvres from countries you visited throughout Asia or five-foot heros from the local pizzeria, your friends always remember the pleasure of your company. Conversation in your home is spicy and lively—the latest gossip, the funniest story, the most extraordinary adventure. Conversation is a perfect way for you to forget about the assortment of Italian pastries you have bought for your guests. Since you love to find out the latest news, ask your friends about their job or love life or Christmas vacation plans. Amuse them—you know you have the gift. Charm and cleverness never added an ounce of fat to anyone. Be careful though that while recounting one of your hilarious anecdotes that keeps everyone in stitches, you are not simultaneously finishing the entire bowl of corn chips and guacamole dip.

Sometimes, Gemini, you have a way of forgetting what and how much you are eating. I know that it may bore you to pay attention when your tastebuds are exploding with a new discovery of chocolate-covered pretzels and your mind is engaged in flirtatious repartee, but unless you exercise some self-monitoring, you won't like what your talking digital scale has to say the next morning.

Although friends think they understand your unpredictable twists and turns, only those there to witness it realize the ability you have to create a top-notch gourmet masterpiece with hardly any preparation. Unless you can make it quickly, you lose interest.

Walk into a Gemini kitchen twenty minutes before guests are expected and you'll find a fast-moving chef, chopping, boiling, simmering, all with lightning speed and efficiency. Underneath the endearing, seemingly scatterbrained Gemini is a highly efficient person, whose kitchen gleams with the latest cookware and whose Plexiglas cabinets are filled with dehydrated, instant lunch and instant snack to make cooking (and life) simpler and faster.

Gemini, you also have a remarkable knack for combining foods, which continually amazes everyone, including you. At this point, you are probably used to the slightly bewildered reactions you get when you casually mention that the unusual dip your guests have been complimenting you on all evening is made from four jalapeño peppers and a half a can of orange juice concentrate whipped together in a blender.

One constant in your ever-moving life: an evening at home with you promises to keep your friends lightly off guard, always on their toes, delighting in your uniqueness and thoroughly entertained.

Food Shopping

If you had your druthers, Gemini, you would probably never set foot in a supermarket. In fact, to you food shopping in general is a colossal waste of your precious creative time. You continually wish that someone would invent a way to shop for food by computer—after all you have never stood on a bank line ever since you began banking at home with your Apple II.

You much prefer to frequent little markets—the local butcher, the fish store around the corner, the neighborhood fruit stand, the "mom and pop" bakery. Fewer people, less hassle, much more personal—even if you find yourself buying fewer items at one time, more frequently, maybe two or three times a week.

When you do shop in a three-block-long monstrous supermarket, you would love to whiz down the aisles on roller skates, a Walkman filling your head with disco sounds. According to you, high-flying Gemini, eating like everything else should be fun, and what is more fun than popping into your shopping cart all the frozen, instant and snack foods that happen to strike your fancy. Frozen mini pizzas you can drop in the toaster, cinnamon pop tarts you devour untoasted, barbecued smoked almonds, heat-and-serve tacos, ready-to-eat lasagne. Health food or junk food, your interest in nutrition fluctuates daily. As long as food tastes good, that is what counts.

Next to taste, Gemini, a clever advertising campaign influences your food selections to a remarkable degree. A well-marketed product tastes better, you joke, but your kidding is not far from your true beliefs. For Gemini, mind and mouth can turn a phrase with dazzling dexterity, to enjoy a slogan or jingle as much as what it sells.

As you stand before the cash register, your shopping cart looks as if you are stocking snacks for a blizzard or hurricane, and you have probably forgotten that in your refrigerator at home you already have half the items you are about to buy. But maybe that is an excuse for a party, and what could be a better way for efficient, social Gemini to combine both and make sure every bit of food is enjoyed.

Social Dining

Wherever you happen to dine, fun-loving Gemini, you want to enjoy yourself. For you, that means being with people whom you keep laughing and who make you laugh, frequenting at least four different restaurants, bars and discos on one given night and discovering the most unique, the most exotic each has to offer. Even if you don't actually get to all four, planning to go can be very pleasurable for many of you.

A typical Gemini evening might begin by your convincing a "small" party of ten friends to try a new Tex-Mex high-tech bar/restaurant you heard was terrific from someone at work. Word of mouth continues to be your richest source for sniffing out the most unusual or hottest places to go. Your taste buds began to tingle when you heard about the ten-foot-long chrome bar of Tex-Mex tidbits served smorgasbord-style. When you arrive, you are delighted by the variety—smoked chicken strips with avocado and papaya, blue corn chips and spicy red pepper dip, cream of mango soup, barbecued beef chunks with shredded coconut and hot sauce. You really begin to take off, sampling everything, talking to everyone—the people you are with, the people at the tables on either side of you, the waiters and waitresses, the people you meet at the food bar as you spoon tomato, onion, and olive salad onto your plate.

An evening for you has as many stops as courses of your favorite buffet and for phase two of your evening, you may decide to transport the moveable feast of friends, fun, and food to a BYOB New Orleans jazz club. Before you leave, though, you invite the couple at the next table to join your retinue. The musical breather gives you just enough space in your stomach for dessert, and after an hour or two of Dixieland and ragtime, off you go again for Chinese pastry at a tea house you always wanted to try. While less energetic signs may show flagging energy, a shot of Gemini verve perks everyone up for reggae dancing in a converted warehouse downtown. By 5 A.M., you may have lost most of your original crowd, but you have collected a whole new group of people, and just as the sky is turning pink, you find yourself arranging a trip to the all-night deli for bagels, cream cheese, and coffee for a picnic breakfast at dawn on somebody's terrace. Careful, Gemini, the impulse to enjoy the moment may end up with several inches on your hips as a reminder of the fun you have had earlier. Even if you want to eat it now, remember, the food will be there tomorrow. Pace yourself.

For the following evening, you may plan an intimate dinner for you and that delectable new person you met the night before. You decide to begin this romance at the revolving tower-top restaurant with the panoramic view. As long as you are having a good time, which means good conversation, you are happy to spend an evening—or at least a large part of it—in one place.

You can turn the simple act of ordering a meal into a memorable, joyful experience, and you have a charming way of deciding what you and your partner will eat. Tactfully you might suggest the steak tartare, which you have heard is prepared particularly well at this restaurant, or maybe, you add, your companion would prefer the squid with scallions, sherry, and fresh ginger. You handle these arrangements so diplomatically, only you know you are secretly satisfying your dual Gemini appetite—trying two specialties that appeal to you equally. Also, you just adore taking a taste from every dish at the table—it's much more exciting to you than merely eating your own choice.

Your wonderful sense of humor makes you very appreciative of a good comedian and nothing pleases you more than clever cabaret that allows you to eat and giggle at the same time. You also love spacious three-tiered bars with balcony after balcony, so you can see everyone and be seen, while catching the most interesting bits from the conversation at your table. You love to watch people as much as you love talking to them. Trust Gemini to appear at the chicest places in town. You have a real nose for the best—no new undiscovered spot escapes your ever-receptive ears— from the number-one hamburger joint to the most futuristic ice cream parlor to the most soul-satisfying Creole restaurant.

Although you love to try new pubs, bars, coffee shops, and cafés, after an evening of carousing during which you wend your way from one end of town to the other, you find it hard to remember the names of the places you have been. You can recount with entertaining detail who said what to whom, whom you saw, who you just happened to bump into, who you flirted with—but what you ate exactly and where it was—those answers evade you. For social Gemini, company and conversation come first. And like lightning, Geminis rarely return to the same restaurant twice. Why should they, they ask, when there are so many new places to try!

Special-Occasion Dining

Every day is a special occasion for a Gemini, and along with the great excitement you create celebrating any event, big or small, generally you are constantly nibbling. A Sunday trip to the zoo turns into a safari with a Gemini at the head. But you love to feed yourself (and the friends you bring with you), as well as the furry animals. A peanut for the elephant, a peanut for me—a pretzel for the monkey, a lick of soft ice cream for me. . . . Sound familiar?

When traveling, Gemini, your round-the-world jaunts are filled with once-in-a-lifetime adventures and lots of exotic food. Somehow, you seem to leave your diet resolutions on the airline ticket counter right before you board your first plane. From Kenya to Turkey to Italy, no native delicacy is left untried, no matter how fattening or how many you munch.

Not counting the spontaneous get-togethers, too many to count, that make your social calendar glitter, you love to celebrate the holidays you enjoy. For July 4th, you arrange a backyard barbecue for fifty friends, over-stocking franks, hamburgers, cole slaw. To avoid waste, you spend the rest of the week personally finishing the leftovers. What would Halloween be like without your now-legendary annual party. But no matter how conscientiously you try, you can never resist the tiny chocolate bars and candy corns you supposedly bought for trick-or-treaters.

Gemini Health

Gemini, you are among the lucky signs endowed with the gift of youthful appearance, natural slenderness, and good health. You have an agile and active mind but sometimes you have a tendency to push yourself to the limit, which results in extreme nervous tension, as well as physical and mental exhaustion. An overtaxed mind and body will certainly result in health problems. At those times, you may be either too preoccupied to eat, or you fashion a diet of cigarettes, coffee, and continuous junk food snacks for an instantaneous sugar boost. Erratic eating patterns can be particularly disastrous for Gemini's already frazzled nerves. You need to slow your pace, relaxing your ever creative, ever thinking brain.

Make sure though that when resting, you avoid boredom, it can actually make you ill. Learn a new language, take scuba diving lessons, go mountain climbing (you need lots of fresh air), create a new salad combining arugula, cashews, and orange slices, and invite a friend over to share it with you.

Each sign of the zodiac rules certain parts of the body, which are usually the most sensitive and vulnerable areas for those people born at that time. Gemini rules all of "tubular system," such as the bronchial, fallopian, and eustachian tubes; as well as the windpipe, esophagus, apex of the lungs, the pulmonary artery, the pulmonary veins, the thymus gland, larynx, arms, fingers, second rib (which affects asthma), wrist bones, and eyesight. In addition, another sensitive spot for you, Gemini, is the dorsal spine area. As the arms and shoulders are particularly vulnerable parts, make sure, Gemini, that you keep your body posture erect so that you do not put added pressure on these two areas. Also a perpetually agitated emotional state can play havoc with your defense system, makes you susceptible to upper respiratory infections like bronchitis, laryngitis, and even pneumonia.

The dual nature of the Gemini sun sign can cause two diseases to manifest at one time.

Diseases to which Geminis are subject to include:

Accidents to shoulder, collar, clavicle bone, and hands	Pleurisy
Asthma	Rheumatism in arms, hands and shoulders
Bronchitis	Sciatica pain in the hips and thighs
Diseases of trachea and esophagus	Speech problems
Hay fever	Thymus gland
Mental depression and exhaustion	

Potassium chloride is the Gemini cell salt. Cell salts are naturally occurring minerals that are normal constituents of the body cells. They are found in trace amounts in foods, and plants, animals, and human beings require these compounds for proper nutrition. And, like vitamins, cell salts get used up. Potassium chloride enables the body to assimilate other nutritional substances found in a variety of foods. It is also the cell salt responsible for the formation of fibrin. Fibrin is an essential constituent of every tissue and organ in the body; it is a filament protein which aids in blood clotting and general coagulation. Fibrin also plays a role in maintaining the proper shape of cells. A deficiency of potassium chloride can cause colds and congestion of the chest as well as malnutrition. Potassium chloride is one preventive measure Geminis can use to help protect themselves against sore throats, tonsilitis, dandruff, and psoriasis.

The best source of potassium chloride is found in the following foods and should be included in your daily plan after you have lost your desired weight and are on maintenance menus.

FOODS RICH IN POTASSIUM CHLORIDE

Apricots	Oranges
Asparagus	Peaches
Carrots	Pears
Cauliflower	Pineapples
Celery	Plums
Green beans	Sweet corn

Usually Geminis are too involved developing their many interests and ideas simultaneously to pay much attention to nutrition and vitamins. Grabbing a bite while you are on the go may be the life-style you prefer, Gemini, but it is not what your body needs. The sugar you regularly infuse into your system can induce or aggravate a depressive state, the endless supply of coffee you drink serves to make you more tense, and chain smoking puts a terrible strain on your lungs, bronchials, and larynx. You need a calming diet, rich in all the B vitamins, especially vitamin B-1 (thiamin), as well as such minerals as calcium and magnesium, which are natural tranquilizers. Eating foods rich in vitamins A and D will protect your lungs from infection.

Restless Gemini, many of you have difficulty sleeping at night. Your supercharged brain seems to work overtime all too frequently. To help you get a peaceful night's rest, you might try taking 500–660 mg of the amino acid L-tryptophan, one-half hour before bedtime. Take a tablet with water or juice only; do not ingest it with milk or any milk products. L-tryptophan is considered by many nutritionists to be the body's most effective calming agent. You will find that the edginess and depression that insomnia often causes will disappear with a good night's sleep. Anxious Geminis can also take one tablet during the day to calm those supersensitive nerves.

Above all, Gemini, use your fine intelligence to control yourself when nervous energy propels you to the refrigerator. Relaxation comes not with compulsive, mindless, neurotic eating, but with heightened self-regard. Turn the care and concern you have for others inward, and take some time concentrating on yourself. Curb your impulse to rush. Good health takes time to develop, and I guarantee that you will feel better sooner than you imagine.

Gemini Daily Nutritional Supplements

- One general multivitamin with minerals
- One super B-complex
- 2,000 mg vitamin C
- 600–800 mg Os-Cal (calcium carbonate from oyster shells)

Remember, Gemini...

This diet is uniquely prepared to address your sun sign and *should not be interchanged with any other Sun Sign Diet.* It has been prepared to meet your biological, chemical, nutritional and behavioral needs. For optimum weight loss, follow the diet exactly as it appears. Before starting your Gemini diet, carefully read "General Diet and Maintenance Guidelines for All Sun Signs," at the beginning of this book. Remember, drink 8 glasses of water daily.

You will note that even though your Gemini diets are each only three days long, they include the necessary vitamins and minerals to help you maintain your good health. The above supplements will ensure that you are getting nutritional requirements even when your erratic eating patterns cause you to follow an inbalanced diet.

Good luck, and *go for it.*

Gemini Three-Day Reducing Diets A and B

Restless Gemini, you who quickly lose interest in dieting, here at last is a program tailored to meet your needs. It is as fun and varied and exciting as you are.

I have prepared two simple three-day diets. (I can't imagine a Gemini reading one sentence further if I did not include two diet programs. Even you, impatient Gemini, can follow anything for three days.) You may choose to start with Diet A for three days and then follow with Diet B for three days. Or, you may decide to reverse the order. However, under no circumstances should you mix menus from diets A and B. If you really dislike a particular food on your daily menu, just leave it out—but do not substitute.

You may repeat the diet(s) until you have achieved your desired weight loss. If you plan to use both Diet A and Diet B throughout the month, you are entitled to have a "binge" day when you feel that you just cannot go on any longer without pulling your hair out. Use a binge day no more than four times a month. (You will find binge day instructions at the end of the Three-Day Reducing Diets.)

Approach the following diet as a new adventure and challenge. Though it may appear to be a bit unorthodox, it is designed specifically to support your nutritional needs, body chemistry and fast-paced style of living. In this diet you eat the tasty exotic foods you love—you will even find wine and champagne included, and as many snacks as calorically possible. All foods are easy to prepare, so you can adapt the menus to your busy schedule.

Rich in the B vitamins, as well as vitamins A and C, and the minerals calcium and magnesium, this diet will make you feel lighter, livelier, and clearer. In fact, you will have more bubbling Gemini energy than you probably have ever had before.

At the end of your reducing diets, you will find "Notes for Gemini Three-Day Reducing Diet A/B." In this section I explain the nutritional effects of foods included in your diet and why they are so important for the Gemini constitution.

To speed weight loss and suppress your appetite, you may choose to try a dietary fiber called Glucomannan, which is extracted from the Japanese konjac root. A final monograph on its effectiveness has not yet been established by the FDA, as it has no history of use in the United States before 1958; however, the konjac root has been cultivated and eaten in Asia for over a thousand years. Glucomannan aids in decreasing cholesterol and triglyceride levels, and in maintaining low-density lipoprotein levels. It acts as a dietary fiber to increase viscosity and moisture content of food, helping it move easily through the intestinal tract. Two capsules taken three times a day may cut your appetite in half!

GEMINI THREE-DAY REDUCING DIET A

DAY ONE

BREAKFAST

½ cup unsweetened applesauce stirred into 8 oz. plain yogurt or 4 oz. skim-milk ricotta cheese

LUNCH

Gemini Jalapeño Orange Yogurt Dip* over crudities

and

1 hard-boiled egg

or

4 oz. sliced cold roast beef*

6 water-pack artichoke hearts* flavored with Dijon mustard

tea or no-sodium seltzer with lime.

MIDAFTERNOON SNACK

20 grapes*

DINNER

1 cup durum wheat spaghetti* mixed with ¼ cup Aunt Millie's spaghetti sauce, and 2 Tbsp. grated Romano or Parmesan cheese (add 2 oz. water-pack tuna if you desire)

salad of watercress,* parsley,* fresh spinach, and lettuce seasoned with lemon juice and garlic pepper

espresso coffee with lemon peel

EVENING SNACK

20 grapes and 1 can Yoo-Hoo diet chocolate drink

Remember, drink 8 glasses of water every day.

DAY TWO

BREAKFAST
>1 bran muffin with 2 tsp. diet margarine
>
>decaffeinated coffee with a little milk

MIDMORNING SNACK
>4 oz. unsweetened grapefruit juice* mixed with 4 oz. no-sodium club soda

LUNCH

>### *Asparagus Pistachio à la Gemini* *
>Cook up to 1 lb. fresh or frozen asparagus. Top with 15 pistachio nuts and ¼ cup guacomole dip (La Victoria brand)...delicious!

MIDAFTERNOON SNACK
>2 cups hot tea

DINNER
>4 oz. unsweetened grapefruit juice with 4 oz. no-sodium club soda
>
>½ baked or broiled chicken with Mexican salsa sauce
>
>as much fresh or frozen broccoli or cauliflower you want with 1 oz. Swiss cheese
>
>salad of arugula, cabbage, watercress, and 2 Tbsp. sunflower seeds seasoned with 2–3 Tbsp. no-oil Pritikin salad dressing
>
>no-sodium Perrier with a twist of lime

EVENING SNACK
>2 cups unsalted air-blown popcorn
>
>*Remember, drink 8 glasses of water every day.*

DAY THREE

BREAKFAST

6 almonds or pecans

⅔ cup Dannon lemon yogurt*

tea with lemon

LUNCH

pita sandwich of tofu,* onion, tomato, bean sprouts, and alfalfa

or

4 oz. cottage cheese or ricotta cheese* with 1 chopped apple, 2 tsp. raisins on a slice of pumpernickel bread

iced decaffeinated coffee or no-sodium seltzer with lime

MIDAFTERNOON SNACK

20 grapes*

DINNER

1 glass dry white wine (optional)

2 broiled or baked veal chops*

½ jar roasted peppers* in natural juice

1 cup raw spinach sprinkled with lemon

juice and garlic

D-Zerta diet gelatin—all you want

Remember, drink 8 glasses of water every day.

GEMINI THREE-DAY REDUCING DIET B

DAY ONE

BREAKFAST
>1 whole papaya,* 1 mango,* or 2 oranges

LUNCH
>8 oz. bowl of brown rice* with 2 tsp. diet margarine topped with 1 poached egg
>
>Chinese, herb, or regular tea
>
>1 Chinese fortune cookie

MIDAFTERNOON SNACK
>3 fresh apricots or 1 tangerine

DINNER
>8 oz owl of brown rice* with 2 tsp. diet margarine topped with 1 poached egg
>
>1 Chinese fortune cookie

EVENING SNACK
>3 fresh apricots* or 1 tangerine
>
>herbal tea

>*Remember, drink 8 glasses of water every day*

DAY TWO

BREAKFAST

¼ honeydew, ½ cantaloupe, or 1 orange

1 slice rye toast

MIDMORNING SNACK

1 tangerine

LUNCH

Avocado or Tomato Tuna Salad

½ avocado or tomato stuffed with 3 oz. water-pack tuna, served with alfalfa sprouts, cauliflower, watercress, 5 black olives and topped with 2 tsp. caviar.

no-sodium seltzer with a twist of lime

MIDAFTERNOON SNACK

10 pistachio nuts

1 can Yoo-Hoo diet chocolate drink

DINNER

1 cup fresh or canned (Campbell's) gazpacho soup

2-egg omelette of either broccoli, spinach, or watercress, made with a little butter

tea, no-sodium diet soda or seltzer

EVENING SNACK

1 peach or 1 cup fresh strawberries

Remember, drink 8 glasses of water every day.

DAY THREE

BREAKFAST

*Banana Milk Shake**
In blender, mix until frothy, 8 oz. skim milk, 1 small banana, 2 Tbsp. wheat germ, and 2–3 ice cubes.

LUNCH

4 oz. Tofutti,* any flavor

1 small banana

or

4 oz. white wine (optional)

1 bowl French onion soup

MIDAFTERNOON SNACK

1 oz. sunflower seeds

DINNER

6 oz. package Mrs. Paul's frozen light natural sole filets*

large salad of spinach, endive, arugula, mushrooms, watercress, and green peppers*

(at least 2 cups) seasoned with 2 Tbsp. Pritikin no-oil salad dressing and/or garlic pepper

no-sodium diet soda

EVENING SNACK

1 35-calorie strawberry Jell-O frozen pudding pop

Remember, drink 8 glasses of water every day.

Notes for Gemini Three-Day Reducing Diet A

Gemini Diet A Notes—Day One
This is a very well-balanced day of proteins and carbohydrates. Breakfast is rich in calcium and the B vitamins, so that nerves will remain calm even with your hectic pace.

* Jalapeño peppers have been referred to as a "Mexican chicken soup." They have an antibiotic property, are an excellent source of vitamins A and C, and when combined with egg yolk, provide an excellent high-protein lunch.

Jalapeño Orange Yogurt Dip
5 fresh jalapeño peppers
8 oz. plain yogurt
1 package diet orange Tang
Mix the above ingredients together in blender for 1 minute.

* Roast beef and artichokes are both low-calorie, high-protein, and high-energy foods.
* Durum wheat spaghetti is lowest calorie pasta available, and is the only type that you should use on your diet. A quick, readily absorbed carbohydrate meal.
* Watercress and parsley must be included where indicated in your diet, because of the rich source of calcium these foods provide. It is not necessary to drink glasses of milk if you include other sources of calcium.

Gemini Diet A Notes—Day Two
* Unsweetened grapefruit juice mixed with no-sodium seltzer or club soda goes into the bloodstream quickly and provides an instant lift.
* Asparagus is an excellent diuretic vegetable. It provides vitamins C, B-1, and folic acid. In addition, it is rich in the enzyme asparagine, which helps to break up accumulated fats in the cells.
* Pistacho nuts are rich in phosphorus, iron, potassium, and magnesium. Another excellent Gemini food for quick energy.
* Guacamole is one of Gemini's favorite foods, and a diet for you would not be complete without it!
* Chicken is naturally high in vitamin B-6 and low in calories. B-6 helps minimize water retention and is essential to the utilization of protein.

Gemini Diet A Notes—Day Three
*Yogurt and almonds or pecans are packed with B vitamins and calcium. Slow to metabolize and with great staying power, this breakfast is a nice relaxed way to start your day.
* Tofu and pita bread sandwich, as well as cottage cheese/raisin salad are naturally light and easily digested combinations. Tofu is an excellent vegetable protein and a natural nutritional source for the Gemini constitution.
* Grapes are an excellent snack for you. The natural fructose is quickly absorbed in the blood stream, and the natural silicon in the grape has a very calming effect on the constitution.

* Veal chops and roasted peppers are rich in all the B vitamins as well as vitamins A and C.

You should be very proud of yourself, Gemini . . . how much have you lost? Why not go ahead and try for the next three days.

Notes to Gemini Three-Day Reducing Diet B

Gemini Diet B Notes—Day One
* Papaya and mango are rich in vitamin C and accelerate the enzyme production in your body.
* Rice is not only rich in the B vitamins and a perfect carbohydrate, but it is an important food for balance, within yourself and the universe. It is also a highly alkaline food, which will help to balance your more acid constitution.
* Apricots have the highest level of iron in the fruit kingdom.

Gemini Diet B Notes—Day Two
A perfectly well-balanced Gemini day of low-calorie dieting, while incorporating all the essential maintenance requirements for Gemini's optimum health, and in accordance with your very special taste preferences. You should certainly not feel as though you are dieting today!

Gemini Diet B Notes—Day Three
* Bananas and milk are a soothing and wonderful way for you to start your day. The potassium-rich banana and calcium-rich milk are important for your nervous system. It tastes like a milkshake. If not sweet enough for you, add 2 packets of sugar substitute.
* Tofutti is made from tofu. Although it has many sweeteners and is not in its pure tofu form, it is an acceptable deviation from your dieting fare. It will make you feel as though you are "almost cheating." And there are those times when this is just enough for you.
* Mrs. Paul's frozen light natural filets are easy and convenient to prepare. Cooking fish is not always your favorite chore, Gemini, and you will find this dish a delight.
* Spinach, endive, mushrooms, and green pepper salad. Your system needs the high in folic acid and B and C vitamins.

End of your diet . . . now step on the scale. I am sure you will be delighted. Repeat your Gemini diet for continued weight loss.

GEMINI TOTAL BINGE DAY

Gemini, in the midst of all your social flutter, scheduled and spontaneous activities, you sometimes find yourself in such a frenzied state that you are unable to continue your diet. If you have stayed with your two Gemini diets for the total six days you are entitled to have a binge day. Use it only when necessary and never more than four times a month. Read the following rules carefully.

Before You Binge
1. Drink water.
2. Drink water.
3. Drink water.
4. Rest.
5. Brush your teeth and rinse with your favorite mouthwash.
6. Chew sugarless gum for 20 minutes.

You may find that the desire to binge has passed. However, if you are still suffering from intense food frustration, follow these basic binge rules:

Rule One
Under no circumstances should you ever binge before completing Day Six of your reducing diet. This will ensure a maximum weight loss with a minimum of food frustration.

Rule Two
If, for example, you binge on the seventh day of your diet, resume your diet the following day (Day Eight) with the menu for Day Seven. If you binge for just one meal, such as lunch on Day Seven, resume your reducing diet with dinner on Day Seven of your reducing diet.

Rule Three
Bingeing is for when you get that creepy, anxious feeling, when you feel like pulling out your hair—strand by strand—and you cannot endure dieting for even one more moment. Before you climb the walls, give yourself a binge day. It's hoped that this will not be necessary more than four times a month.

Rule Four
After you have lost your first 10 pounds, you may vary your binge day with the binge day of the sun sign opposite yours, which is Sagittarius.

Remember, an occasional binge day—when necessary—will still allow you to lose weight (without guilt). Here, Gemini, is your binge day menu.

Binge Day Menu

BREAKFAST

4 oz. orange juice or 1 whole orange

1 whole wheat or pumpernickel bagel
1 Tbsp. cream cheese

café au lait with 2 Tbsp. Cool Whip dessert topping

LUNCH

frankfurter on roll and loads of sauerkraut and mustard

or

2 Mexican tacos

or

1 slice pizza

no-sodium diet soda or light beer

MIDAFTERNOON SNACK

2 cups air-blown popcorn

1 strawberry or cantaloupe Frozfruit pop

DINNER

4 oz. glass white wine or champagne (optional)

6 oz. any broiled or baked fish (no butter)

1 cup linguine mixed with 1 tsp. olive oil, garlic pepper, and 2 Tbsp. grated Parmesan cheese

1 sliced tomato with fresh basil

no-sodium Perrier with a twist of lime

1 cup fresh strawberries with 1 oz. rum

Maintaining Your Ideal Weight

Gemini Maintenance Foods for Optimum Health

When you have achieved your desired weight goal, you should follow a maintenance diet rich in the specific nutrients that you, Gemini, need each and every day.

The B Vitamins

The B vitamins are essential in maintaining the health of the nervous system, and are used by the body to help synthesize enzymes. The B vitamins aid the body to break down proteins, carbohydrates, and fats. A deficiency can lead to heart ailments and an overly sensitive nervous system. Poor eating habits and excessive alcohol consumption can drastically deplete the body's supply of these vitamins. To keep your nervous system in tiptop shape, Gemini, reach for foods rich in this vitamin.

FOODS RICH IN THE B VITAMINS

Alfalfa sprouts	Egg yolk
Avocados	Fish
Bananas	Green peppers
Beets	Lamb
Cabbage	Liver
Chicken	Peanuts
Cottage cheese	Potatoes

Rice	Tuna
Salmon	Veal
Skim milk	Yogurt
Sunflower seeds	

Vitamin B-1 (Thiamin)

Vitamin B-1, or thiamin, is crucial for proper metabolism of carbohydrates. When combined with pyruvic acid, it forms an enzyme that breaks down carbohydrates into glucose, which produces "energy." Thiamin also helps stabilize the nervous system. Frenetic Gemini, thiamin can help to relax you and alleviate your insomnia. The body's supply of thiamin is depleted by smoking, alcohol consumption, and excessive sugar ingestion, so make sure you include thiamin-rich foods in your diet.

FOODS RICH IN VITAMIN B-1 (THIAMIN)

Asparagus	Pistachio nuts
Avocado	Radishes
Beef liver	Rice
Egg yolk	Sweet corn
Grapefruit	Wheat germ
Okra	Whole wheat flour

Vitamin C

Vitamin C is very important in helping the body resist dangerous bacteria and infection. It also aids in the formation of collagen. Collagen constitutes about 35 to 40 percent of the body's protein. It fortifies cells, keeping them in their natural formations and allowing them to resist any invading infections. Vitamin C is also critical in the production of white blood cells, which protect the body from invading bacteria, reducing Gemini's proclivity to colds, bronchitis, and allergies.

FOODS RICH IN VITAMIN C

Alfalfa	Blueberries
Almonds	Broccoli
Apples	Brussels sprouts
Asparagus	Cantaloupe
Bananas	Carrots
Beets	Celery

Chicken	Orange juice
Cranberries	Paprika
Currants	Parsley
Grapefruit	Pineapple (fresh only)
Green peppers	Skim milk
Jalapeño peppers	Strawberries
Lemons	Tomatoes
Oranges	Watercress

Vitamins A and D

Your lungs need vitamins A and D to resist infection. It is of particular value to fight against upper respiratory infections and other virus-caused illnesses. I recommend that you include the following foods as often as possible for future healthy eating and nutrition.

FOODS RICH IN VITAMINS A AND D

Bananas	Oranges
Broccoli	Parsley
Cantaloupe	Peaches
Carrots	Red chili peppers
Cheese	Shrimp
Egg yolk	Squash
Herring	Sunflower seeds
Mangos	Watercress
Milk	Yogurt
Mushrooms	

Magnesium

Magnesium is one of the minerals essential to maintain a proper balance within the body of calcium and phosphorus. Magnesium is also necessary for a healthy nervous system, as it helps to carry messages from the brain to the muscles. Magnesium plays a role in the regulation of the heartbeat; a deficiency can lead to heart palpitations.

FOODS RICH IN MAGNESIUM

Almonds	Avocados
Apples	Beets
Asparagus	Broccoli

Buckwheat
Cabbage
Carob
Cauliflower
Cherries
Chicken
Corn
Cucumbers
Dried beans
Egg yolk
Figs
Grapes
Green peas
Kidney
Lamb

Lemons
Lettuce
Limes
Liver
Mushrooms
Olives
Onions
Peaches
Pears
Pistachio nuts
Plums
Radishes
Red wine
Sesame seeds
Spinach

Calcium

About 99 percent of the body's calcium is found in the bones and teeth, fortifying the skeletal tissues. It helps to maintain vitality and physical endurance. Calcium is vital in the manufacturing of certain enzymes.

FOODS RICH IN CALCIUM

Alfalfa
Almonds
Avocados
Beets
Broccoli
Carrots
Cauliflower
Celery
Chick peas
Chicken livers
Dried apricots
Green beans
Lemons
Lettuce

Lobster
Onion
Parsley
Peaches
Plums
Sardines
Shrimp
Skim milk
Soy beans
Spinach
Sunflower seeds
Tomatoes
Watercress

Gemini Sample Maintenance Menu

When you reach your desired goal, please follow the maintenance eating hints found in "General Diet Maintenance Guidelines for All Sun Signs" at the beginning of this book for proper calculations of caloric intake.

I'm including a sample maintenance menu based on your sun sign for optimal Gemini maintenance. When creating your own menu for yourself, try to choose many of the foods you eat from your Gemini Maintenance Foods lists.

2,000 CALORIES PER DAY

BREAKFAST	CALORIES
6 oz. orange juice	83
½ cup lowfat yogurt with	72
1 diced apple	80
1 slice whole wheat toast	59
1 Tbsp. diet margarine	34
coffee or tea	0
	328

MIDMORNING SNACK	
1 small slice Sara Lee blueberry ring	133
4 oz. tomato juice	20
	153

LUNCH	
1 taco (shell, beef, cheese, raw vegetables)	317
small garden salad with	
2 tsp. low-calorie dressing	100
iced tea	0
	417

MIDAFTERNOON SNACK	
1 oz. Edam cheese	101
4 saltine crackers	52
	153

BEFORE DINNER SNACK

4 oz. glass white wine (optional)	83
1 oz. sunflower seeds	157
	240

DINNER

4 oz. glass white wine (optional)	83
3½ oz. lamb chop	339
1 large artichoke with	44
2 tsp. melted butter	72
½ cup rice	90
	628

EVENING SNACK

½ cup vanilla ice-milk	92

TOTAL DAILY CALORIES

	2,011

Remember, drink 8 glasses of water every day.

Restaurant Eating the Gemini Way

Perhaps you have seen the following dishes on restaurant menus. Both the dishes and the types of restaurants chosen will appeal to your Gemini palate and satisfy your nutritional needs. Note that all of the recommended dishes contain the nutrients specified in your Gemini maintenance food lists. In all menus, one appetizer plus one entrée equals approximately 600–700 calories.

Indian Restaurant

APPETIZERS

Vegetable soup flavored with skim milk, herbs, and spices

Indian-style salad, made with tomatoes, onions, cucumbers, and green peppers

ENTRÉES

Mixture of minced lamb, onions, and herbs roasted on skewers

Shrimps sautéed in a sauce of herbs and spices

Lamb cooked with fresh tomatoes in a spicy curry sauce

Saffron rice mixed with chicken and herbs

Japanese Restaurant

APPETIZERS

Filet of thinly sliced fresh, raw fish, served with exotic vegetables and a piquant soy sauce

Chopped squid, broiled and seasoned with sea chestnuts

ENTRÉES

Tuna broiled with green onions

Chicken prepared with Japanese white wine, bamboo shoots, and other Japanese vegetables and spices

Casserole of meat, fish, and vegetables

A platter of thin slices of assorted raw fish, served with ginger and a piquant soy sauce

Mexican Restaurant

APPETIZERS

Mexican chicken salad

Guacamole

ENTRÉES

Corn tortillas filled with king crabmeat, baked in a tomato sauce

Layer of tortilla with shredded chicken and cheese in a spicy tomato sauce

Peppers stuffed with three cheeses topped with Creole tomato sauce

Fresh shrimps in a green parsley, wine, and garlic sauce

Gourmet Health Food

APPETIZERS

Fresh tropical fruit bowl

Shrimp cocktail

ENTRÉES

Almond turkey salad (turkey breast tossed with almonds, apples, raisins and celery, served with avocado slices and fresh vegetables)

Artichoke linguine with shrimps and scallops

Chicken broccoli and walnut salad in a sesame seed dressing

Vegetable lasagne (fresh vegetables mixed with skim-milk ricotta cheese, marinara sauce, and eggplant)

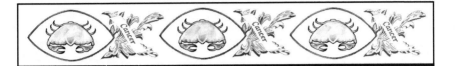

CANCER

June 22–July 23

The Cancer Personality

"I'm in the mood to eat."

For you, Cancer, there is no place like home. And the best place at home is the kitchen. If you are not a caterer by profession, you are one at heart. Nothing pleases you more than setting a bountiful table for your family and friends. With food you communicate, console, celebrate. Your childhood memories carry the aromas and flavors of long-ago meals, and when you prepare fudge brownies, or hearty chili for your own children, you feel you are enriching their own future memories of their time with you. When you make sure the silver candy dish in the living room is always full and the large ceramic bowl in the kitchen is always heaped high with fresh fruit, you are telling your friends they are always welcome in your home; you are always ready to receive them.

With food so symbolic of well-being for you, Cancer, you wonder how on earth you can stay on a diet. How can you deprive your family of ice-cream desserts? Harder still, how can you resist joining them for a midnight snack? So many of your closest moments occur over the kitchen table; a tall glass of milk and a generous chunk of chocolate cake seem to make everyone relax. So if you deprive yourself of food, won't you also be depriving yourself and your family of love?

These questions show your essential nature: You want to be the best you can be, but never at the expense of your home, family, friends. Cancer is a deeply sensitive sign, moody as the moon; blues songs must have been written with you in mind. You try to do all you can for the people you love, but you also take seriously your professional responsibilities. You are well-organized, hard-working, goal-oriented, and trying to do justice to both work and family absorbs all your available energy.

Food means much more to you than just nourishment. When you feel terrific, you celebrate your happy time with an éclair . . . or two. When you are feeling low, you might comfort yourself by hunkering down by a rock on the beach, sipping a malted, downing a bag of potato chips while staring at the rhythmic ocean waves.

You also eat out of sentiment. You have seen every heart-wrenching, tearjerking movie ever made, and upon its tragic ending you've run out of the theater clutching your bag of M&M's and chocolate bonbons you purchased in the lobby. Oh, you needed that. What a sad movie. It made you feel so much better.

Cancers are real softies at heart. You've probably saved every birthday card, love letter, and theater program you ever got. You press flowers from proms and weddings and mount them in albums. You become very attached to memories involving friendships and emotions. You cry over every pop of a champagne cork. And you may find many special occasions to celebrate.

You also use food to help you make decisions, including what diet to go on. While munching on a creamy Milky Way candy bar, you read all about this month's latest diet. And, you probably have every diet book ever written, including *The Neurotic Diet Book* and *The Indian Quick Weight Loss Program.*

You have really tried everything in the dieting game, including eating matzoh balls with chopsticks. But no diet has ever really *felt* right to you, a necessary requirement for intuitive Cancer. Juice fasting, for example, seemed absurd: Why drink calories when you can eat them? You need something to sink your teeth into!

The problem with most diets is that they fail to take into account that Cancer's weight often fluctuates as much as 3 to 4 pounds from one day to the next as the moon changes phases. (Cancer is ruled by the moon and is often referred to astrologically as the "moonchild.") Your moods are greatly affected by the moon, and in order to counteract moodiness and fluctuation of food cravings I have addressed these important issues.

Some Cancers do well in diet groups, where they welcome the opportunity to open up about their feelings. But many other Cancers feel much too private to join a group, and a bit too proud, too. You may feel that you are able to handle so much else in your life so competently by yourself—why not dieting as well?

Surrounded by a thousand diet books, you give up, grab your coat, and take off for a party where you will savor fine wine, sample several cheeses, and try to forget about the diet dilemma. But one chance remark someone makes about your weight will bring you back down to earth. Cancer likes to look good. Clean, well-groomed, clothes always well-pressed and stylish, you look fashionable and finely tuned. But a chunky Cancer is not a happy one. It's hard for you to break such childhood habits as eating everything on your plate and not wasting any food. But it is even harder for a Cancer to look in a mirror and face the unrelenting fact of flab.

Many a Cancer has had to hit rock bottom before acknowledging that the time has really come to lose weight. You promised yourself many times that you would not steal Halloween candy from your children or let your spoon find its way to the carton of ice cream in the freezer. Maybe you woke up one morning to find you'd fallen asleep on a bed sheet littered with corn chips and pretzels. Or maybe you realize you could only pull on your jeans by lying down flat on the floor and gyrating into them.

And then there's the story of the Cancer woman who ate so much cake batter that her daughter's birthday cake could barely support two candles! And the icing had to be spread thinner because most of it was eaten.

But you tend to be too hard on yourself, Cancer. It's time to start getting rid of your guilt. But from now on, if you miss a dental appointment or sleep later than you'd planned to one morning, don't feel guilty. If the reception on your TV isn't good and your babysitter can't watch her favorite program, don't feel guilty.

Think about how many times you may have eaten to assuage guilt feelings.

You also need to understand that there is another being that affects you deeply: the moon. Just as ocean tides respond to the moon's pull, so do your moods, your nerves, and yes, your stomach. Lunar changes and cycles are a celestial version of your own mood swings, tension, and digestive well-being. The full silvery moon is your own laughing self, brightening any party lucky enough to have you, beaming on those you love.

The vanishing moon is your other extreme. That barely discernible curved line in the sky is like you when you turn away from the world, bitter, gloomy, pessimistic. Fears knot your stomach, worries distract you from all you are supposed to be doing. Inability to concentrate fills you with guilt. The world seems noisy, hostile, fraught with peril for your loved ones. At times like this, you have two sources of private comfort: Water, of course—any will do. A visit to a quiet lake or ocean beach, even just imagining yourself at the seashore helps you to restore serenity. Your other comfort is food. But will even the most splendid goodies really make you feel better?

No one describes food better than a Cancer. You are likely to come home from a stroll on Main Street saying, "I saw such gorgeous plums today, and the strawberries looked just like rubies. The filet mignon in the butcher's window was magnificent . . . the best cut of meat I ever saw."

Your diet needs to allow for your mood swings, water retention problem, and occasional need to binge. And the diet must free you from the notion that if you haven't slaved over a hot stove, your meal lacks that nurturing touch. Certainly dieting shouldn't create extra pressure in your life.

Okay, Cancer, I realize you've always found an excuse to blow your diet because of an emotional crisis in your life. I know that you are sensitive but also so very strong. Look at how many people lean on you. Now muster that strength you give others for your own benefit, and get going.

It's time for you to mother *you.*

Sexual Appetite

Cancer, you are a poet, and love brings out the most lyrical you. You're sensuous and sentimental, and nobody is more wholehearted and romantic in courtship than you. You write songs for your new love, invent silly limericks, and ply your lover with champagne, oysters, and bonbons. You seem almost to live for love; when you find it, you can hardly believe it. After you serenade your love, you look up quickly after the last strum of the guitar, seeking response, reassurance, appreciation. You give and give but any tango you dance had better have two equally committed partners.

Nobody copes terribly well with unrequited love, but Cancer has an even harder time with it than many. Love is Cancer's nourishment; when you lack someone to give to, to protect, to take care of, you question the very meaning of your life. You even tend to question your own value. That is the danger for Cancer, especially when the moon pulls you into a darkly introspective phase. At these times, you are quick to imagine slights and rejections, often unintended, and you can become self-pitying and bitter. Your anxiety flowers like a toxic weed. You often use food to console you. Sometimes you've tried to compensate for unmet sexual needs by downing a couple of chocolate donuts. Learn to reach for your mate instead of your plate! Cancer tends to gain more weight when out of love.

But take heart. Cancer also loses weight more easily when in love. In the warm nest Cancers crave, food subsides in importance and Cancer's highly sexual and demonstrative lovemaking burns calories and steams the air. Emotional Cancer, you spill your feelings and listen to your lover's every word, every breath. When your lover reciprocates, hugging and caressing you, drawing you out, remembering every day to ask how you are, nurturing you, you feel on top of the world.

Sometimes, Cancer, you have a hard time accepting your looks and regarding yourself as sexy. Often losing weight or exercising or changing your hairstyle will make you feel better about yourself, but sometimes your self-deprecating prevents you from acknowledging your strengths. Your sensitivity, compassion, and total involvement with love are very sexy. Your laughter is a joy and your sense of humor is delicious. You arouse tender, giving feelings in others.

Being fussed over, snuggled, prized, and doted on will help you love yourself. Every Cancer's mate should know that the Cancer's secret voice is saying, "Love me and make me feel nurtured, and that I belong to you."

You, Cancer, do not look for a quick conquest. You seek to love for the long-term, and when you finally find it, not even a few extra pounds should interfere with your reveling in love. Lose the weight you can, but don't obsess about it to the point where you lose sight of what is most important to you—a warm home, glowing with love.

Eating/Entertaining at Home

Cancers take great pride in their homes, and keep them clean, comfortable, and covered with photos of family and friends. Amid this gallery of portraits, other mementos stake their claim to fame. Carved boxes hold seashells collected on family vacations. Children's fingerpainted masterpieces transform the refrigerator into a psychedelic sculpture. Treasures you've picked up at flea markets and garage sales represent great bargains as well as someone else's memories. Colorful bowls, bought at a roadside antique sale, hold cuttings from your garden.

And Cancer's garden is a beautiful sight to behold. Nobody appreciates nature's beauty more than a Cancer. The poet in you comes out when you give a tour of your garden. You are so very proud of your home-grown tomatoes, your plentiful cucumbers, and the shape your squash is in.

If you are invited to a Cancer's home for dinner, don't eat breakfast or lunch that day: Show up starving. Cancer's menu often includes appetizers and soup as well as entrée, dessert, and a lovely liqueur. Portions in a Cancer dinner are always generous; no one ever leaves hungry.

To produce such feasts, you feel happiest and most in control in an extra-large kitchen with lots and lots of storage space. Because food symbolizes a sense of security for you, cupboards are always well-stocked, and special treats like chips and cookies are squirreled away behind the mile-high stacks of canned tuna and cream of mushroom soup. (Not that you'll ever *need* forty cans of the stuff, but it *was* on sale and just too good a deal to pass up. Besides, you reason, what if there were a flood or just a group of unexpected guests? Cancer likes to be prepared.)

Cancer enjoys experimenting with many types of ethnic foods. Your cans of tuna and soup coexist peacefully with a veritable United Nations of condiments: Mexican salsa, Japanese sukiyaki sauce, imported French tarragon vinegar, Szechuan Chinese hot sesame oil. Many Cancers sign up for cooking classes in exotic new cuisines. For you, cooking is entertainment and you take pride in award-winning performances.

Just the same, Cancer, your best friends know your secret vice: fast food. You like basic burgers, fried chicken, a frankfurter loaded with mustard and sauerkraut. Tied into these foods' basic appeal is, again, the security factor. Any time of day or night, you can walk into a fast food joint, plunk your money down, and get just what you order—no surprises, no disappointments.

Whether you cook prime rib and potatoes or order in a pizza, you make eating at home an occasion every night.

Food Shopping

What a tantalizing experience food shopping is. And Cancer does not like to be rushed. You like to select the finest produce at your leisure, gently prodding avocados and scrunching a head of lettuce to make sure it is fresh and crisp. After all, you are not shopping just for food. You are choosing culinary gifts for your family. Chicken soup was probably invented by a nurturing Cancer; you eye each chicken carefully. Which one is good enough? You allow only the freshest carrots, parsnips, dill, and onions into your soup. Soups must satisfy and to Cancer, a chicken soup made right is a most worthy achievement.

Cancers like comforting foods. Creamy, homey dishes like macaroni and cheese, baked ziti with mushrooms, all-American apple pie. Lots of cups of yogurt, flavored with sweet preserves. A glance into Cancer's shopping cart reveals your fondness for childhood favorites. Bananas and peanut butter, bran muffins, and blackberry jam. Big bottles of apple and orange juice. And there, tucked shyly behind the wholesome oatmeal, is a box of the sugary kids' cereal you still don't have the heart to resist.

If your favorite brands are on sale, all the better. Frugal Cancer likes to reap all the benefits of leisurely food shopping. And it is not just money you like to save. You save everything! Cancer is a hoarder. The item in the reusable container has greater odds of making it into Cancer's shopping bag than the throwaway alternative. One Cancer I know, buys only one brand of applesauce, for the jar as much as the taste. She spray-paints the jars different colors and has collected a pretty array of holders for pencils, paper clips, nails, screws, diaper pins, buttons, and chopsticks. It runs in the family, by the way—her Cancer dad used marmalade crocks as coffee mugs.

Social Dining

Spartan eating is not for you, Cancer, and you like a restaurant that gives you your money's worth. Ambiance is important, but food is the deciding factor.

The fancy French restaurant that serves one precious square-inch of filet mignon, four peas, and a single stalk of white asparagus topped with a tablespoon of chic sauce is not for you. But a fancy restaurant that doesn't forget that diners are *hungry people* will get your business time and time again.

Cancer likes to choose one of two types of restaurants, depending on your mood. A romantic dinner out will be at an elegant bistro that serves good-size portions of delicious food. Cancer is fond of soft jazz piano or sentimental violin as background for your special evening. Good service is as important to you as the cuisine. You believe that things should be done properly, and you are willing to pay for it. If you have a good waiter who doesn't rush you from course to course, you always tip generously. You are likely to return to the restaurant for business lunches. You enjoy yourself most at a restaurant where you are known.

Cancer's other choice of restaurant couldn't be more different. A Cancer who finds a cheap but dependable coffee shop or fast food place is in seventh heaven. Here, you can relax and dig into roast chicken and salad or into a thick juicy hamburger. If this restaurant does cheap food right, it will become your home away from home.

Special-Occasion Dining

Cancer, you are involved in so many activities that there always seems to be some special occasion coming up—and you wouldn't think of missing it. You RSVP enthusiastically to the many invitations and announcements that come your way—Cub Scout barbecue, wedding, PTA coffee hour, company picnic, and your favorite, the family reunion.

Dieting on these occasions seems difficult to you, because you want to participate fully in all the festivities, and you don't like to be the only one turning away a piece of cake. To further hinder your diet, you are often involved with food preparation or serving. Try delegating some of this to others; your talent for organization should help you organize a kitchen management team that will get the work done and keep you out of nibbling range. Don't forget to assign a clean-up crew that will throw out the leftover cheesecake or take it home themselves. This will help break your own habit of rescuing food that is too good to waste—and devouring it in the car on the way home.

You have so many special occasions on your calendar that you can't dare go off your diet "just this once" or even treat them like "binge days." One Cancer male thought he had a solution to special occasion temptations. As a guest at a small party at an expensive Chinese restaurant, he surveyed the menu then announced to his host, "I'm not that hungry. I'll just have a little of everything." And he wasn't joking.

Try to remember it's your company people seek out—not your appetite.

Having your boss over for dinner? Your impulse is to spend days preparing a banquet of all the dishes that have been in your family for generations. You look forward to basking in the boss's praise for a job well done. But stop! Before you begin the three-day stint in your kitchen, reconsider. It is perfectly fine to serve a simpler, less fattening meal that will show off your selection of the best-quality ingredients while keeping you on your diet. Or take your boss out to dinner. You can order foods allowed on your diet, and your boss can indulge in the high-calorie dishes—or surprise you by joining you in more prudent fare.

Your Health

The sun sign Cancer is ruled by the moon. And just as the moon affects the oceans and tides, so it affects the mood of Cancers.

Sensitive Cancer, your stomach is the barometer of your emotions. Whenever you are in a stressful situation or undergoing emotional upheaval, that stomach starts to churn.

As a child, you would often stay home from school because of stomachache, and you were doted on and pampered. In adulthood, you still tend to lapse into self-pity and sometimes compound your misery by trying to soothe yourself with food. *Avoiding* food when your stomach is upset would be far more beneficial.

Your emotions can often be a menace to your health. You repress anger and bear grudges. This can lead to self-destructive mental and emotional syndromes. Compulsive eating and escape-oriented drinking can ruin your health and make you even more gloomy.

Your turbulent emotions show you are in touch with your feelings, but your endless cycle of ups and downs wreaks havoc with your nerves and your pretense of being cool and in control doesn't fool your digestive organs. The moon exerts a strong influence on you and it is hard for you to stay even-tempered for long.

As a water sign, you tend to retain a good deal of water, which often results in weight gain and bloat. It is absolutely essential that you eat many of the foods indicated on your Cancer diet, which will serve to maintain a good sodium/potassium water balance. Keep your system flushed out by drinking eight glasses of water every day. It will help you lose weight too.

Keep your diet as light as you can. Eat more low-starch foods. If you crave in-between meal snacks, munch on fruit instead of cookies. Stay away from very spicy foods.

Cancer rules the stomach, breasts, solar plexus, pancreas, epigastric region, diaphragm, thoracic duct, upper lobes of the liver, alimentary canal, glycogen storage, and body fluids. Diseases to which Cancer are subject include:

Arthritis and rheumatism	Gastritis
Digestive disturbances	Nervous stomach
Dropsy	Nervous tension
Dyspepsia	Sclerosis
Flabby fatness	Tumors
Gastric fever	Ulcers

The Cancer diet must be rich in calcium and magnesium. They will stop the sugar cravings experienced by most Cancers.

Calcium fluoride is the Cancer cell salt. Cell salts are naturally occurring minerals that are normal constituents of the body cells. They are found in trace amounts in foods, and plants, animals, and human beings require these compounds for proper nutrition. And, like vitamins, cell salts get used up.

Calcium fluoride is an important constituent of all connective tissues, such as bones, teeth, and fingernails. Calcium fluoride is the elasticity cell salt; it maintains elasticity in the connective tissue. A deficiency of calcium fluoride will cause your bones to be brittle and possibly crack. Calcium fluoride also protects skin and lips from chapping and cracking, as well as protecting the hard tissues and skin. Calcium fluoride is needed to avoid hardening of the arteries and veins.

FOODS RICH IN CALCIUM FLUORIDE

Cheese	Pumpkin
Egg yolks	Raisins
Kale	Red cabbage
Lemons	Rye bread
Milk	Savoy
Onions	Watercress
Oranges	Yogurt

Try to avoid alcoholic beverages, they do you no good at all. Because of your active stomach and digestive juices, your body may seem to be asking you for alcohol—but it's really wanting sugar. Satisfy that need with natural sugars found in fresh fruits and vegetables. Nerve-calming foods include vegetable juices, asparagus, carrots, celery, watercress, coconut, and pineapple. Phosphorus, very important for Cancer, can be found in cabbage, cucumbers, and endive.

Cancers should learn to have variety in their diet plans to adjust for the often moody feeling experienced every 48 hours by the movement of the moon.

Cancers should also understand that your pseudo-independent style denies your feelings of dependency. Presenting yourself as overly strong and independent makes you prone to ulcers. Let your friends help you more. If you're worried or afraid about something, say so. You don't need to always appear self-sufficient. Your friends and family will be glad for a chance to reciprocate for all the times you have given them a shoulder to cry on.

You must find ways to release the pressure cooker inside you and increase your emotional equilibrium. Meditation and yoga are marvelous for you, and swimming is the exercise of choice. Walk more instead of driving. A sedentary life is too stultifying for you.

Throughout your life, you have probably not enjoyed truly robust health or strong recuperative powers. But sticking to the Cancer diet will improve your health, fortify your ability to combat illness, and help lower your tension level. And your stomach will thank you.

Cancer Daily Nutritional Supplements

- Super B-complex multivitamin to keep nerves in good shape
- 2,000 mg vitamin C to help combat stress
- 400 mg vitamin E per day to maintain healthy, young-looking skin
- General multivitamin with minerals to ensure good health

Remember, Cancer...

This diet is uniquely prepared to address your sun sign and *should not be interchanged with any other Sun Sign Diet.* It is important that you follow the diet exactly as it appears, for optimum weight loss and assimilation. Before starting your Cancer diet, carefully read "General Diet and Maintenance Guidelines for All Sun Signs" found at the beginning of this book. Remember, drink 8 glasses of water daily.

You will never have to have a dieting problem again, dear Cancer, because this diet has been prepared to meet your biological, chemical, nutritional, and behavioral needs.

Get set for success.

The Cancer
Seven-Day
Reducing Diet

(with two optional days)

The diet has been specifically designed for the Cancer constitution: to counteract sugar and carbohydrate cravings, to eliminate excess water weight and speed up your sluggish metabolism, and to keep your body fortified with calcium, magnesium, potassium, and all the B vitamins. The B vitamins are especially important to the dieting success of a Cancer because they help calm you as well as stabilize your mood swings during the 48-hour transit every other day of the moon. Remember, Cancer, your dieting problems are very different than those of any other sign in the zodiac, for you are ruled by the moon, which flips to a different place every two days, often changing your moods, metabolism, water retention level, anxiety, and nerve centers...all of which play such a vital role in successful eating control.

For the first time in your life, you will have a diet prepared to address this unique manifestation. You finally will feel in control. Your diet has a high vitamin and mineral content, and will ensure you that you are getting more than the maximum content, and will ensure you that you are getting more than the maximum RDA requirements while consuming few calories. The diet will follow the changing chemical and metabolic needs and mood swings common to some Cancers. The next time anyone complains that you are "moody," just explain that you are "orbiting."

The Cancer diet starts with a cleansing day, called the Cancer Creamy Day, then proceeds with the Cancer Fish Day, Cancer Potassium Day, Cancer Sweet Day, Cancer Calcium/Magnesium Day, All-Carbohydrate Day, with special options, and of course, the Cancer Total Binge Day.

To further speed up your weight loss and suppress your appetite, you may choose to try a diet aid known in the United States as Glucomannan. It is extracted from the Japanese konjac root, a tuber that is very high in fiber. A final monograph on its effectiveness has not yet been established by the FDA, as it has no history of use in the United States before 1958; however, the konjac root has been cultivated and eaten in Asia for over a thousand years.

Glucomannan contributes to a decrease in cholesterol and triglyceride levels, and aids in maintaining low-density lipoprotein levels. It acts as a dietary fiber to increase viscosity and moisture content of food as it is digested, so that it forms a smooth, soft mass that moves easily through the intestinal tract. Digestion is slowed, so normal blood sugar levels are maintained after a meal. Two capsules taken three times a day may cut your appetite in half!

Please note the asterisks (*) which appear after certain foods listed in your menu plan. You will find a detailed explanation of their vitamin and mineral content, and direct information as to why they are essential components of your successful diet regimen, located in the section "Notes to Cancer Seven-Day Reducing Diet."

Follow the diet exactly as designed. Do not mix your menus. Eat what is scheduled for that day. (If you do not want something, leave it out, but do not substitute.) This diet is nutritiously balanced so as to allow you to use it for the duration of your entire weight loss.

Last but not least, Cancer, this diet is written with the understanding that your weight can fluctuate by as much as 5 pounds in two days, even though you stayed on the diet. Don't feel that you have to convince anyone that you did not cheat.

For optimum results, start your diet on the first Monday after a full moon. How do you know when it is a full moon? Many inexpensive calendars indicate the phases of the moon.

CANCER CREAMY CRASH DAY— DAY ONE

You, Cancer, have always binged on all sorts of goodies before you started your diet. Well, now you can start your diet with the same feeling, and tomorrow morning when you step on the scale you will be at least 1 pound lighter. And brighter. The food for today is rich in calcium and potassium and will keep you feeling more satisfied. Use buttermilk if you can, because the fermentation of the milk will have a greater enzyme action on your metabolism. However, you will also have excellent results if you choose to use skim milk, so do not despair.

On this day there are no deviations. You may have all the herbal tea, black coffee, or regular tea you want. No diet soda today.

BREAKFAST, LUNCH, AND DINNER

    1 qt. no-sodium buttermilk* or 1 qt. skim milk*

    4 cups of fresh strawberries*

    sugar substitute to taste

    Blend the buttermilk (or skim milk) and strawberries with ice cubes in a blender and drink throughout the day for each one of your meals. You will find it to be thick, luscious, creamy, and very, very soothing. It will taste like something sinfully rich. But what is truly wonderful is that you will have lost at least one pound by the next day. Drink lots of water in between. *Absolutely nothing else is allowed.*

Remember, drink 8 glasses of water every day.

CANCER FISH DAY—DAY TWO

Each zodiac sign conveys a preference for the type of foods that not only appeal to the palate of people born under that sign, but which their bodies need and demand. Cancers, ruled by the water and sea, love seafood. *It is the best source of protein* for you, and you should try to incorporate as much fish into your menus as possible.

After yesterday's hard work, nourish your body today with high levels of protein derived mostly from linoleic and polyunsaturated sources.

BREAKFAST

2 scrambled eggs (in 2 tsp. diet margarine)

1 oz. smoked salmon (lox)*

1 Wasa Crisp Bread or 2 melba toast

or

2 oz. water-pack tuna* with 2 oz. cottage cheese (mix together) and spread on 2 Wasa Crisp Bread or 2 melba toast

LUNCH

4 oz. water-pack tuna, filet of sole, flounder, halibut, codfish, shrimp, or lump crabmeat*

very large mixed salad of endive, watercress,* parsley, cabbage, cucumbers,* radishes, scallions, served with 2 Tbsp. reduced-calorie dressing or lemon juice with garlic pepper

coffee, tea, herbal tea, or mineral water

DINNER

6 oz. broiled, steamed, or baked fish* (consider striped bass, tile fish, etc.)

large salad of cucumber, parsley, and watercress,* with lemon juice and garlic

½ cup cooked carrots

or

Lean Cuisine Filet of Fish Florentine or Fish Jardinière

coffee, tea, no-sodium diet soda

Remember, drink 8 glasses of water every day.

THE CANCER POTASSIUM DAY— DAY THREE

The wonderful thing about being a water sign is that you are so sensitive, warm and caring. The difficult part is that you do tend to retain water more than some other zodiac signs. For this reason, to keep energy levels high and to flush out excess water, include the Potassium Day in your diet.

BREAKFAST
>1 cup yogurt* with medium-size banana
>(Excellent source of calcium and potassium.)

MIDMORNING SNACK
>water, water, water

LUNCH
>3 oz. breast of turkey*
>
>large tossed salad with 2 Tbsp. reduced-calorie dressing
>
>2 prunes
>(Few people know, Cancer, that turkey and prunes are absolutely loaded with first-quality potassium.)
>
>water, water, water

DINNER
>4 oz. sardines

or

>4–6 oz. fresh baked or broiled salmon
>
>tossed green salad with lemon juice
>
>½ cantaloupe

(Both salmon and cantaloupe are packed with potassium.)

Remember, drink 8 glasses of water every day.

CANCER SWEET DAY—DAY FOUR

Is a diet week without a sweet day worth experiencing? Of course not. Using the richness of fructose (natural fruit sugar) you will experience a wonderfully uplifting feeling and sense of satisfaction.

BREAKFAST

> banana shake—in a blender combine 1 ripe banana, 1 cup skim milk, ½ tsp. vanilla extract, 2 packets sugar substitute; blend until smooth

or

½ cantaloupe* and 2 tsp. raisins and 4 oz. orange juice

or

1 orange, 4 oz. apple juice, and 2 tsp. raisins

LUNCH

> fresh fruit salad*—up to 3 heaping cups of any type of fresh fruit
>
> herbal tea, regular tea, or black coffee

MIDAFTERNOON SNACK

> 1 whole papaya, orange, apple, or 20 grapes

DINNER

> 6 oz. lean roast beef or steak
>
> large tossed salad with 2 Tbsp. reduced-calorie dressing or lemon juice with garlic pepper
>
> large serving of fresh or frozen steamed asparagus with basil
>
> coffee, tea, or no-sodium diet soda
>
> *Remember, drink 8 glasses of water every day.*

CANCER CALCIUM/MAGNESIUM REDUCING DAY—DAY FIVE

It's time to fortify the nervous system with a good deal of the calming nutrients of calcium and magnesium. I am sure that you will even be calmer and more composed about your dieting after you step on the scale tomorrow. By now you should be feeling pretty good about yourself.

BREAKFAST

4 oz. skim-milk ricotta cheese or low-fat cottage cheese*

1 sliced apple or 1 peach

black coffee, tea, or herbal tea

LUNCH

3 oz. canned sockeye salmon*

1 large portion of broccoli

mixed green salad with lemon juice and garlic pepper

coffee, tea, no-sodium Perrier, or no-sodium diet soda

MIDAFTERNOON SNACK

3 almonds* and water, water, water
(Almonds are one of the richest sources of calcium.)

DINNER

Cancer à la Japanese

1 serving of bean curd soup or Lipton Trim Soup

8–10 oz. of tofu,* either plain or stir-fried with broccoli and scallions in a clear bouillon soup
(Tofu bean curd is one of the richest sources of magnesium in the most easily digested form. You can be sure you have had a fine supply of low-calorie calcium and magnesium.)

or

6 oz. stir-fried veal scallopine for those who do not like tofu

mixed green salad seasoned with lemon juice and garlic pepper.

Remember, drink 8 glasses of water every day.

ALL-CARBOHYDRATE DAY— DAY SIX

Cancers crave carbohydrates. Just accept this about yourself. But now you will be able to work with this craving. It really hits you approximately every fifth day because the moon has now traveled into another sign. Usually by this day on a traditional diet, you would feel like you just wanted to bite into something soft and breadlike. You will do just that.

BREAKFAST

1 frozen waffle topped with 3 Tbsp. light pancake syrup

or

1 bran muffin with 1 tsp. diet margarine and 1 tsp. diet jam

coffee with milk, tea, or herbal tea

or

½ cup bran cereal with ½ cup skim milk

or

12 almonds and 1 large orange

(All these breakfasts are high in fiber.)

LUNCH

1 huge baked potato* seasoned with ½ cup plain yogurt (if you absolutely cannot get yogurt, use 1 Tbsp. of sour cream) sprinkled with scallions, chives, and basil

1 dinner roll with 1 tsp. butter

coffee, tea, no-sodium Perrier, or no-sodium diet soda

(You will find that the carbohydrate slow digestion of the potato coupled with the high potassium level will keep you satiated for hours and hours. You also will notice that your mood is elevated.)

DINNER

¼–½ baked, broiled, or barbecued chicken* (no skin)

1 large ear of corn*

1 baked apple with 1 dollop of Cool Whip dessert topping

black coffee, tea, no-sodium Perrier, or no-sodium diet soda

Remember, drink 8 glasses of water every day.

ALL-PROTEIN DAY—DAY SEVEN

BREAKFAST

6 oz. skim-milk ricotta cheese or low-fat cottage cheese topped with sugar substitute and cinnamon

black coffee, tea with lemon, or herbal tea

LUNCH

6 oz. canned tuna in water sprinkled with a little fresh lemon juice, garlic pepper, and chives

water, water, water*

MIDAFTERNOON SNACK

3 pecans and water, water, water

DINNER

one grapefruit

6 oz. minute steak or roast beef or broiled clams or fish

watercress, tomato, cucumber, and green pepper salad with oregano and lemon juice

water, water, water

Remember, drink 8 glasses of water every day.

THE ALL-AROUND CANCER REDUCING DAY— DAY EIGHT

May be substituted for Day One if it seems too rigorous.

BREAKFAST
    ½ fresh pineapple*

or

    1 large peach and 4 oz. orange juice

or

    up to 10 oz. unsweetened fruit juice

LUNCH
    asparagus* or artichoke or mushroom omelette (2 eggs)

    mixed green salad with tomatoes with 1 tsp. butter

    1 Wasa Crisp Bread or 2 melba toast

MIDAFTERNOON SNACK
    1 apple

DINNER
    1 cup whole wheat spaghetti or macaroni* with ¼ cup spaghetti sauce

    2 slices veal or 1 veal chop*

    large salad of watercress, spinach, parsley, radishes, and 1 sliced tomato

or

    1 cup stuffed macaroni shells with 4 oz. skim-milk ricotta cheese and ¼ cup Aunt Millie's Spaghetti Sauce

Remember, drink 8 glasses of water every day.

CANCER SUBSTITUTE REDUCING DAY

Can use in place of any other day, so there are no excuses.

BREAKFAST

6 oz. orange juice and ½ orange

black coffee, tea, or herbal tea
    (This is a particularly high-enzyme potassium breakfast that will prepare your metabolism to burn stored fat and quickly absorb fructose in bloodstream. Try to have 2 glasses of water before lunch.)

LUNCH

Salade niçoise: ¼ head of lettuce, 2 oz. water-pack tuna, 1 hard-boiled egg, 1 tsp. capers, 1 sliced raw green pepper, seasoned with lemon juice and garlic pepper

coffee, tea, or no-sodium diet soda

MIDAFTERNOON SNACK

½ fresh lemon squeezed in no-sodium seltzer, no-sodium Perrier, or water (Have at least 2 glasses; you may choose to add sugar substitute.)

DINNER

½ baked, broiled, or barbecued chicken without the skin

1 cup diced papaya or fresh strawberries

1 large tossed salad of spinach, lettuce, and green pepper, seasoned with 1 Tbsp. reduced-calorie dressing

coffee, tea, no-sodium seltzer, or no-sodium diet soda

10 grapes

Remember, drink 8 glasses of water every day.

Notes to Cancer Seven-Day Reducing Diet (with 2 optional days)

Cancer Diet Notes—Day One

* If you use buttermilk, you must use only the no-sodium kind. Fermented foods, such as buttermilk, have high-quality enzyme power, which can help dissolve carbohydrates and rid the body of extra water weight. If you do not care for buttermilk, substitute liquid or powdered skim milk. The high calcium content of the milk will keep you calm, a must for first day Cancer dieting jitters.

* Strawberries are rich in vitamin C and also have excellent enzyme properties. This liquid day allows the digestive system to take a rest and slow down. Its rich and satisfying taste will fool your taste buds. You may space your meals to fit your own schedule.

Cancer Diet Notes—Day Two

* Fish nourishes your body with high levels of protein derived mostly from polyunsaturated sources. You should always have as much seafood in your diet as possible. After all, your sun sign is ruled by the crab ... found in the depths of the water.

* The cucumber has high levels of silicon and phosphorus, which are extremely important for keeping the nervous system calm.

* The watercress and parsley have extraordinary digestive enzymes and act as superb internal cleansers. They also act as energy boosters to get you going for the next day.

Cancer Diet Notes—Day Three

* The yogurt is a good source of calcium and B vitamins, especially B-12, which act to calm your nervous system.

* Turkey—just 3½ ounces of turkey supplies you with a hefty 31 grams of protein, 320 mg of phosphorus, and 367 mg of potassium.

Cancer Diet Notes—Day Four

By now you are hankering for something creamy and sweet, and so your wish is my command.

* The banana supplies you with 370 mg of potassium, 8 mg of calcium, and 33 mg of magnesium. You will feel calm, satiated, and content.

* Cantaloupe yields only 50 calories per half but has 251 mg of potassium. It supplies you with vitamin A and folic acid. The choice is up to you.

* Fresh fruit salad—must be eaten alone for proper assimilation, digestion, and weight loss. You must not have any milk or milk products with this meal, because the milk lactose will inhibit the production of enzymes.

* Herbal tea ... Cancers should become herbal tea connoisseurs. First, you are very oral people and need to be eating or drinking something. The water rulership requires that you drink a lot of liquids, and herbal tea is both soothing and warming as well as comforting.

Cancer Diet Notes—Day Five

* Salmon is an excellent source of high-quality low-cholesterol protein, resplendent with vitamins A, B, and E. Choose the sockeye brand, whenever possible, because of the high calcium content. (Provides more than 500 mg of easily digestible calcium.)

* Tofu is an excellent food for Cancers. Get a recipe book and start learning about the 200 ways to prepare this wonderful low-calorie, high-protein food creatively. If you want, you may use the powdered bean curd soups sold in various supermarkets. Tofu has long satiety power. But if you do not like tofu you may substitute 6 oz veal scallopine.

Cancer Diet Notes—Day Six

Cancer, the carboholic. You really crave these little devils and so I have included a variety of no-guilt healthy options, for today.

* Potatoes are very rich in potassium, which serves to give you abundant energy, and acts as a good diuretic for water-retentive Cancers.
* Chicken is high in vitamin B, especially B-6. B-6 has now been found to be the "diuretic vitamin." It is also rich in B-2, B-12, and folic acid.
* 3½ oz. of corn has 165 mg of potassium and supplies you with 18 grams of carbohydrate.

Calorie for calorie and carbohydrate for carbohydrate ... it is a nutritional bargain day, my Cancer friend.

Cancer Diet Notes—Day Seven

Today is a low-carbohydrate, high-potassium day. It is just the opposite of yesterday's menu. This has been planned to jolt your "set point" for optimum weight loss. It is important to alternate each day's menu and calorie count so that your metabolism is always activated.

* Water ... it is absolutely imperative, with all high-protein menus, that you have 8 glasses a day of water. The more you have, the more you will lose!

Cancer Diet Notes—Day Eight

* Pineapple is chock full of a great digestive enzyme called bromelin, which helps break down fatty deposits. It is also rich in chlorine, which has an invigorating effect upon the liver, and has excellent diuretic properties.

* Asparagus is yet another diuretic vegetable, containing the enzyme asparagine, which also helps to break up accumulated fats. Expect breakfast and lunch to produce a lot of urination.

* Spaghetti or macaroni—use only durum wheat or vegetable pasta. It digests more quickly, is easily assimilated, and much lower in calories.

* Veal is low in cholesterol, low in calories, and rich in phosphorus.

Cancer Diet Notes—Substitute Reducing Day

This day has been included in your regimen so that you will have no excuses for any digression. You can substitute this day for any day in your diet. Everything on this day's menu is readily accessible and easy to prepare.

CANCER TOTAL BINGE DAY

Cancer, with all the temptations of food in your life, you sometimes need to let go. I have given you that option with a binge day. Now remember, Cancer, don't go overboard. This is for one day only.

Before You Binge
1. Drink water.
2. Drink water.
3. Drink water.
4. Rest.
5. Brush your teeth and rinse with your favorite mouthwash.
6. Chew sugarless gum for 20 minutes.

You may find that the desire to binge has passed. However, if you are still suffering from intense food frustration, follow these basic binge rules:

Rule One
Under no circumstances should you ever binge before completing Day Five of your reducing diet. This will ensure a maximum weight loss with a minimum of food frustration.

Rule Two
If, for example, you binge on the sixth day of your diet, resume your diet the following day (Day Seven) with the menu for Day Six. If you binge for just one meal, such as lunch on Day Six, resume your reducing diet with dinner on Day Six of your reducing diet.

Rule Three
Bingeing is for when you get that creepy, anxious feeling, when you feel like pulling out your hair—strand by strand—and you cannot endure dieting for even one more moment. Before you climb the walls, give yourself a binge day. It's hoped that this will not be necessary more than four times a month.

Rule Four
After you have lost your first 10 pounds, you may vary your binge day with the binge day of the sun sign opposite yours, which is Capricorn.

Remember, an occasional binge day—when necessary—will still allow you to lose weight (without guilt). Here, Cancer, is your binge day menu.

Binge Day Menu

BREAKFAST

½ cantaloupe or 4 oz. orange juice

1 English muffin, bagel, corn or bran muffin with diet margarine and diet jam

1 frothy chocolate Alba 77 skim-milk drink

or

4 oz. orange juice

¼ cup granola cereal with skim milk and 1 tsp. raisins

or

The Cancer Cheater Drink

1 ripe papaya or ½ fresh pineapple cut in chunks, juice of 1 orange, 1 big strawberry, and 1 ice cube. Beat in blender . . . sinful and delicious.

½ toasted bagel with diet margarine

coffee

LUNCH

1 all-beef frankfurter (on bun) loaded with sauerkraut and mustard

1 Carvel Thinny-Thin or Weight Watchers ® frozen treat

no-sodium diet soda

or

1 slice of pizza

1 scoop vanilla, chocolate, strawberry, or coffee ice cream

no-sodium diet soda

DINNER

1 cup spaghetti or linguine with 3 oz. flaked tuna and 2 Tbsp. caviar seasoned with basil, oregano, grated Parmesan cheese, with a scant tablespoon oil and garlic pepper

20 frozen grapes for dessert (place in freezer 6 hours earlier)

or

any broiled or baked fish

large house salad with 1 Tbsp. dressing

2 pieces garlic bread

Maintaining Your Ideal Weight

Cancer Maintenance Foods for Optimum Health

The B Vitamins

The B vitamins are extremely important in maintaining the body's metabolism, especially of protein and fats. If proper precautions are not taken, dieting can drastically decrease your vitamin B intake. A healthy nervous system is also dependent on an adequate supply of B vitamins. Insufficient amounts of the B vitamins can lead to both heart ailments and an overly sensitive nervous system. Stress can really take its toll on you, Cancer, therefore you *must* include the B vitamins in your diet to avoid heart and neural problems.

FOODS RICH IN THE B VITAMINS

All seafoods	Green peas
Avocados	Liver
Bananas	Skim milk
Beets	Sunflower seeds
Chicken	Tuna
Cottage cheese	Yogurt
Eggs	

Vitamin C

Vitamin C cannot be internally synthesized, and therefore *must* be included in your diet. Vitamin C is essential to the body's production of hormones. With a deficiency of vitamin C, the body's glands may hemorrhage, drastically reducing hormone production and leaving the body internally taxed by stress. Another concern for you, Cancer, is that the body's supply of vitamin C is depleted by stressful situations, of which you are too often the victim. This deficiency can be repaired only by external sources, so it is absolutely necessary that you include foods rich in vitamin C in your diet. Vitamin C also enables vitamin E to function as an anti-aging agent and allows iron to be broken down and used properly by the body.

FOODS RICH IN VITAMIN C

Alfalfa	Currants
Almonds	Grapefruit
Apples	Green peppers
Asparagus	Lemons
Bananas	Oranges
Blueberries	Paprika
Broccoli	Parsley
Brussels sprouts	Pineapple
Cantaloupe	Skim milk
Carrots	Strawberries
Celery	Tangerines
Chicken	Tomatoes
Chicken liver	Watercress
Cranberries	

Vitamin E

The most important task of vitamin E is that of an anti-aging agent. One of your more sensitive areas, Cancer, is the skin. Vitamin E maintains the skin's health and youthful glow by slowing cellular aging. Vitamin E also helps to prevent the development of scar tissue. As well as protecting and enriching the skin, vitamin E can alleviate fatigue and help reduce blood pressure.

FOODS RICH IN VITAMIN E

Apples	Milk
Asparagus	Mushrooms
Avocados	Oats
Broccoli	Parsley
Cabbage	Peanut butter
Carrots	Salmon
Cheeses	Shrimp
Chicken	Spinach
Corn	Sunflower seeds
Eggs	Sweet potatoes
Halibut	Turkey
Liver	Wheat germ

Calcium

Most of the body's calcium is found in the bones and teeth. Because old bone cells break down and the body must develop new bone cells, 20 percent of an adult's bone calcium must be replaced every year. Proper calcium intake should help with Cancer's knee problems. Calcium also soothes your nervous system, Cancer, and alleviates stress.

FOODS RICH IN CALCIUM

Alfalfa	Lobster
Almonds	Onion
Avocados	Parsley
Beets	Peaches
Broccoli	Plums
Carrots	Sardines
Cauliflower	Shrimp
Celery	Skim milk
Chick peas	Soy beans
Chicken	Soy products
Chicken livers	Spinach
Dried apricots	Sunflower seeds
Green beans	Tomatoes
Lemons	Watercress
Lettuce	

Magnesium

Magnesium works in cooperation with calcium, and should be taken in proper proportions (two parts calcium to one part magnesium). The two minerals work together to regulate your heartbeat. A magnesium deficiency may cause the heart to skip beats. Magnesium is also absolutely necessary to ensure the proper functioning of the nervous system and can have a calming effect on the nerves.

FOODS RICH IN MAGNESIUM

Apples	Figs
Asparagus	Grapes
Beets	Lemons
Buckwheat	Peaches
Cabbage	Pears
Carob	Plums
Cauliflower	Radishes
Cherries	Sesame seeds
Corn	Spinach
Cucumber	Watercress

Potassium

Potassium regulates your body's balance and fluid distribution. Water signs —including Cancer—tend to retain water due to a sodium excess. Potassium and sodium must be kept in balance to prevent bloating, cramping, and moodiness. Potassium also functions very much like magnesium, only it is much more effective in relieving stress and promoting relaxation.

FOODS HIGH IN POTASSIUM

Almonds	Green leafy vegetables
Apples	Lemons
Asparagus	Pineapple
Bananas	Potatoes
Beets	Prunes
Broccoli	Salmon
Buttermilk	Sardines
Cantaloupe	Sesame seeds
Coconut	Skim milk

Strawberries	Tuna
Sunflower seeds	Turkey

Cancer Sample Maintenance Menu

When you reach your desired goal, please follow the maintenance eating hints found in "General Diet and Maintenance Guidelines for All Sun Signs" at the beginning of this book for proper calculations of caloric intake.

I'm including a sample maintenance menu based on your sun sign for optimal Cancer maintenance. When you create your own menus for yourself, try to choose many of the foods you eat from your Cancer Maintenance Foods lists.

2,000 Calories Per Day

BREAKFAST	CALORIES
1 cup orange juice	120
1 bagel	165
1 Tbsp. cream cheese	50
2 oz. smoked salmon	100
6 oz. coffee	3
2 oz. milk	25
	463

LUNCH	
1 cup mushroom soup	135
1 cup low-fat cottage cheese	165
1 Tbsp. wheat germ	25
1 cup dried peaches and raisins	420
8 oz. tea	0
	745

MIDAFTERNOON SNACK	
¼ cup sunflower seeds	205

DINNER

1 glass sauterne wine (optional)	85
¼ lb. scallops	127
1 cup spaghetti with 1 Tbsp. corn oil, 1 tsp. garlic powder, ½ tsp. oregano	287
1 cup spinach	41
	540

EVENING SNACK

2 ginger cookies	45

TOTAL DAILY CALORIES   1,998

Remember, drink 8 glasses of water every day.

Restaurant Eating the Cancer Way

Perhaps you have seen the following dishes on restaurant menus. Both the dishes and the types of restaurants chosen will appeal to the Cancerian palate and satisfy your nutritional needs. Note that all of the recommended dishes contain the nutrients specified in your Cancer Maintenance Foods lists.

However, a good Cancer diet must not deny your love of fast food. It is much too difficult to kick old habits when dieting and you should not have to totally deprive yourself of something that gives you so much pleasure. The fast food menus listed here let you indulge while lowering your calorie intake.

In all menus, one appetizer plus one entrée equals approximately 600–700 calories. The fast-food menus do not include appetizers; all calories are included in the entree.

One last bit of advice, Cancer. Nearly all Cancers feel compelled to take home "doggie bags." Go right ahead—as long as the food you take home will be fed to a *real* doggie.

Seafood Restaurant

APPETIZERS

Clams on the half shell

Plate of steamers—no butter

154

ENTRÉES

Shrimp-stuffed sole

Clam casserole

Broiled shrimp with garlic and pepper

Chicken flambé with baked cranberries

Boiled lobster with lemon juice (Sorry, Cancer, no butter; lemon juice will do the trick.)

Italian Restaurant

APPETIZERS

Assorted antipasto in vinegar

Slice of melon and anchovy

ENTRÉES

Eggplant parmigiana

Lasagne

Boneless shell steak, with spicy sauce of tomatoes, capers, and anchovies

Linguine in red or white clam sauce

Chicken with prosciutto and cheese

American Restaurant

APPETIZERS

Fresh fruit salad

Chilled tomato juice

ENTRÉES

Sliced prime filet of beef

London broil with grilled tomato

Salade niçoise

Baked chicken with herbs

Fast Food

Believe it or not, Cancer, you can still have your fast-food fix. Here are some safe bets:

ENTRÉES

Fried chicken (one breast and one drumstick) and coleslaw

Hamburger (not too much mayonnaise or ketchup) and one *small* order of french fries
(If you are craving a double cheeseburger, Cancer, have one, but skip the french fries.)

Chicken chunks (6-pack) and one *small* order of french fries

Slice of pizza and an Italian ice

Drink no-sodium diet soda, in moderation, or as much water as you like while you wolf down that burger.

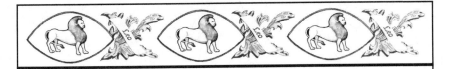

LEO

July 24–August 23

The Leo
Personality

"Let's go out to eat."

A ll the jungle watches the lion slink by, the undisputed king—or queen —of the primal kingdom. Leo, your jungle may be asphalt instead of tropical, but you capture awed admiration just like your feline namesake. You are never one to fade into the scenery; there is no mistaking Leo's commanding presence. With a toss of your mane, you enter any room and find yourself taking over the show.

Leo, you are not only royal, you even have attendants. True, your friends may not actually call themselves ladies-in-waiting, but they are a doting entourage, nonetheless. And how they praise you: Leo's friends know that you like—you *need*—to be appreciated and reassured of your eminent worthiness. They keep their flattery frequent. But don't for a moment think that the quantity of compliments lessens their quality. For there is much to admire in proud, ebullient Leo. You are great fun, a great friend, and a dramatic force in whatever you do.

But the Leo who has much to be proud of wants to be proud of it *all*. Partial perfection is not enough for you.

You crave recognition for achievement, for your consummate sense of style, for your charismatic leadership. You want your party invitations to be the most coveted. And oh, Leo, you want to look so good.

And there is your Achilles paw. You want the sleek body of a lion, and nothing exasperates you more than excess pounds that refuse to come off —*fast*. Your enormous energy makes you restless when you don't find an immediate outlet, and you may have accumulated some pudginess from

159

munching late at night when you couldn't sleep. Now what do you do? You don't have time to pussyfoot around with timid little diets. You simply don't have the patience to wait for the offending pounds to decide to disappear. You'll give a diet one week to prove itself; if it fails to give quick results, off with its head! You want to be Cat Woman or Cat Man, *now*. You want your admirers to note your polished claws, glossy hair, and shapely, jungle-ready body.

Fat is so depressing to the—let's admit it—rather vain Leo. But who said vanity need be a bad trait? Leo, you regard your pride in your appearance as integral to pride in yourself. You are inclined to say, "Looking good makes me feel good, and when I am happy I make everyone else feel good and warm." In other words, you are sure your entourage will *thank* you for buying that gold necklace, splurging on that designer suit, or dropping some pounds at an expensive spa. Anything that boosts Leo's morale lets everyone around you bask in your glow.

Credit cards must have been invented for Leo. When a silvery bauble beckons, you can't bear to turn frugally away. Being broke is chronic for you, Leo, but it is all for a worthy cause—yourself.

Your hair is truly your crowning glory. You'll hunt all over town for the hairdresser who will cut it just right, and will pay whatever it takes to attain the mane you deserve. If your hair looks terrific, your day goes well; but let a drizzle frizz your hair and all is chaos. You'll sometimes reschedule appointments for a drier day when your hair will be back to looking its best.

And what shows off a mane better than a great tan? You like to look as tawny as that big cat we all know and love. You smooth on suntan lotion in February to get a head start for summer, and may even invest in a little home sunlamp. A study of tanning salons would probably reveal that most customers are Leos, toasting themselves to a perfect golden hue.

Your closet is full of striking, unusual clothes. Appliquéd vests, vivid prints, sensuous fabrics. When you are overweight, you try to distract the viewer's eye by favoring long, loose sweaters and tunics, and sweeping caftans. One Leo woman bought cigarettes in a rainbow of colors and matched them to her outfits—the better to distract you, my dear.

The Leo who loses weight, however, takes pride in showing off a sleek body once it's finally achieved. Off come the oversize T-shirts, and, in fact, off comes a lot else, too, as you choose simple, sometimes skimpy styles that let the tanned skin gleam through.

Through thick and thin, Leo is always anointed with intriguing adornments from your extensive (and always growing) jewelry collection. You are an inveterate shopper for accessories as well as clothes, and sometimes collapse when you get home from the sheer strain of deciding which window displays you'll allow to lure you into the store.

Leos love furs. Snuggled in a sable, you purr with pleasure. One Leo woman demurred to buy her own fur coat out of sympathy for the skins' original owners. But she readily confessed that she would not hesitate to accept a fur coat as a gift.

And Leo has a weakness for presents. When you are sick in bed with the flu, your friends know to forget the chicken soup and show up with a silk robe instead. That will put the sparkle back in your eyes.

If you and a friend have argued, you just might accept a week in Acapulco as a peace offering. A gold bracelet should suffice to mend a serious quarrel, while a mere tiff can be resolved with a box of imported chocolates.

But you are not likely to bear lasting grudges in any case, Leo. When you get angry and the lion in you growls, a little cooling-off time calms you down and has you playful as a kitten again. You tend to be quick to take offense at unintended slights, but your warm, bubbly smile returns quickly.

Leo's friends are lucky people, the beneficiaries of your huge heart and considerate nature. You pamper your friends, Leo, just the way you like to be pampered yourself. You keep the U.S. Post Office solvent by sending a steady stream of greeting cards and funny notes to your pals. You never forget a kindness, and repay it many times over. Your expensive tastes make you want the best for your friends as well as yourself, and you remember birthdays with carved jade, silk scarves, or just the right book for a special friend.

Leo is an idea person, ready and able to help friends find answers to all kinds of problems—from wardrobe to love to work. Professionally, Leo is a "do-er," a proud and self-sufficient leader who encourages coworkers to do their best. Leo helps shy people emerge from their shells and insecure people to rediscover the expressive, happy child within them. The team headed by creative Leo will be a record-breaker, with team members fired up by Leo's enthusiasm.

What does Leo want in return for that magnanimous friendship? *Appreciation.* Leo, who appears to be so very independent, is really hungry for constant reassurance. The best way to show a Leo your love? Try building a seventy-five-foot monument carved out of stone, and place it right in the middle of Leo's living room. That might get the message across.

Leo's natural habitat may well be the party. What better opportunity for Leo rightfully to claim center stage? You make the most of your grand entrance by wearing what is sure to be the party's most sensual and dramatic garb. The Leo man who has recently dropped some pounds will show off in a sexy ultrasuede shirt that just happens to be casually unbuttoned. The Leo woman often diets with parties in mind, for she longs to wear a clingy sheath of silk that will show off the curves that are finally all in the right places.

When Leo throws a party, money is no object. Imagination reigns supreme. Leo's friends never know what to expect, for Leo seeks the unusual: a cruise to nowhere... an evening of mystery, magic, and costume... an intimate dinner for ten or a blowout bash for a thousand. Whatever the number of guests, Leo's parties are theatrical events.

Leo, your theme song might be, "Let the Good Times Roll." You throw yourself into a party spirit like a seal thrown into a pool of water, with squeals of pleasure and lots of splash. Balloongrams, bellygrams, and singing telegrams were probably created by Leos. And you may be sure that many of the world's great magicians and video performers are Leos. You love to be entertained and to be the entertainer yourself. The spotlight feels so natural to you, the applause so deserved.

Your refrigerator may offer slim pickings much of the time (though you can always find *something* to snack on) but at party time your kitchen gets to show off its full potential. You are a good cook but you prefer to hire a caterer so you can lavish all your attention on your guests, and let them lavish attention on you.

Leo is a sign of the zodiac that retains the charm of childhood. You have mastered the fine art of guileless, innocent flirtation. In a restaurant, a drink in your hand, you play absent-mindedly with your straw as a child might, clinking the ice cubes against the side of the glass. Your childlike moods are refreshing—but the cat's eyes that glance across the table are filled with an allure that is definitely adult.

You come across to the outside world as dominating, gregarious, and full of life. You hide the vulnerable, sensitive part of your nature because you'd much rather be adored than pitied. You are so aware of your "public" that you even get dressed up to take out the garbage.

Let down your guard, dear Leo. Be human, and people will like you even better. And life without love is no life at all to a Leo. True, you seek always to be admired and desired. You need constant reassurances, and your lover must constantly find new ways to express love for you. Don't ask too much, Leo, or you might find your evenings spent cuddling up to a box of chocolates instead. And sugar is no substitute for the true sweetness of love.

Sexual Appetite

One of the most beautiful things you bring to a relationship, Leo, is your ability to throw yourself into love spontaneously and with great joy. Leos know that a life without mystery and risk is a life half-lived. You give yourself completely to the rich possibilities of the unknown and unplanned in a loving relationship. No halfway, half-hearted romances for you, Leo.

A Leo in love is a splendid sight to behold. You lavish your beloved with hugs, kisses, cuddles, and giggling. Love brings out the playful, romantic child in you that is hiding behind that strong, proud façade. When you are in love, you light up like sunshine. You want the whole world to participate in your joy, and you demand that all your friends admire your mate, and know that this person is yours.

But your need for complete devotion, constant admiration, and praise may be difficult for an ordinary mortal to satisfy. And your expectations are so high that your disappointment is all the greater. Your one failing in love may be your ability to sabotage a fine relationship. You question your lover's power, intelligence, looks, style. The more you analyze, the less you are able to appreciate your love's strengths and concentrate on what attracted you in the first place. But you also have doubts about your own worthiness. After reading "Slim Legs in Five Minutes" or "Even Thinner Everything—Instantly," you become so self-conscious about how you look in bed that you forget why you are there.

When there are setbacks, your sense of privacy comes into play, and you don't reveal your frustrations. But they take their toll, and may be damaging to your pride. Be aware that your ego is huge, but fragile.

You tend to seek comfort in the refrigerator or candy box. Don't use food as a solace for hurt pride. Reason with yourself. Sometimes you overdramatize your emotions, feeling devastated when your "image" has been tarnished. Recover your dignity! Turn that hurt pride into ambition. Move on to another position of leadership.

Set up some guidelines for handling your ego, pride, need for flattery, and the resulting discontent. The following advice from Leo Buscaglia's book *Loving Each Other,* seems tailor-made to you, Leo: ". . . to bring another into our life in love, we must be willing to give up certain destructive tendencies." For example:

- The need to be always right.
- The need to be first in everything.
- The need to be constantly in control.
- The need to be loved by everyone.
- The need to change others for our needs.
- The need to reign supreme.

If you can manage to give up those tendencies, you'll be less frustrated. You often are attracted to people who are different from you. Enjoy them and don't try to remold them in your own image. Let the people you love keep their own identities; trust them. They can value you and still have separate interests of their own.

Above all, keep your sense of humor and you won't need such constant reassurances of faithfulness and love.

And here's a suggestion for keeping both your mate and your diet. Next time you feel like saying, "Let's go out somewhere to eat, now," say instead, "Let's go someplace where we can be alone, now." That's the real food for romance.

Eating/Entertaining at Home

Gracious entertaining is your trademark. It gives you pleasure to bring together a group of friends at your home for an evening of good food and conversation. It's important to you to maintain your friendships, and you regularly take the time and make the effort to strengthen those bonds. Often, you have a potpourri of unusual guests at one of your little dinners, and each time you try to vary both the menu and the mix of people. It makes for interesting, stimulating exchanges.

Chances are you issued the invitation by telephone, your favorite household appurtenance. Those who have visited you before know they can look forward to a magical evening, because they've received a royal invitation to an enchanted world.

Everything in your home has magnificent visual appeal. Drama and romance are your decorating themes. You set your table with fine china, ornate sterling flatware, and sparkling crystal bowls, all set off by a magnificent linen tablecloth. You love flowers, and you'll nest potted African violets in baskets to use as centerpieces.

When your guests arrive, you're cool as a cucumber, perhaps with a drink in your hand, and ready to give each guest a share of your undivided attention. You've done all your planning and preparation in advance, and you're proud that the effort it took doesn't show.

You are very imaginative, Leo, and your entertaining is creative, artistic, and in good taste, whatever the size of your budget. You have a way of using condiments to turn simple foods into sublime treats. You experiment with unusual seasonings like lime mustard, chili vinegar, lemon garlic sauce, or sesame sauce, and you know how to use malt vinegars, red wine vinegars, and fine herb vinegars to enhance more mundane fare. You flavor your foods with little touches of dill, fennel, or mint, and decorate platters with parsley, radishes cut into roses, or little carrot curls.

The hors d'oeuvres might include *pâté de foie gras,* sweetbreads, and an assortment of cheeses, from Brie to Edam to Neufchâtel. And your fruit platters—yum ... they are unmistakably Leo-designed; large, lavish, and lovingly prepared. They may have a large scooped-out pineapple in the center, filled with exotic fruits. Masses of strawberries, blueberries, and tiny clusters of grapes surround it. And you can sculpt marvelous watermelon baskets too, filled with perfect little melon balls.

Champagne and caviar will probably appear during the course of the evening. Fine imported chocolate you bought from a chocolatier in a boutique will punctuate the end of a lovely meal. Your chocolate expertise is beyond reproach, and you will go far out of your way for just the right chocolate nut balls, chocolate éclairs, chocolate mousse, or chocolate pinwheels. Watch out, Leo: All that chocolate will be your undoing!

Food Shopping

You are a great shopper, Leo, for crystal, clothes, cruises, adornments, jewelry, perfumes, and shoes. But food? That is really not your cup of tea . . . or should I say, champagne?

But you are very good at knowing the best place in town to order up, one that delivers right on time and sends up something that looks like you slaved over it in the kitchen for hours. A dear friend of mine is particularly ingenious with barbecued chickens from the fast food take-out service. She places the lovely darlings on an elegant cut-crystal serving platter, surrounds them with pickled apples, olives, and artichokes (a spectacular array of colorful delicacies), and then just opens a can of sweet and sour sauce, drips the whole bottle over the chicken, throws an orange slice on top, and voila, who would know? Now *that* is class.

Leos know the best caterers in town, and how to make reservations at any restaurant. You know where the best food in town is, so why shop for food?

However, when you do go food shopping (if you can't avoid it), you buy only what *you* like to eat. In fact, you don't care as much about the inside as the outside. You buy what looks appealing . . . and often it will be an array of goodies that are not terribly good for you. High-cholesterol foods, like potato chips, ice cream, and delicatessen meats (already prepared). And, of course, no self-respecting Leo will leave without a box of raisins, ripened by the Leo sun.

You are not terribly fond of standing in long lines and will not bother to hunt for bargains if the neighborhood supermarket will deliver. Service is your middle name: You deserve it.

The place to shop that makes you happiest is the neighborhood specialty store that carries the most delicious delicacies prepared by the pound. Many of the specialties are flown in from all parts of the world and not exactly inexpensive. There you'll shop for pâté, fine aspic gelatins, special blends—anything, from coffee to chutney fit for a king or a queen.

When you start a diet, you will go up and down the supermarket aisles looking for aids. You buy swell-up pills, vitamins, fat-burning items, and copies of magazines with the newest diets. If the headline is "Kill Cellulite

Forever," you optimistically grab it up. And, at the same time, you pick up diet candies, sugarless chewing gums, diet sodas, and a new beauty product to reward yourself in advance and make you feel it's all worth it.

Social Dining

You love elegant restaurants with exotic, romantic appeal, especially those with flattering candlelight and expensive decor. The drama of waiters in white gloves bustling around to serve you puts you in bubbling good spirits, like the champagne you love. An atmosphere of splendor and excitement, good food, fanfare, and activity all put you in your best mood.

You enjoy spicy foods that are served either very warm or hot. You prefer your meat rare and surrounded by colorful little delicacies. Eye appeal is important. Cholesterol counts are the furthest thing from your mind when you order, and you care little about balance or nutrition.

When you go out to dinner, you are conscious of proper dress and makeup, so you want to know beforehand what the lighting is like. Will it be soft lights, bright lights, candlelight? All this counts to a Leo. Leos tend to dine at supper clubs with a special ambiance. If influential people congregate there, so much the better.

Even when you dine at a friend's house, you are concerned with wearing just the right dress for the occasion, so you give the matter much thought. Sometimes you try on half the clothes in your closet before you reach that important decision of what to wear.

Whenever you are invited out, you go, even if you know that the circumstances will ultimately do in your diet. How could they manage without you? Who would keep the laughter going and the evening gay if you are not there?

Really, Leo, can you ever find a reason to stay at home?

Special-Occasion Dining

Leo, you have to be particularly careful about special occasion events. You do love parties. As the song says, you can dance all night and still have room for more. Your social life is very busy, because you love people, leadership, and activity, and you join so many groups. Some months you have so many engagements it can really wreak havoc on your diet.

If you have a career, you may be involved in entertaining clients at lunch or dinner, or, worse yet, traveling to conventions. Conventions are your complete downfall. You are everyone's friend and are forever joining people for food or drink. You may find yourself at 5 P.M. in the hotel lobby bar buying drinks for everyone. Leo, for the sake of your diet, please try to keep a lower profile.

You like romantic places that are sumptuous and elegant. You lure your lover into weekends of magic, preferably some place once frequented by royalty. A castle feels like home to you, because underneath it all, you are a monarch and nothing is too grand for you.

Remind yourself that all those special events can be very costly...in calories. Those restaurant lunches and dinners will start to show up in the mirror. Now's the time to use those great leadership qualities on yourself. Before your weight gets out of control.

Your Health

As you know, Leo, your constitution is extremely robust by all measures. Notice how your energy level remains high long after your friends have run out of steam. Your vitality is one of your charms.

You are seldom ill, a fortunate circumstance, because illness represents weakness and you identify with strength. Leo has rulership over the heart, blood, circulatory system, gall bladder, back and dorsal region of the spine. Diseases to which Leos are subject include:

Aneurysms	Obesity
Arteriosclerosis	Poor blood circulation
Backache	Rheumatic fever
Eye trouble	Sleep disturbances
Heart and muscle strain	Spinal problems
Heart disease	Tachycardia
High fevers	

To prevent illnesses like these, your diet should be high in vitamins A, C, D, and E, and lecithin. It is very important that you eliminate high-cholesterol saturated fatty foods from your diet and substitute lecithin-rich and polyunsaturated foods. Remember, Leo, you must take care of your heart, and heavy fats can damage the arterial walls of the heart muscle, creating plaque and fat deposits within the interior heart wall.

Since you are a fire sign, Leo, a sign of strong vitality, you just seem to burn up protein. Your diet regimen should be generous in high-quality protein, but low in starch and sugar. In addition, you need foods high in iron, magnesium, and iodine. The Leo diet includes bioflavonoids to help you maintain good blood circulation.

Magnesium phosphate is the Leo cell salt. Cell salts are naturally occurring minerals that are constitutents of the body cells. Plants, animals and humans all require these compounds for proper nutrition, and they are found in trace amounts in many foods. But, like vitamins, cell salts get used up. Magnesium phosphate is known as the "anti-pain" or the "anti-spasmodic" cell salt. It acts upon the white fibers of the muscles and the nerves to ease cramping and pain. Inadequate magnesium phosphate can cause the liquid in the nerves and muscles to become inflamed, resulting in cramps, headaches, and pain. An example of a severe spasm which may occur from lack of magnesium phosphate is angina pectoris, a spasm of the heart. As you know, Leo, the heart is a sensitive area for you. Include in your daily diet foods rich in magnesium phosphate, and it will make you a healthier Leo.

FOODS RICH IN MAGNESIUM PHOSPHATE

Almonds	Lemons
Apples	Lettuce
Blueberries	Onions
Coconut	Plums
Cucumber	Rye
Figs	Walnuts

Cinnamon tea has a special effect on Leos, on whom it serves as a mild stimulant.

Make sure to include garlic in your daily menus, and lots of fruit, fish and soy products in place of red meat. Above all keep your weight under control.

Leo, you are a lover of life and you want to lead it to the fullest. Do it the healthy way. You are about to embark on a diet regimen that is not only healthy and nutritious, but actually supplies you with the essential nutrients your body has been demanding for years.

Temper your eating and drinking, Leo, and you will keep that good health. I know that you like to entertain. I know that you like to dine well, and with great ceremony. But temper it, my good friend. Most of the time I can count on you to do this, because your pride and vanity ultimately win out and you simply get yourself in control. You cannot stand not looking your very best.

Leo Daily Nutritional Supplements

- 400 mg vitamin E
- 2,000 mg vitamin C
- One general multivitamin with minerals (make certain multivitamin includes vitamins A and D, 10–25,000 units)

Remember, Leo...

This diet is uniquely prepared to address your sun sign and *should not be interchanged with any other Sun Sign Diet.* It is important that you follow the diet exactly as it appears, for optimum weight loss and assimilation. Before starting your Leo diet, carefully read "General Diet and Maintenance Guidelines for All Sun Signs," found at the beginning of this book. Remember, drink 8 glasses of water daily.

You will never have to be a member of the yo-yo team again, dear Leo, because this diet has been prepared to meet your biological, chemical, nutritional, and behavioral needs.

Good luck, and *go for it.*

The Leo
Seven-Day
Reducing Diet

(with options)

I've given special attention to your diet, Leo, to help you meet your busy social schedule of dining out with friends for lunch and your special someone for dinner. Notice that to meet those needs I have included a Restaurant Socializing Day, so you will not have to digress from your diet. It furnishes all the vitamins, minerals and essential nutrients that you require by nature, Leo.

I have also included an Alternate Day menu. This is to ensure variety and additional choices for you and to eliminate any boredom you might experience when you repeat the diet for the duration of your weight reduction program. I am leaving no room for excuses.

For the first time you have a diet that was prepared for your own physical makeup. When the combinations are followed as listed, a specific dynamic action takes place. Therefore, except where noted, no substitutes are permitted. If you do not like a particular food, just omit it. At any time, if you wish to exchange lunch with dinner, or vice versa, you may do so as long as you do not use a lunch or dinner from another day's menu.

Although I am opposed to "crash dieting," I know that as a Leo you always want everything to happen yesterday, and that if you don't see an instant result you can easily become discouraged. Patience is not one of your virtues. For those of you who are especially impatient, I have included three types of two-day crash diets to get you started. However, you should never crash diet more than two days per week. Remember, crash dieting is

170

unhealthy. Reserve it only for getting you into that fabulous dress for a special occasion.

I have found that Leo, a fire sign, needs a low-cholesterol, high-protein diet. You will also notice the inclusion of dry red or white wine. It is optional. If it is not important to you, just skip it. It has been carefully calculated in your dieting regime, should you desire it.

Stir one teaspoon of apple-cider vinegar into an 8-ounce glass of water as an excellent diet aid. It will help tame your robust appetite for starchy bread products. The potassium/phosphorus balance in the apple-cider vinegar will definitely help cut down your appetite. Have it with meals and perhaps once midday for optimal effect.

You may choose to try a diet aid known in the United States as Glucomannan. It is extracted from the Japanese konjac root, a tuber that is very high in fiber. A final monograph on its effectiveness has not yet been established by the FDA, as it has no history of use in the United States before 1958; however, the konjac root has been cultivated and eaten in Asia for over a thousand years.

Glucomannan aids in decreasing cholesterol and triglyceride levels, and in maintaining low-density lipoprotein levels. It acts as a dietary fiber to increase viscosity and moisture content of food as it is digested, so that it forms a smooth, soft mass that moves easily through the intestinal tract. Digestion is slowed, so normal blood sugar levels are maintained after a meal. It is especially beneficial, Leo, for its laxative capabilities, since regularity can sometimes be a problem on a high-protein diet. Two capsules taken three times a day may also cut your appetite in half!

And when Leo, you feel you have reached your absolute limit of will power and that you cannot go on any longer without some sinful, wonderful food, you may use a binge day. Just make sure this does not happen more than four times a month. You will find all instructions for your binge day at the end of the Leo Reducing Diet.

After just one week, you will notice how good you look and how well you feel. I am sure you will be receiving compliments from your friends and neighbors.

Please note the asterisks (*) that appear after certain foods listed in your menu plan. You will find a detailed explanation of their vitamin and mineral content, and direct information as to why they are essential components of your diet regimen, located in the section "Notes to the Leo Seven-Day Reducing Diet," which follows your programmed diet.

DAY ONE

BREAKFAST

> hot water with 2 tsp. lemon juice
>
> 1 whole orange or 1 apple

If hungry, you may have another orange or half a grapefruit before lunch.

LUNCH

> fresh fruit salad—you may have 3 cups of any combination of seasonal fresh fruit, plus 2 Tbsp. sunflower seeds or 5 almonds
>
> (The specific dynamic action of the fruit enzymes will start your metabolism burning for the day.)

DINNER

> 4–6 oz. sautéed chicken livers or broiled beef liver (Sauté in non-stick pan with red or white wine instead of oil.)
>
> ½ cup broccoli and ½ cup carrots with ½ onion.
>
> (Liver is an excellent source of lecithin and vitamins D and B. However, those of you who dislike liver may use the following dinner as a substitute.)

or

> ¼–½ broiled or baked chicken (no skin), seasoned with paprika and cayenne pepper.
>
> 1 cup fresh or frozen asparagus seasoned with lemon juice and garlic pepper

Follow this diet precisely and you should see a good weight loss by the first morning.

Remember, drink 8 glasses of water every day.

DAY TWO

ON RISING

2 tsp. lemon juice in 1 cup water

BREAKFAST

1 whole orange or 1 apple or ¼–½ fresh pineapple

coffee, tea or herbal tea, water

LUNCH

Leo Borscht Soup*

1 cup low-calorie borscht served with ½ cup plain yogurt, ½ cup sliced cucumber, 1 chopped scallion, and 2 hard-boiled eggs (slice and float in soup).

2 melba toast

DINNER

¼–½ baked or broiled chicken with Mexican salsa*

½ can of artichokes (canned in water) seasoned with paprika

(Salsa warms the body and is very rich in vitamins A, C, and potassium. It will help you to feel energized and satisfied.)

Remember, drink 8 glasses of water every day.

DAY THREE

BREAKFAST

4 oz. tomato juice

3½ oz. Pacific sardines* drained of oil on 1 slice pumpernickel or black bread

black coffee or tea

(Sardines are a major source of low-cholesterol protein. They are filling, and will keep you from feeling hungry until lunchtime.)

LUNCH

asparagus*—as much lightly steamed fresh or frozen asparagus as you want; sprinkle with lemon juice and 2 Tbsp. grated Parmesan cheese

iced tea with cinnamon

DINNER

1 or 2 large baked potatoes,* seasoned with ¼ cup plain yogurt mixed with basil, dill, and chives

green or black olives

½ cup raspberry sherbet

apple-cider vinegar and water

black coffee, tea, Red Zinger herbal tea, or black coffee with cinnamon

Extremely low-calorie day which will result in extraordinary weight loss.

Remember, drink 8 glasses of water every day.

DAY FOUR

BREAKFAST

strawberries, strawberries*—up to 2 cups fresh strawberries or 1 cup *unsweetened* frozen strawberries

LUNCH

3½ oz. Chinook salmon*

1 cup fresh strawberries (or ½ cup frozen unsweetened strawberries)

black coffee, tea, no-sodium Perrier, apple-cider vinegar and water, or no-sodium diet soda.

(Salmon is an excellent source of a class of fats [Omega 3s] that have far-reaching effects on the metabolism. It is very powerful at lowering cholesterol levels and important for the Leo diet.)

DINNER

6 oz. broiled, baked, or steamed salmon* with dill

1 cup fresh strawberries (or ½ cup frozen unsweetened strawberries)

unlimited quantities of D-Zerta diet gelatin with 4 Tbsp. Cool Whip dessert topping

black coffee, tea, herbal tea, or apple-cider vinegar and water

The combinations of today's foods will produce excellent loss of weight and will keep energy high.

Remember, drink 8 glasses of water every day.

DAY FIVE

BREAKFAST

1 container plain yogurt sweetened with ½ cup dietetic applesauce

black coffee, tea, herbal tea, or water

LUNCH

The Leo Iron Punch Salad

Fresh spinach, parsley, 8 oz. tofu, mixed with raisins and 1 cup water-pack mandarin orange sections; toss with juice from orange sections.

2 Wasa Crisp Bread

no-sodium sparkling water with a slice of lemon

(This salad is just packed with the highest quality of readily available iron. It is also very low in calories. Note that parsley is an excellent diuretic food.)

DINNER

4 oz. white wine (optional)

1 apple 20 minutes before dinner*

Pasta with Clam Sauce

1 cup vegetable pasta; durum or whole wheat, mixed with 1 small jar pimientos; use the liquid from pimientos plus 1 Tbsp. olive oil to stir-fry broccoli, zucchini, and spinach; sprinkle with 2 Tbsp. grated Parmesan cheese; season with fresh basil, oregano, and garlic pepper.*

no-sodium Perrier with a twist of lime

Remember, drink 8 glasses of water every day.

DAY SIX*

BREAKFAST

> 1 packet vanilla or strawberry Alba 77 skim-milk drink, mixed in blender with 2 ice cubes, 1 medium-size banana, and 2 Tbsp. wheat germ
>
> (Powerful, energizing breakfast.)

LUNCH

> 1 large baked potato seasoned with ½ cup plain yogurt mixed with basil, dill, and chives
>
> 6 green or black olives
>
> no-sodium Perrier with a twist of lime

DINNER

> 4 oz. dry white wine (optional)
>
> 6 oz. broiled or baked lean veal, chicken, or fish
>
> all the steamed asparagus you want with lemon juice and garlic pepper
>
> unlimited D-Zerta diet gelatin

EVENING SNACK

> 1 35-calorie Jell-O frozen pudding pop

(An incredibly high-powered, nutritious day of Leo dieting.)

Remember, drink 8 glasses of water every day.

LEO REDUCING DIET
DAY SEVEN

BRUNCH

1–2 glasses champagne or dry white wine (optional)

two-egg spinach, broccoli, or asparagus omelette*

or

8 oz. unsweetened grapefruit juice

DINNER

4 oz dry wine (optional)

steamed lobster, shrimp, crab legs* (no butter—use lemon juice, garlic, and pepper)

tossed salad of lettuce, tomato, and watercress (1 tsp. oil and vinegar)

no-sodium Perrier

or

¼–½ baked or broiled chicken* (no skin)

¼ cup canned red peppers or pimientos
salad as above

black iced coffee or iced tea

This seven-day plan can be repeated week after week until you reach your ultimate goal weight. If, during the long haul of dieting, you want a change, you may substitute the following "Alternate Day."

Remember, drink 8 glasses of water every day.

ALTERNATE DAY*

BREAKFAST

> ¾ cup water-pack canned mandarin orange sections
>
> black coffee, tea, water, or herbal tea

LUNCH

> 3½ oz. Pacific sardines or sardines in mustard sauce (drained of oil)
>
> ½ head of lettuce seasoned with lemon juice and garlic pepper
>
> iced black coffee with cinnamon
>
> herbal tea, or apple-cider vinegar and water

DINNER

> 1–2 cups low-sodium Herb-Ox chicken or beef bouillon
>
> 4 oz. pickled herring in wine sauce
>
> large salad of lettuce, tomato, cucumber, parsley, and watercress, seasoned with lemon juice

or

> 4 oz. sliced roast beef
>
> salad as above
>
> black coffee, tea, no-sodium diet soda, water

EVENING SNACK

> 1–2 Tbsp. natural unprocessed sunflower seeds

Cinnamon is very important to Leos and makes them feel exceptionally peppy. You may have it any time in your tea or coffee.

Remember, drink 8 glasses of water every day.

"SOCIALIZING"*
RESTAURANT MENU DAY

BREAKFAST
>
> choice of 1 whole grapefruit
>
> > *or*
>
> 2 oranges
>
> > *or*
>
> 1 cup blueberries
>
> > *or*
>
> ½ cantaloupe
>
> > *or*
>
> ¼–½ fresh pineapple
>
> tea, black coffee
>
> *Nothing but water until lunch.*

LUNCH
>
> 4 oz. dry red or white wine (optional)
>
> large tomato stuffed with lump crabmeat, solid tuna, chunks of chicken, or 2 hard-boiled eggs

MID-AFTERNOON SNACK
>
> 1–2 glasses Crystal Light diet drink

DINNER
>
> 4–6 oz. filet of flounder or sole (broiled with lemon juice, no butter)
>
> 1 cup fresh or frozen asparagus
>
> 1 cup sliced cucumber, parsley, or watercress; 1 Tbsp. yogurt sprinkled with basil for dressing

EVENING SNACK
>
> as much D-Zerta diet gelatin as you want
>
> *Remember, drink 8 glasses of water every day.*

Leo Emergency Crash Days

The Pineapple Day

For two days just eat a total of 10 pounds of fresh pineapple, and herbal tea, water, black coffee, or very light tea. You will lose 4 pounds in two days . . . *only for emergencies.* (Not for other sun signs—only Leo.)

The Apple Day

Up to 3 pounds of apples for the entire day. One apple and a glass of water for breakfast, midmorning snack, lunch, midafternoon snack, dinner, and/or late evening snack. That's it.

My Favorite Crash—The 36-Hour Vegetable Break

From 8 P.M. on any evening until 8 A.M. thirty-six hours later (for instance Monday evening at 8 P.M. until Wednesday morning at 8 A.M.) you will have nothing but the following: all the raw vegetables you want, all the D-zerta diet gelatin you want (you may even blend them in a vegetable mold), black coffee, tea, water, or no-sodium diet soda. *That's all.*

Notes to Leo Seven-Day Reducing Diet

Leo Diet Notes—Day One

This is a high-powered Leo vitamin-packed day that will yield a good weight loss. Follow it exactly.

Leo Diet Notes—Day Two

* 3½ oz. of beets supplies you with 207 mg of potassium and fights fat buildup. Borscht is rich in vitamins A, B, and C, as well as sodium chloride, phosphorus, selenium, and calcium. Start to enjoy beets, my Leo friend.
* Mexican salsa . . . you can either make your own, or purchase any brand in a health food store. If you wish you may also purchase, La Victoria brand salsa, sold in most supermarkets. Mexican salsa is made from the Jalapeño pepper, and has been referred to as "Mexican chicken soup."

Leo Diet Notes—Day Three

* Sardines are a major source of low-cholesterol protein, and chock full of calcium and vitamin E.
* Asparagus is an excellent diuretic food. It also contains the enzyme asparagine, which helps to break up accumulated fats in the cells.

* Potato, carbohydrate, fiber, and bulk will make you feel as though you have eaten a 10 oz. steak. If you are comfortable and satiated with one potato, stop.

Leo Diet Notes—Day Four

* Strawberries have a good deal of potassium, and vitamin C. You will feel an instant lift, which should last until lunch.
* Salmon is an excellent low-cholesterol, high-level protein food that is extremely high in vitamins A and B, and calcium. When using canned salmon, purchase Sockeye. It is richer in calcium than other brands, because they have crushed the bones into the salmon meat.

Leo Diet Notes—Day Five

* The apple must be eaten twenty minutes before you eat your pasta meals so that the stomach enzymes produced from the digestion of the apple will work on the pasta. You may substitute crabmeat, lobster, shrimp, or tuna for the clams.
* No self-respecting Leo can really live without some starch. I have given you an easy way to prepare a first-class pasta dish, which will truly excite your taste buds and nourish your body.

Leo Diet Notes—Day Six

* An excellent, low-calorie, high-energy day. You will be smiling when you step on the scale tomorrow morning.

Leo Diet Notes—Day Seven

* Eggs are rich in vitamins E, B-12, folic acid, phosphorus, and chlorine. In combination with the broccoli and spinach, your calcium intake is increased, and with the asparagus water retention is reduced.
* Lobster—you may have up to 2 lbs. steamed or broiled lobster or 8 oz. shrimp or 6 crab legs.
* Chicken is a real bargain for Leos. It is low in cholesterol, low in calories, and can be prepared 100 different ways.

Leo Diet Notes—Alternate Day

I have included this day so that you have more variety when eating.

Leo Diet Notes—"Socializing" Restaurant Menu Day

I have lunched with enough Leos to know what you like to order, what you like to be seen eating, and what socially appeals to you. This has been especially prepared for you so that you will have no excuses for any digressions.

LEO TOTAL BINGE DAY

Leo, with all your social commitments and pressures, you are bound to succumb to so many temptations. When that day arrives, and you really cannot go on any longer, lest you collapse, you may switch to your binge day. Remember, you have a tendency to go overboard so be careful and follow the rules.

Before You Binge

1. Drink water.
2. Drink water.
3. Drink water.
4. Rest.
5. Brush your teeth and rinse with your favorite mouthwash.
6. Chew sugarless gum for 20 minutes.

You may find that the desire to binge has passed. However, if you are still suffering from intense food frustration, follow these basic binge rules:

Rule One
Under no circumstances should you ever binge before completing Day Five of your reducing diet. This will ensure a maximum weight loss with a minimum of food frustration.

Rule Two
If, for example, you binge on the sixth day of your diet, resume your diet the following day (Day Seven) with the menu for Day Six. If you binge for just one meal, such as lunch on Day Six, resume your reducing diet with dinner on Day Six of your reducing diet.

Rule Three
Bingeing is for when you get that creepy, anxious feeling, when you feel like pulling out your hair—strand by strand—and you cannot endure dieting for even one more moment. Before you climb the walls, give yourself a binge day. It's hoped that this will not be necessary more than four times a month.

Rule Four
After you have lost your first 10 pounds, you may vary your binge day with the binge day of the sun sign opposite yours, which is Aquarius.

Remember, an occasional binge day—when necessary—will still allow you to lose weight (without guilt). Here, Leo, is your binge day menu.

Binge Day Menu

BREAKFAST
½ grapefruit or ½ orange

1 Aunt Jemima french toast with 2 Tbsp. diet maple syrup

or

½ cup Life cereal and ½ cup milk

MIDMORNING SNACK
1 cup unbuttered popcorn

LUNCH
1 serving Sara Lee cheesecake

or

1 slice pizza

no-sodium diet soda, coffee, tea, 8 oz. light beer, Yoo-Hoo diet chocolate drink or 4 oz. white wine (optional)

or

1 cup Tofutti frozen dessert or 1 cup Light & Lively caramel nut ice

MIDAFTERNOON SNACK
1 cup unbuttered popcorn

or

20 pistachio nuts

DINNER
lobster bisque followed by poached salmon with 2 Tbsp. caviar

or

lemon sole with 1 slice Bellacicco frozen garlic bread

or

any 3 oz. Lean Cusine with 1 slice Bellacicco frozen garlic bread

½ cup raspberry sherbet, ½ cup Tofutti frozen dessert, or any flavor FrozFruit fruit pop

EVENING SNACK
1 cup unbuttered popcorn

Maintaining Your Ideal Weight

Leo Maintenance Foods for Optimum Health

Vitamin A

You need vitamin A to help maintain clear, bright, healthy eyes. Vitamin A also protects your skin from premature aging. It is of particular value, also, in deterring infections like recurring colds and other virus-caused illnesses, and reducing the incidence of coronary heart disease. Therefore, I've planned a Leo diet rich in vitamin A.

FOODS RICH IN VITAMIN A

Bananas	Oranges
Beets	Parsley
Broccoli	Peaches
Broiled liver	Potatoes (sweet or yams, not
Cantaloupe	white)
Carrots	Red chili peppers
Chicken liver	Salmon
Egg yolk	Squash
Mangos	

(Think of yellow and orange-colored fruits and vegetables.)

Vitamin C

Vitamin C is one of the vitamins the body cannot manufacture for itself or store from day to day. Therefore, it is important that your diet supplies adequate amounts of vitamin C every day.

One of vitamin C's main functions is to help the body to form collagen, which constitutes approximately 40 percent of the body's protein. If collagen is weak because of insufficient vitamin C intake, cells in the bones may lose their supportive strength, and Leos are prone to back problems. Vitamin C also keeps the capillaries, veins, and arteries elastic, thus preventing hemorrhaging.

FOODS RICH IN VITAMIN C

Alfalfa	Grapefruit
Almonds	Green peppers
Apples	Lemons
Asparagus	Oranges
Bananas	Orange juice
Beets	Paprika
Blueberries	Parsley
Broccoli	Pineapple
Brussels sprouts	Skim milk
Cantaloupe	Strawberries
Carrots	Tomatoes
Celery	Watercress
Currants	

Vitamin D

Without adequate vitamin D, the body could not properly assimilate calcium. The result would be soft bones. Scoliosis (or spinal curvature) is one of the more serious problems resulting from a lack of vitamin D. Your back and spine may be problem areas for you, Leo, so you must be doubly sure to have an adequate intake of vitamin D.

Insufficient calcium absorption due to lack of vitamin D also can negatively affect your heart and increase your already high susceptibility to heart disease, Leo.

FOODS RICH IN VITAMIN D

Bass

Butter

Cheese

Herring

Liver

Mackerel

Milk

Mushrooms

Oysters

Salmon

Sardines

Shrimp

Sunflower seeds

Tuna

Watercress

Yogurt

Vitamin E

Vitamin E's most important function is to serve as an antioxidant. It prevents red blood cells from combining with toxic peroxide and instead promotes their combining with oxygen. Vitamin E also helps to dissolve blood clots and dilates the blood vessels so that oxygen-rich blood is freely carried to all parts of the body.

Many of your specific health problems, Leo, result from impaired circulation—varicose veins, for example. Because of vitamin E's positive effect on circulation, it both prevents and relieves varicose veins. Vitamin E is so crucial for you that you may wish to memorize the following list.

FOODS RICH IN VITAMIN E

Apples

Asparagus

Avocados

Broccoli

Cabbage

Carrots

Cheese

Chicken

Eggs

Halibut

Liver

Milk

Mushrooms

Parsley

Peanut butter

Salmon

Sardines

Shrimp

Spinach

Sunflower seeds

Sweet potatoes

Turkey

Wheat germ

Bioflavonoids

Bioflavonoids act with vitamin C to maintain "clean" blood; they prevent cholesterol buildup and clot formation. Because of their anticlotting effect, bioflavonoids can also be quite effective in preventing varicose veins. Varicose veins are the external manifestation of unhealthy circulation—a problem to which Leos are susceptible.

Leos always need to look their best. Adequate bioflavonoids will certainly help keep you from developing those unsightly varicose veins.

FOODS RICH IN BIOFLAVONOIDS

Apples	Grapefruit
Apricots	Green peppers
Blackberries	Lemons
Black currants	Oranges
Blueberries	Parsley
Buckwheat	Prunes
Cherries	Rose hips
Grapes	Spinach

Lecithin

Lecithin is an emulsifying agent. It breaks down large fat globules into microscopic bits. This helps prevent cholesterol plaque from forming on the walls of your arteries. Since cholesterol plaque can cause hardening of the arteries, lecithin's cholesterol-combating function is very important if your are to maintain healthy arteries and prevent heart disease.

FOODS RICH IN LECITHIN

Avocado	Rice
Barley	Sesame Seeds
Beef	Tuna
Chicken	Turkey
Liver	Veal
Milk	Wheat

Leo Sample Maintenance Menu

When you reach your desired goal, please follow the maintenance eating hints found in "General Diet and Maintenance Guidelines for All Sun Signs" at the beginning of this book for proper calculations of caloric intake.

I'm including a sample maintenance menu based on your sun sign for optimal Leo maintenance. When you create your own menus for yourself, try to choose many of the foods you eat from your Leo Maintenance Foods lists.

2,000 Calories Per Day

BREAKFAST	CALORIES
1 whole wheat bagel	163
2 oz. cottage cheese	58
1 oz. lox	50
4 oz. unsweetened grapefruit juice	48
	319

LUNCH	
1 cup French onion soup	57
1 slice garlic bread	150
Caesar salad with 3 oz. tuna fish (in water)	375
	582

MIDAFTERNOON SNACK	
6 oz. apple juice	38

DINNER	
4 oz. dry red or white wine (optional)	84
1 cup pasta shells stuffed with	216
4 oz skim-milk ricotta cheese	108
tossed green salad with 1 Tbsp. blue cheese dressing	160
6 oz. veal scallopine	300
½ cup raspberry sherbet with 2 Tbsp. Cool Whip dessert topping	118
	986

EVENING SNACK
   1 apple   80
                                                 ——

TOTAL DAILY CALORIES   2,005

Remember, drink 8 glasses of water every day.

Restaurant Eating
the Leo Way

Perhaps you have seen the following dishes on restaurant menus. Both the dishes and the types of restaurants chosen will appeal to your Leo palate and satisfy your nutritional needs. Note that all of the recommended dishes contain the nutrients specified in your Leo Maintenance Foods lists. For example, the guacamole appetizer on the Mexican menu, made of avocados, is rich in vitamin E, a requirement for the Leo circulatory system. All of the dishes are enticing and prepared with elegance to fit Leo's glamorous style.

In all menus, one appetizer plus one entrée equals approximately 600–700 calories.

Mexican Restaurant

APPETIZERS

Guacamole

Nachos

ENTRÉES

Shrimp in spicy sauce

Three cheese-stuffed peppers with Creole tomato sauce or piquant sauce

Chicken enchiladas

Corn tortillas filled with king crabmeat, baked in a tomatillo green sauce

Chinese Restaurant

APPETIZERS

 Prawns with sesame

 Stuffed eggplant

ENTRÉES

 Diced chicken with peanuts in hot pepper sauce

 Lobster with chili sauce or garlic sauce

 Shredded beef with hot pepper sauce

 Curry shrimps with water chestnuts

Continental Restaurant

APPETIZERS

 Smoked brook trout in horseradish sauce

 Caviar

ENTRÉES

 Planked steak tartare

 Steak with peppercorns, flambé

 Veal scallops with wild mushrooms

 Calves liver sautéed with onion and white wine

American Restaurant

APPETIZERS

 Fresh lump crabmeat

 Avocado and pineapple cocktail

ENTRÉES

 Baked fresh oysters stuffed with crabmeat

 Medallions of venison in wild mushroom sauce (not cream)

 Sautéed baby chicken with tarragon vinegar

 Calves liver—sautéed with green and black peppercorns

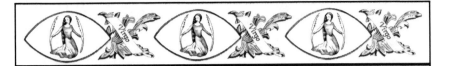

VIRGO

August 24–September 23

The Virgo
Personality

"I want the perfect solution to weight control."

Virgo, "perfection" is your middle name. It is what you seek in everything and everyone, and above all, it is what you demand of yourself. Overweight bothers you more than anyone else. You do want your body to look perfect, feel perfect, and act perfect. And you worry about it, if it is not so.

An overweight friend, who used to drag herself on occasion to an early morning aerobic workout, once confided in me her utter frustration caused by the presence of a trim and shapely woman in the class. "No matter what day of the week I show up, there she is, seven o'clock sharp and wide awake, sweating and working harder than anybody. She looks just perfect to me."

My guess is her dedicated classmate was a Virgo. To others she may look like Bo Derek's double, but in her own eyes she will never measure up to a "10."

Virgo tends to keep slim not due to vanity, but because you strive to be the pink of perfection in everything you do. You size yourself against the toughest standards: your own. There are times when you do get discouraged, however. You will never admit it to me, but it is difficult to find fulfillment in this imperfect world, and living only on salads, as much as you love them, can be a sparse existence.

Despair, overwork, and worry can send you into a tailspin of mental depression. You sometimes do not know where to draw the line in your life. Perhaps Virgo, you have to learn the difference between "servitude and slavery." And you must come to terms with what guilt is, what guilt does if allowed to continue, and how to cope with guilt. Learning to *work for yourself first,* making the choice to help others second, will ensure Virgo a more peaceful state of mind. You will be less likely to drown your sorrows with food, piling pounds on the otherwise slender Virgo frame. Can I count on your self-discipline not to really let things get out of hand? Let's hope your sharp, inquisitive intellect will discover your way back on track. The road to perfection isn't easy, but hard work never scared you away, Virgo.

Virgos are thinkers and problem-solvers. Especially for their friends. You look like you carry the weight of the world on your mind sometimes, and probably you do. Ragged nerves is a common source of Virgo health problems. Tension is your most insidious diet enemy. As serious as you are inclined to be, I do not mean to imply that you cannot have a good time, Virgo. You are not the wild and crazy type, to be sure, but you have a surprising sense of humor, a lightening-quick wit, and are a lively conversationalist *when you* have something to say. In fact, I know many Virgos who have such an accomplished sense of humor that they make their living telling jokes and are some of the world's best comedians. Comedy covers up all the strains in life, doesn't it? Keep cultivating your ironic outlook on the world and learn to transcend worries through humor, and you can avoid the stress-related disorders the Virgo flesh can be heir to.

Your health is one thing you do tend to worry about. I am sure your friends think you are a hypochondriac. No doubt the term "health nut" was first coined to describe a September person (not as common for my August friends). Virgo rules the health house in the zodiac. The symbol of the virgin connotes purity, but also healing and wholeness. You take this domain very seriously and tend to be obsessed with it in some or all its forms: diet, fitness, nutrition, hygiene, psychotherapeutics, preventive medicine.

Need I say, your goal is perfect health. You can be a walking compendium of medical facts and health-related information. You know more about drug reactions than your doctor or pharmacist. There isn't a holistic health treatment you haven't read about and maybe tried. A good number of Virgos are vegetarians. Even the carnivorous kind prefer lentil burgers, vegetable salad, or fruit and yogurt as an entrée once in a while. Though others might regard your daily rituals (mixing and drinking the concoction of brewer's yeast and protein powder every morning) to be a form of asceticism, you know it for what it is: taking good care of yourself as any sound, sensible person would do. How could we accuse you, Virgo, of self-denial! A trim, healthy body is just what you want.

Not surprisingly, Virgo is likely to legitimize this obsession and become a health professional. (Any service profession is a natural for helpful Virgo.)

But even *without* the diploma, you like to play nurse, doctor, or nutrition-ist, and do a good imitation of it. In addition to your complete personal inventory of home remedies and pharmaceutical cures, at times you are a portable drugstore, especially when traveling.

Speaking of vacationing, a week at a super spa is your dream spot. There you can be sure of eating healthy foods, maybe even getting in a few days' cleansing fast. And you can exercise to your heart's content—all the better if the facility staff puts you on a routine. Back at home you will keep up your own physical fitness regimen. Of course, in the office you can practice isometric exercises at your desk a few minutes every hour. I have seen you tightening those buttocks for three or four seconds when you thought no one was looking.

Even Virgo's clothes have a look that says, "I'm into making a new body." Running suits, leotards, warm-up socks, and big, baggy sweaters worn down over the knees are your favorite leisure wear. You are not into designer labels; *your* identity is more important than Calvin's or Ralph's. But what-ever you wear, even at your most casual, it is neat, fresh and, oh yes, made of natural fibers. You like most things unadulterated, the way Mother Nature intended them. *She* might have created spring water, but I suspect you, Virgo, were the first to bottle it for drinking.

Your motto is, "Cleanliness is next to Godliness." Entropy of any sort—dirt, loud noises, even sloppy thinking or crudity—is nervewracking to Virgo, the zodiac's great organizer, systematizer, and logician.

By now you might be thinking that all Virgos are neat and tidy and organized. Well, you couldn't be farther from the truth. The fact is that inwardly Virgos resent their secret compulsion to be organized and neat and it often manifests itself . . . you guessed it . . . in the extreme opposite. So the next time you make note of someone's sloppiness take heed . . . it might just be a Virgo "letting it all hang out."

You are well-read and favor do-it-yourself and self-help books, dictio-naries, encyclopedias, and all kinds of reference books that impose order on diverse facts and forms of information.

You derive a deep sense of security and peace of mind through the perfection of the intellect. Knowledge, particularly that which brings money and status, is power to practical, prudent Virgo.

You like to have a regular paycheck each week and would find freelanc-ing to be very stressful to your delicate nerves. You are exacting and tend to be drawn to those fields which demand precision; you are apt to become highly specialized within your area of expertise. Your work is *perfectly* done. You are achievement-oriented and skilled at establishing goals and objectives and at designing plans to reach them. You also love to keep track of your daily progress. Nothing gives you greater satisfaction than ticking off items on a "to-do" list as each is completed. Each check mark is like a gold star along the path to perfection.

You do thrive best on routine, and good habits develop spontaneously out of your desire to be better, or best . . . and perfect.

That is why you are the ideal candidate for success on my weight loss program, Virgo; it will meet your high standards, it will spell out everything to the last detail. I will tell you how to follow your diet regimen exactly, day by day, and because it addresses all your bodily needs I know that you will be *perfectly* content with the marvelous results you will soon see! I also know, Virgo, I can count on you to follow it P - E - R - F - E - C - T - L - Y .

Sexual Appetite

The literal-minded might be surprised to hear about the sexual appetite of one whose sign is the virgin. In fact, many have been misled by superficial appearances with respect to you, Virgo. You can seem pretty aloof and self-controlled at times, as though you have rid yourself of any feeling quite so messy or entangling as desire. You often have your life so meticulously organized, it does indeed look like you have no need, or even room, for love.

You and I both know, Virgo, that nothing could be further from the truth. The Virgo reserve and self-containment often masks a great gaping emptiness smack in the middle of the soul. It is that very vulnerable place inside you that nearly screams out for completeness. It is the same emptiness that, for lack of love and physical affection, you will sometimes seek to fill by stuffing yourself with food.

What was the person thinking who ever called you a realist? When it comes to romance, you can be extremely unrealistic, Virgo. The truth is, you crave perfect love. And your conviction that only this can make you whole leads to much disappointment, frustration, rejection, and loneliness in life, sensitive Virgo. And all those unhappy feelings lead you straight to the refrigerator door.

Your feeling that your loved one must be your soulmate tends to keep you in relationships which would drive other members of the zodiac wild. On the other hand, your naturally critical nature makes it almost impossible for you to overlook a fault, no matter how minor. And yes, I know you genuinely believe that giving feedback to another serves that individual's personal quest for perfection. It is just that sometimes your nitpicking makes you difficult to live with. What *you* have to realize is that you dish out criticism so well, people naturally assume you can take it, too. Others do not always understand that you are least forgiving of your own faults, Virgo. If you are judged harshly you feel it confirms every bad thing you hold true about yourself. Your emotional mechanism snaps shut tight as a clam, and your eating mechanism goes into high gear.

Virgo, if you truly want to be a winner in the game of love—and a weight loser—you will have to start by changing the rules. Number One: No one is perfect, not even you. Number Two: Virgo, that's okay. You are starved for love because deep in your heart you fear no one could love someone as flawed as you believe yourself to be. Well, Virgo, love thyself. No one else can really make you whole and happy anyway. Begin to accept your own imperfections and those of others and you will be well on your way to success in relationships as well as weight control.

Learn to give yourself credit for all the wonderful things you already are. You have a great capacity for caring and loyalty. Those who have you for a friend are fortunate indeed. Learn to toot your own horn more and to seek feedback from those who love you. Learn to pay compliments just as you enjoy receiving them, and you will soon find you receive more in kind— and watch that empty feeling in the stomach begin to disappear.

You need to build up some emotional muscle. Don't be afraid of rejection, cautious Virgo. Say to yourself, "Well, you win some, you lose some," then ask someone to join you for an evening at the theater. You won't meet anyone sitting home, brooding and eating.

And forget about finding the perfect mate. Just find someone willing to work at a relationship as hard as you are. Work—emotional, mental, or physical—is sexy to you. Someone who shares your intellectual interests and aptitudes and your fascination with health and exercise—someone you can share your nuts and sprouts with, and your daily workout routine— that person turns you on.

But be careful, Virgo, that you do not let your number-one enemy— stress—zap your sex life. You need your weekly quota of affection. If you have to, schedule sex into your busy life just the way you schedule everything else—mark it into your datebook. Seriously, it may take some pressure off, and what is wrong with setting aside some special time for you and your lover? Also, cut down on your coffee, tea, cola, and chocolate consumption because caffeine can act as a sexual depressant.

Virgo, you are known for being discriminating in your sexual life. But this reserve should not be mistaken for a lack of passion. Virgo's shyness often exists to protect a very sexy creature who feels things deeply and takes intimacy extremely seriously. But if you protect yourself too dearly, Virgo, others might think you September people really prefer to remain untouched.

Eating/Entertaining at Home

Friends and family are always welcome in the Virgo home, especially for breakfast, lunch, or dinner. After all, you know better than anyone that it is virtually impossible to get a nutritious, well-prepared, meal anywhere except your own kitchen. Indeed, this or some variation on the food and diet theme will likely be the topic of conversation at your table any time of day. You will inform your guests of the number of laps in the pool it takes to burn off the calories they have consumed or talk at great length about the vitamin content of steamed vegetables as compared to boiled ones. You, of course, cook vegetables only in a steamer, pressure cooker, or wok.

Your recipes aren't the 25-ingredient kind, but you do like to cook from scratch using natural foods and preparing them in simple, classic ways that don't obscure their original taste. You will add a spice or two, as long as the natural flavor and juices are retained, but no thick gravies or rich sauces. When served, everything will be at its proper temperature: piping hot or well-chilled. The arrangements on the plate will be colorful, attractive and crisp as the lettuce in your famous salad, a Virgo staple.

Simple, elegant, functional: that is the Virgo style of home entertaining. These adjectives describe everything from your interior decoration to the placesettings on the table to the food you will put on your company's plates. Your home is impeccably neat, of course. You don't trust "help" to get into every corner with the mop or to dust every slat on your Levolor blinds. There is nothing more chaotic to you than dirt, so you'll do the straightening up yourself, thank you. Every piece of furniture will have a place and a purpose. You do like rooms to be well-lit, and prefer earthy, muted tones. No cutesy, frilly things in shocking colors for you, Virgo. Your homefurnishings are likely to include a selection of leather, rattan, hand-woven baskets and natural fiber rugs, dried or fresh-cut flowers, macramé, earthenware, and plants—all very understated and tastefully chosen. You may have collectibles on display, which add some feeling of clutter to an otherwise spare look, but even these, whatever they may be, will be dust-free and precisely arranged.

The overall effect is charming and practical at the same time. It may look costly, but knowing you, thrifty Virgo, whatever furniture you didn't make yourself, you probably bought at warehouse sales. You love to get unfinished furniture you can finish yourself, or take a thing and make it into something else. You read *Good Housekeeping, Home Carpentry,* and others for do-it-yourself decorating tips, and derive great satisfaction from redoing an entire room for under $1,000.

As much as you enjoy home entertaining, it is hard for you to relax, Virgo. You want everything to be just right, including the combination of people you invite to your home. Your concern in certain areas can be overbearing at times. You expect your guests to show up on time. If you call dinner at eight, you do not mean eight-ish, and Lord help the soul who arrives a few minutes late or early. You also tend to hover about your guests as they are taking the final sip of coffee. You just can't wait to get every last dirty cup into the dishwasher. It's not a way to make your company feel comfortable, Virgo, so do try to take it easier. Everyone will have a better time, including you. Besides, when you are tense, you tend to eat unconsciously and it doesn't help your sensitive digestion, either.

Food Shopping

The Virgo food shopper would not think of entering a supermarket without a list. It is basic to your organization. If you are familiar with the store, the list is arranged according to the order of items on the supermarket shelves, starting at Aisle 1 where you enter and end at Aisle 10 near the checkout counter.

It is a good thing you are so methodical, Virgo, otherwise it might take you even longer than you already do to shop. You prefer to take your time because you read every word on every label before you purchase an item. First you peruse the ingredients. You avoid foods containing chemical additives and preservatives. You absolutely draw the line at processed and convenience foods like TV dinners, whipped toppings, and frozen desserts. But you are not fooled by headlines like "All Natural" and "100% Pure," either. Not you, sharp-eyed Virgo. For example, take a popular spaghetti mix that touts "all natural blended Italian flavors." You read the fine print: Sugar is the number one ingredient? Salt, number two? That box goes right back on the shelf where it came from.

Value-conscious Virgo, you are a comparison shopper and price evaluator. You calculate unit costs to ferret out the real bargain brands. No one is going to sell you a bill of goods. You know when a sale is really a sale. You will use coupons, but only to purchase items you would buy anyway. You buy in quantity to save money, but you will never sacrifice quality. On the other hand, you consider the prices at gourmet stores to be quite unreasonable and would not shop at one as a matter of economic principle. Your high standards and consumer know-how, Virgo, ultimately benefit all the shoppers who are not quite so demanding.

Where you do spend lots of money is in the drug and household sections of your supermarket. Costly disposable items like tissues, paper towels, and cotton swabs are popular with you because they are useful for cleaning, and they are sanitary at the same time. Then there are the drug items in your cart: antihistamines, anti-inflammatories—anti, anti, anti. You are extremely fussy about germs, Virgo, and buy every available type of household soap, disinfectant, deodorizer, and scrub on the market. Of course, you only shop in the neatest, brightest, best-kept supermarkets. You wouldn't be found within 100 feet of a dirty, unkempt store, no matter how good the prices.

By the same token, Virgo, you love to wrap your food in plastic bags. Lots of bags, one for each item. All the fresh produce. And the dairy products. And the meats. This protects them, keeps them fresher and neater (if you say so, Virgo). You also like to bag your own groceries at the checkout because you can pack them according to the order in which you plan to empty them back home in your kitchen: dairy in one bag, frozen foods in another, canned items in the third.

Basically, you know how to shop well and wisely, Virgo. You lean toward natural, organic foods, and patronize health food stores regularly. Farmers markets and roadside stands are Virgo favorites, too. You love buying fresh garden cucumbers, and especially carrots and beets with the greens left on. Crocks of bees honey and fresh fruit preserves in glass jars are what you go for when you buy yourself a special treat. If it's a six-pack of beer you want, well, its got to be Coors, made from fresh mountain spring water.

Your healthy, methodical shopping habits, Virgo, will be a boon to your diet because they reduce the chances of you buying tempting, off-the-program foods on impulse.

Social Dining

Dining out is one of the rare times you let yourself relax, nervous Virgo—once the important details have been attended to, that is. For instance, the reservation. You would never show up at the door of a restaurant without one, and you will expect your table to be ready promptly since you've made one. You probably will have specified the table you want—that quiet one in the well-lit corner, with a lot of privacy and good vantage point for people-watching (your favorite pastime), too. The restaurant itself will be one of your regulars, or one that has come highly recommended by a trusted friend. Nothing ruffles your neat feathers more than paying good money for bad food or bad service. You won't make a scene if it is not up to par, but you won't return to the restaurant, either.

Whatever restaurant you select, it undoubtedly will have a widespread reputation for Caesar salad made to order or, at the very least, have an appetizing salad bar. A meal's not a meal without your fresh salad, Virgo. A vegetarian restaurant is usually a hot meal ticket for you, especially if it serves delicacies like zucchini fritters with tomato sauce and sliced avocado or swiss chard and spinach soup with parsley cream chantilly. Family-style, homecooking establishments which convey a sense of wholesomeness and purity also appeal to your tastebuds, Virgo.

Your main course is always "the special of the day." Your rationale: It has to be fresher. You abstain from things like crabburgers or vegetable pot pie or anything that might be called "mystery meat." You like to be able to see, analyze, and know what's in the food you eat. You like to dissect. However, the same crabburger offered on the menu under a heading: "We serve only local crabs" will definitely entice you, Virgo. The native dish is always a safe bet: lobster in Maine, steak in Texas, and Key Lime Pie in Key Largo.

Now, if everything is in order, you can really enjoy quite a pleasant evening out. It is times like these when your dazzling wit really has an opportunity to shine. Not that you'll take centerstage; you're generally not the stand-up comedian type. Instead, you sit back and listen and watch until your practiced senses discover some heretofore unnamed quirk of human nature; then you humorously name it for your delighted friends. You may also wear their patience thin with your discourse on the lethal effects of alcohol on brain cells and of preservatives on the nervous system. But you really are, in the main, an adorable, charming companion. You never talk with your mouth full or chomp noisily on your food or eat with fingers when a fork and knife will do. To watch you spread jelly on toast—right up to the corners but never over the edges—is to see an artist at work.

At times you find the civilized pleasures of fine dining and conversation so fulfilling, all tensions dissolve and the vague, ubiquitous inner hunger almost fades away.

Special-Occasion Dining

As long as the invitation comes well in advance of the event, and you can mark it on your calendar, Virgo really enjoys a special occasion. A last-minute, spur-of-the-moment invitation can send you into a dither, however. You absolutely must have time to prepare.

Since you can be rather particular about your food, even when not on a special diet, you have learned to take little CARE packages whenever you go visiting—a crockpot of stew, a bottle of your homemade salad dressing. This way you get to eat the foods you like, and you don't have to impose upon your hosts to prepare a special dish for you "without this and without that." You do not feel comfortable with all that attention, and "bringing your own" seems less conspicuous.

Special occasions let you test your diet strength, Virgo—you like the challenge. You will map out your eating strategy for the day, you will promise yourself not to divert from it one morsel's worth no matter what, and . . . you know what? You won't. And you feel good about having this strength of will, Virgo.

Your Health

The Virgo body is generally very healthy—despite or perhaps because of your preoccupation with it and all its workings. (One reason many of you Virgos become nurses and doctors is that you like to get the answers for yourself.) You often are able to avoid serious illness due to the fact that, like the princess and the pea, you are sensitive to the slightest signs of irregularity or abnormality that other members of the zodiac would never notice. You rule the health house, and your sign is associated with mental activity, worry, and overstrain.

Virgo rules the intestines, the alimentary canal, the abdominal cavity, the spleen, the lower lobe of the liver, and the duodenum.

Diseases to which you are subject include:

Afflictions of digestive tract	Nervous breakdowns
Allergies	Old-age maladies
Appendicitis	Pancreatitis
Asthma	Peritonitis
Cholera	Tapeworm
Colitis	Typhoid
Hypochondria	Ulcers
Hypoglycemia	Weak intestines
Malnutrition	

Your finicky eating habits are not entirely without basis, Virgo. You do tend to have quite a delicate digestive system which needs to be treated respectfully if you are to avoid problems in this area. So don't be embarrassed when your friends call you a "health nut" or accuse you of being more picky than Morris the Cat. Due to your nervous nature it is important to keep your diet free of heavy fats and proteins which are especially difficult to digest when the system is uptight. Natural foods including whole grains, yogurt, and seeds are indicated for Virgos. It really is best for you to avoid refined foods and follow a natural, simple diet free of additives and preservatives.

Cell salts are naturally occurring minerals that are normal constituents of the body cells. They are found in trace amounts in foods, and plants, animals and human beings require these compounds for proper nutrition and, like vitamins, cell salts get used up. Potassium sulfate manufactures and distributes oily secretions which prevent pores from the skin from clogging. It can be thought of as the "cleanser" cell salt. A deficiency of potassium sulfate will cause the oils in the skin to become viscous thus clogging pores, acne, and dandruff. Potassium sulfate also regulates the level and distribution of oils in the body, and is therefore known as the body's lubricant which keeps all the body's parts functioning smoothly. Another of potassium sulfate's duties is that of carrying oxygen to the mucous membranes. One of your more sensitive areas, Virgo, is the lungs. Lack of potassium sulfate can cause respiratory infections, because cells in the mucous membranes will be deprived of oxygen.

FOODS RICH IN POTASSIUM SULFATE

Almonds	Lean meats
Beans	Nuts
Cheese	Onions
Clams	Peas
Eggs	Rye
Fish	Turnips
Fruit and vegetable juice	Watercress
Grapes	Whole wheat

These foods should be included in your diet, Virgo, to ensure healthy skin and to protect mucous membranes. Every machine needs proper lubrication to function.

You will be happy to note that they are included in your reducing maintenance diets.

Often, you tend to suffer the extreme opposite of colitis: constipation. To relieve this problem, and for optimum health, be sure to include fiber foods in your diet, too. If you are especially sensitive to your need for fiber, you may choose to try a diet aid known as Glucomannan. It is extracted from the Japanese konjac root, a tuber that is very high in fiber. A final monograph on its effectiveness has not yet been established by the FDA, as it has no history of use in the United States before 1958; however, the konjac root has been cultivated and eaten in Asia for over a thousand years.

Glucomannan aids in decreasing cholesterol and triglyceride levels, and in maintaining low-density lipoprotein levels in the body. It also increases the viscosity and moisture content of food as it is digested, so that it forms a smooth, soft mass that moves easily through the intestinal tract. Digestion is slowed, so normal blood sugar levels are maintained after a meal. Two capsules taken three times a day may cut your appetite in half, Virgo!

Virgo Daily Nutritional Supplements

- One general multivitamin with minerals
- Super B-complex multivitamin
- 2,000 mg vitamin C
- Fiber foods

Remember, Virgo . . .

This diet is uniquely prepared to address your sun sign and *should not be interchanged with any other Sun Sign Diet.* It is important that you follow the diet exactly as it appears, for optimum weight loss and assimilation. Before starting your Virgo diet, carefully read "General Diet and Maintenance Guidelines for All Sun Signs," found at the beginning of this book. Remember, drink 8 glasses of water daily.

You will never have to be a member of the yo-yo team again, dear Virgo, because this diet has been prepared to meet your biological, chemical, nutritional, and behavioral needs.

Good luck, and *go for it.*

The Virgo Ten-Day Reducing Diet

The Virgo Ten-Day Reducing Diet has been designed to meet all your nutritional needs and to incorporate foods that will help you deal with stress. It is important that you try not to eat processed or refined foods (white breads, white sugar) and that you eat natural, unadulterated foods as much as possible. Do eat plenty of fiber and try to limit the amount of caffeine in your diet. It also includes foods with high concentrations of vitamin B-1 to protect your digestive system and vitamin B-6 for regulating your protein metabolism as well as phosphorus foods, which aid all the assimilation of B-vitamin foods. Remember, Virgo, you may choose to try the diet aid Glucomannan, described on page 205. It is an excellent source of fiber, should you wish to supplement your already fiber-rich Ten-Day Reducing Diet, and will also reduce large swings in blood glucose after meals.

You may repeat the ten-day diet until your proper weight is maintained. Please note, that you will find a binge day at the end of your reducing diet. This day is reserved for the times when you feel, "I cannot go on any longer." Then just use your binge day and enjoy.

You may use the Substitution Day if you feel the Day One reducing diet is too strenuous.

Eat what is scheduled for the day; if you do not want something leave it out, but do not substitute. Please try to get ample rest. Many times you eat in place of needed sleep. Balance work and recreation. The ten-day diet has been prepared for variety and nutrition. If you choose to make it seven days—you may choose those days that are your favorite. You may always repeat a day you particularly like. However, you may not repeat Day Ten more than three times a month or every ten days.

You may choose your beverages as you like with your meals—no sugar and no milk in coffee. Tea, herbal tea, black coffee, no-sodium diet soda, mineral water, club soda, or seltzer. All your menus have been designed for optimum weight loss and for energy and vitality.

You now have the key to success in your hands.

And last, but not least for your nutritional information at the end of your Virgo reducing diet, you will find a section "Notes to Virgo Ten-Day Reducing Diet." It is here, you will find that all the foods marked with an asterisk (*) in your diet plan appear with detailed explanations as to why they have been included in your regimen, along with vitamin, mineral, and nutritional supplementation.

DAY ONE

BREAKFAST

1 large banana*

4 almonds*

LUNCH

fresh fruit salad*—up to 3 cups of fresh fruit salad with 2 Tbsp. sunflower seeds or 6 almonds

(Be sure to include the sunflower seeds or almonds. They are an excellent source of vitamin B-6, calcium, and fiber. In addition, they have high enzyme quality and this combined with the fresh fruit acts to break down stored fat.)

DINNER

1–2 large baked potatoes* seasoned with ¼ cup plain yogurt mixed with basil, dill, and chives.

2 cups mixed salad consisting of alfalfa sprouts, arugula, and scallions mixed with lemon juice

Remember, drink 8 glasses of water every day.

DAY TWO

BREAKFAST

    1 ripe banana, or apple, or orange*

    6 raw almonds

    tea or herbal tea

LUNCH

    ½ avocado* or tomato* stuffed with 3 oz. tuna

    1 Wasa Crisp Bread or 2 melba toast

    tea, herbal tea, or no-sodium Perrier

DINNER

    6 oz. broiled or baked veal or veal chop*

    ½ lb. freshly steamed asparagus*

    1 cup salad of lettuce, watercress* and parsley

    tea, herbal tea, or no-sodium Perrier

    Remember, drink 8 glasses of water every day.

DAY THREE

BREAKFAST

¼ cup cottage cheese with ½ cup unsweetened applesauce* and 2 tsp. raisins

tea, herbal tea, or decaffeinated coffee

LUNCH

1 cup tomato juice

tuna* in a pita pocket: 3 oz. water-pack tuna mixed with 1 tsp. diet mayonnaise, chopped onion, celery, and radishes

DINNER

Chicken-Tofu Stir-Fry*

Stir-fry 6 oz. tofu and 6 oz. chicken with mushrooms in low-sodium chicken broth.

½ lb. fresh asparagus* seasoned with garlic pepper

SNACK

tea, herbal tea, black coffee, or no-sodium Perrier with a twist of lime

D-Zerta diet gelatin—all you want

Remember, drink 8 glasses of water every day.

DAY FOUR

BREAKFAST

½ cup mandarin orange sections* canned in natural juices mixed with ½ cup yogurt* or cottage cheese

LUNCH

all the freshly steamed asparagus you want (frozen may be substituted if you cannot purchase fresh asparagus) with 2 Tbsp. Parmesan cheese seasoned with 2 tsp. lemon juice and garlic pepper

(Asparagus is an excellent diuretic food. It also contains the enzyme asparagine which helps to break up accumulated fats in the cells.)

DINNER

¼ honeydew melon or ½ grapefruit

*Chicken Paprika**

Bake chicken and season with paprika. Cover with ½ cup yogurt* and bake until done. Cover with chives and oregano.

large salad of lettuce, watercress, parsley, and Chinese cabbage seasoned with 2 Tbsp. Pritikin no-oil salad dressing

beverage of your choice

SNACK

D-Zerta diet gelatin—all you want

Remember, drink 8 glasses of water every day.

DAY FIVE

BREAKFAST
>½ grapefruit or orange
>¾ cup Special K
>
>½ cup skim milk

LUNCH
>2-egg spinach omelette* served with parsley and one sliced tomato
>
>iced tea, herbal tea, or no-sodium club soda

MIDAFTERNOON SNACK
>10 grapes*

DINNER
>4 oz. baked or broiled salmon* without any butter with fresh cabbage* and tomatoes sprinkled with 1 Tbsp. reduced-calorie vinaigrette dressing
>
>1 cup sliced cucumbers
>
>beverage of choice
>
>(Virgo, *do not* substitute a different fish for the salmon. Salmon is rich in vitamin B-6 and phosphorus which you require.)
>
>*Remember, drink 8 glasses of water every day.*

DAY SIX

BREAKFAST

½ cup cottage cheese

½ cup unsweetened applesauce

2 Tbsp. wheat germ

(Delicious mixed together.)

LUNCH

salad of hard-boiled egg, 4 oz. sliced chicken breast or turkey tossed in broccoli, cauliflower, mushrooms, watercress, parsley, and grated carrot; mix with ¼ cup yogurt blended with 2 tsp. lemon juice, paprika, and garlic pepper

DINNER

1 cup macaroni* seasoned with 2 Tbsp. Parmesan cheese

½ can artichoke hearts canned in water, pimientos canned in water, parsley, and green peppers; toss with ¼ cup Aunt Millie's Spaghetti Sauce

SNACK

4 oz. unsweetened grapefruit juice (optional)

Remember, drink 8 glasses of water every day.

DAY SEVEN

BREAKFAST

1 slice raisin toast

1 Tbsp. sesame butter or peanut butter*

LUNCH

3½ oz. canned Chinook salmon* in salad of 1 cup alfalfa sprouts with 4 black olives, sprinkled with lemon juice and garlic pepper

D-Zerta diet gelatin—as much as you want

or

Celery Nut Salad*

5 stalks celery, 1 sweet green pepper, 2 tomatoes, ⅛ cup chopped walnuts. Toss salad on endive or lettuce and garnish with ¼ cup plain yogurt or cottage cheese. Season with Sweet 'n Low and cinnamon.

DINNER

baked or broiled salmon without any butter

large salad of fresh cabbage and tomatoes sprinkled with 1 Tbsp. reduced-calorie vinaigrette dressing

SNACK

herbal tea of your choice

Remember, drink 8 glasses of water every day.

DAY EIGHT

BREAKFAST

1 cup tomato juice

½ toasted bagel with 1 tsp. diet margarine

LUNCH

3½ oz. Chinook salmon*

1 cup fresh strawberries (½ cup unsweetened frozen if fresh not available)

or

Virgo Lentil Soup*

2 qts. water and 3 packages Herb-Ox low-sodium beef stock, 1½ cups lentils, 2 stalks celery, 2 sprigs of parsley, 2 medium onions, 1 small shallot. Bring everything to a boil and then simmer for 1½ hours. Have 1 cup (you may freeze the rest for future days).

DINNER

¼–½ broiled or baked chicken, no skin, baked in tomato juice

1 artichoke (may use ½ can of artichokes in water)

1 cup fresh strawberries*

no-sodium seltzer with a twist of lime

Remember, drink 8 glasses of water every day.

DAY NINE

BREAKFAST

½ grapefruit

cheese omelette made with 1 egg, 2 oz. cottage cheese or skim-milk ricotta cheese* with chopped chive—use nonstick pan

LUNCH

½ cup plain yogurt,* mixed with 5–6 pecans*

½ lb. fresh spinach* with 1 cup freshly diced zucchini—steam spinach and zucchini lightly, top with basil, and pour yogurt on top (Absolutely delicious.)

DINNER

Watercress Soup*

½ bunch watercress, mixed with 2 cups plain yogurt, 1 package of Herb-Ox low-sodium chicken broth. Add pinch of nutmeg. Blend in blender. Serve cold.

and

4 oz. sliced flank steak, veal scallopine, or 6 oz. broiled or baked fish (no butter)*

1 sliced tomato* and green salad

Remember, drink 8 glasses of water every day.

DAY TEN*—VIRGO CRASH DAY "THE FERMENTED WAY DAY"

BREAKFAST

> 1 cup plain yogurt (may use Sweet 'n Low sugar substitute)
>
> 1 medium-sized banana

MIDMORNING SNACK

> ½ cup plain yogurt

LUNCH

> 1 cup plain yogurt
>
> 1 medium-sized banana
>
> (Put in blender with 3 ice cubes and sugar substitute—it becomes a cool frothy drink—or just enjoy in its natural state.)

MIDAFTERNOON SNACK

> ½ cup plain yogurt

DINNER

> 1 medium-sized banana
>
> 1 cup plain yogurt

This is a truly cleansing day. You may have herbal tea, regular tea, or water today, *but no other drinks.* The enzymes in the fermented yogurt restore the natural bacteria of the digestive tract and help metabolize weighty substances in the cells. A one-day "fermented way" will help catalyze stubborn weight plateaus and produce excellent diet results.

Remember, drink 8 glasses of water every day.

Notes to Virgo Ten-Day Reducing Diet

Virgo Diet Notes—Day One

* Almonds are rich in protein, potassium, manganese, and phosphorus.
* Bananas are a rich source of vitamin B-6 that Virgos require constantly. Together they are fibrous and have plenty of easily digested staying power which will keep you from hunger until lunchtime.
* Fresh fruit salad has the highest level of enzyme power which is necessary to break up fat accumulation. In addition, it is the most easily

assimilated and quickly digested lunch giving you energy from its natural fructose. You may have less than three cups. The choice is up to you. However, make sure it is absolutely fresh. You may not have any milk products with lunch. Milk lactose will affect the enzyme production.

* Potatoes are a perfect Virgo food. Their rich source of potassium and all the B vitamins plus their superb fiber count supply you with many of your dieting requirements. Combined with the yogurt (B vitamins) you will feel quite full. Have your phosphorus-rich salad with potatoes for optimum nutrition.

Virgo Diet Notes—Day Two

* Either the tomato or the avocado is a good choice. The tomato is full of vitamin C and the avocado, surprisingly to many Virgos, contains a good portion of fiber. Avocado is rich in vitamin B-1 (thiamin).
* Veal is not only low in calories and cholesterol, compared to other meats, but is easily digested by the Virgo constitution, providing a rich source of phosphorus.
* Asparagus is a favorite food for its diuretic qualities and for its natural enzyme called asparagine. Asparagine helps to break up accumulated fat in the cells and is noted for its vitamin C and folic acid content.
* Watercress is a forgotten wonder food, Virgo. Whenever you see it listed on your daily menu, it is important that you include it in your meal plan. Part of the success to your dieting depends on keeping your body nutritionally at its peak. Watercress is also rich in minerals, especially chlorine, and sulfur. Watercress offers a superb option for calcium.

Virgo Diet Notes—Day Three

* Unsweetened applesauce is easily digested and a rich source of phosphorus.
* Tuna is rich in vitamin B-6.
* If you wish to stir-fry your chicken and tofu in very light Kikkoman soy sauce you may.
* The chicken, tofu, and mushrooms provide plenty of protein but maintain a low calorie count. Chicken is also high in phosphorus and vitamin B-6, both of which are essential Virgo nutrients. The asparagus is included to provide Virgo with thiamin (vitamin B-1) and also acts as an excellent diuretic food.

Virgo Diet Notes—Day Four

* Mandarin sections are very low calorie and combined with yogurt gives your body an extra dose of vitamin B-12. Yogurt is also very soothing to the Virgo nerves, and good for your intestinal tract.

* Yogurt is often called "one of the five wonder foods of the world." The healthful bugs work on the harmful bacteria that are present in your intestinal tract. Yogurt can be of great help to a sensitive stomach, because 90 percent is digestible within one hour.
* Chicken is a Virgo wonderfood, chock full of vitamins B-2, B-3, B-6, B-12, and folic acid.

Day four is very low-calorie and you should already start seeing the pounds fly off!

Virgo Diet Notes—Day Five

* Egg and spinach omelette is light but an excellent source of vitamin E, B-12, folic acid, phosphorus, and chlorine.
* Grapes are rich in silicon and quite calming to Virgo nerves. You may freeze the grapes and pop them into your mouth. It tastes just like grape ice cream. Good afternoon pick-me-up!
* Salmon is an excellent source of low cholesterol, high-level lipoprotein with high levels of vitamins A, B, E, C, calcium, and potassium.
* Cabbage is another good source of phosphorus and is very low-calorie.

Virgo Diet Notes—Day Six

* Macaroni is a good complex carbohydrate. Use only durum wheat or vegetable macaroni because they are lower in calories. This is a delicious, light dinner that you will enjoy.

Virgo Diet Notes—Day Seven

* Peanut butter is rich in the B vitamins. If you have a water retention problem, do buy the low-sodium brand, but remember only 1 tablespoon. (You may lick the spoon.)
* Canned Chinook salmon has little bones in it for the good quality calcium it delivers.
* Celery Nut Salad is a light but extremely nutritious lunch. Walnuts are rich in potassium and fiber.

Virgo Diet Notes—Day Eight

* Salmon is an excellent source of low-cholesterol, high-level protein food that is extremely high in vitamins A, B, and E.
* Lentils are a favorite among all my Virgo clients. It is a wonderful light meal, rich in all the B vitamins. Make lots and freeze it.
* Strawberries are truly blood cleansers, rich in vitamin C.

Virgo Diet Notes—Day Nine

* Cottage cheese or skim-milk ricotta may be changed anytime. I prefer Polly-O ricotta cheese because of its creamy taste.

* Yogurt, pecans, and spinach are powerhouse foods loaded with enzymes and all the B vitamins.

* Watercress is a very important food for you. In its soup form, it is soothing and delicious providing vitamin C, calcium, and other minerals, and is an excellent aid in removing toxins from the body.

* You may choose veal or any fish. The choice is up to you. You may use lemon juice on your veal or fish.

Virgo Diet Notes—Day Ten

* I have included this day at the end of your diet, so that your spirits will really be lifted when you step on the scale tomorrow. Not only will you have lost weight, but you will feel so very good. Your digestion will be in top peak and so will your assimilation.

Now, if you wish to continue on, just turn back to Day One. Your Virgo diet, has been programmed for a lifetime and is most healthy and nutritious. Reach for the stars.

VIRGO TOTAL BINGE DAY

Virgo, there are times when you need to let go. I have given you that option with a binge day.

Before You Binge

1. Drink water.
2. Drink water.
3. Drink water.
4. Rest.
5. Brush your teeth and rinse with your favorite mouthwash.
6. Chew sugarless gum for 20 minutes.

You may find that the desire to binge has passed. However, if you are still suffering from intense food frustration, follow these basic binge rules:

Rule One

Under no circumstances should you ever binge before completing Day Five of your reducing diet. This will ensure a maximum weight loss with a minimum of food frustration.

Rule Two

If, for example, you binge on the sixth day of your diet, resume your diet the following day (Day Seven) with the menu for Day Six. If you binge for just one meal, such as lunch on Day Six, resume your reducing diet with dinner on Day Six of your reducing diet.

Rule Three

Bingeing is for when you get that creepy, anxious feeling, when you feel like pulling out your hair—strand by strand—and you cannot endure dieting for even one more moment. Before you climb the walls, give yourself a binge day. It is hoped that this will not be necessary more than four times a month.

Rule Four

After you have lost your first 10 pounds, you may vary your binge day with the binge day of the sun sign opposite yours, which is Pisces.

Remember, an occasional binge day—when necessary—will still allow you to lose weight (without guilt). Here, Virgo, is your binge day menu.

Binge Day Menu

BREAKFAST

1 croissant with 2 oz. skim-milk ricotta cheese

or

⅓ cup granola cereal with 1 cup skim milk

or

1 corn muffin, 4 oz. orange juice and 4 oz. cottage cheese

or

1 cup fresh strawberries and 1 cup plain yogurt

or

1 bagel with 2 Tbsp. cream cheese and 1 orange

LUNCH

2-egg omelette (mushrooms, asparagus, or spinach filling)

1 hard roll or 3 breadsticks

or

1 slice pizza

½ cup vanilla, chocolate, strawberry ice cream, or any flavor sherbet or Tofutti

or

small Greek salad

1 Frozfruit fruit pop

DINNER

4–6 oz. wine, sherry, or sake (optional)

chef's salad with 2 Tbsp. salad dressing

or

1–2 lb. lobster, steamed or broiled (no butter, no stuffing)

large salad with low-calorie dressing

or

any Japanese entrée, not fried.

1 bowl miso soup

tossed salad with lemon juice

very small dish of sherbet with any dinner

EVENING SNACK

    1 chocolate Alba 77 skim-milk drink mixed with 1 can Yoo-Hoo diet chocolate drink

or

1 90-calorie Jell-O chocolate/vanilla frozen pudding pop

or

1 serving any fresh fruit you want

Maintaining Your Ideal Weight

Virgo Maintenance Foods for Optimum Health

When you have achieved your desired weight goal you should follow a maintenance diet rich in the specific nutrients that you, Virgo, need each day.

All the B vitamins, but especially,

Vitamin B-1 (Thiamin)

Vitamin B-1, or thiamin, is crucial for proper metabolism of carbohydrates. Thiamin combines with pyruvic acid to form an enzyme which breaks down carbohydrates into glucose, which is the body's source of energy. Thiamin has also been linked to the nervous system. You, Virgo, who tend to have problems releasing tension, really need thiamin to avoid further digestive problems caused by stress. The body's supply of thiamin is depleted by carbohydrate metabolism and also by smoking, alcohol consumption and excessive sugar ingestion. Since thiamin is necessary for proper digestion, Virgo, you must be careful to replace the body's supply of it every day in your meal plan.

FOODS RICH IN THIAMIN

Asparagus	Peas
Avocado	Radishes
Beef liver	Rice
Egg yolks	Sweet corn
Grapefruit	Wheat germ
Okra	Whole wheat flour

Vitamin B-6

Vitamin B-6 is especially important in regulating protein metabolism. Vitamin B-6 is also crucial for the body's absorption of vitamin B-12, amino acid metabolism, and proper utilization of fats.

More than sixty enzymes in the body depend on B-6 in order to function. B-6 is also required for proper formation and function of red blood cells, bile salts, and many hormones needed for growth; it is an important aid in maintaining energy production and in resistance to stress.

FOODS RICH IN VITAMIN B-6

Alfalfa sprouts	Lentils
Avocados	Mackerel
Bananas	Peanuts
Beef liver	Prunes
Cabbage	Salmon
Egg yolk	Skim milk
Fish	Sunflower seeds
Green peppers	Tuna
Honey	Turkey
Lamb	Wheat germ

Phosphorus

Phosphorus is present in every cell in the body. It works with calcium and magnesium to promote both growth and maintenance of bones. Foot aches and ankle pains can sometimes plague Virgos, so maintain a proper balance of phosphorus and calcium. Remember, without phosphorus, two of the B vitamins (niacin and riboflavin) cannot be absorbed and utilized. The Virgo digestive system is sensitive enough without the additional havoc of deficiencies.

FOODS RICH IN PHOSPHORUS

Almonds	Liver
Apples	Milk
Avocados	Mushrooms
Beef	Nuts
Beef liver	Parsley
Beets	Pumpkin seeds
Cherries	Rice
Chicken	Salmon
Corn	Scallops
Egg yolk	Spinach
Grapefruit	Tuna
Halibut	Veal
Lima beans	

Fiber Foods

Fiber can be helpful in alleviating digestive problems as well as bowel movement problems. For the Virgo, who has such a delicate digestive system, fiber is a must. Fiber also keeps the stools moist and bulky, thus soothing the system's lining. Fiber is an important aid in your weight loss program; it can actually curb weight gain.

FOODS RICH IN FIBER

Avocados	Green beans
Bananas	Okra
Beets	Peaches
Brussels sprouts	Peas
Cabbage	Tomatoes
Carrots	Whole wheat flour

Virgo Sample Maintenance Menu

When you reach your desired goal, please follow the maintenance eating hints found in "General Diet and Maintenance Guidelines for All Sun Signs" at the beginning of this book for proper calculations of caloric intake.

I'm including a sample maintenance menu based on your sun sign for optimal Virgo maintenance. When you create your own menus, try to choose many of the foods you eat from your Virgo Maintenance Foods lists.

2,000 Calories Per Day

BREAKFAST   CALORIES
  ½ cup prune juice   90
  ⅔ cup granola   252
  1 cup skim milk   86
                                                                  ———
                                                                     428

LUNCH
  1 cup tomato juice   41
  chicken and artichoke in large salad bowl with 1 hard-boiled
  egg, lettuce, watercress, parsley, radishes, mushrooms, and
  cut stringbeans with 3 bread sticks   450
                                                                  ———
                                                                     491

MIDAFTERNOON
  1 Weight Watchers® treat   70

DINNER
  6 oz. baked leg of lamb   415
  1 cup cauliflower with yogurt   40
  small baked sweet potato   50
  salad of fresh spinach and bacon bits with 2 Tbsp. of
  no-oil salad dressing   200
  ½ cup raspberry sherbet   115
                                                                  ———
                                                                     820

SNACK
  1 cup fresh strawberries   40

  TOTAL DAILY CALORIES   1,849

  Remember, drink 8 glasses of water every day.

Restaurant Eating
the Virgo Way

Perhaps you have seen the following dishes on restaurant menus. Maybe you have ordered them, and maybe not. You probably already have a list of your favorite local eateries, if I know you, Virgo. Included here are dishes and restaurants chosen to specifically appeal to the Virgo palate. Note that all of the recommended dishes contain the nutrients especially important for you and which are included in your Virgo Maintenance Foods lists.

In all cases, one appetizer plus one entrée equals approximately 500–600 calories.

American/Seafood Restaurant

APPETIZERS

Clams on the half shell

Gazpacho (all vegetable soup)

ENTRÉE

Chef salad (use dressing sparingly)

Avocado, egg, and shrimp salad

Halibut filet with orange sauce and brown rice

Filet of sole almondine with artichokes

Japanese Restaurant

APPETIZERS

Appetizer of vegetables or fish with vinegar sauce

Chicken boiled and seasoned with seaweed, horseradish, and exotic vegetables

ENTRÉES

Broiled chicken marinated in soy sauce with or without red pepper

Casserole with naturally raised tender chicken and fresh vegetables

Salmon broiled with Japanese sauce

Bean curd with vegetable ankake sauce

French Nouvelle Cuisine

APPETIZERS

Plate of green beans and mushrooms

Steamed baby shrimp with aromatic vegetables

ENTRÉES

Sautéed breast of chicken with mushrooms, shallots, and herbs

Broiled sole with herb sauce

Filet of striped bass with cucumbers

Bay scallops sautéed with watercress

Health Food/Gourmet

APPETIZERS

Fresh bean sprouts and mushroom salad

Fresh fruit cup

ENTRÉES

Zen hash (brown rice and vegetables)

Scallops sautéed in fresh tomato sauce seasoned with herbs and garlic

Spinach and mushroom salad

Stir-fried vegetables with long grain wild rice

Omelette with your choice of filling

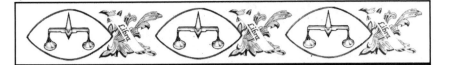

LIBRA

September 24–October 23

The Libra
Personality

"I can't decide what to eat."

Libra, symbolized by the scales, you have been called the peacemaker, the perfect mate, and justice incarnate. One might say you held a rather exalted place in the heavens. Indeed, when you are poised, there is no more gentle, charming, graceful, diplomatic, delightful, and companionable creature in the zodiac. Nor is there a star in the constellations more dazzling than your dimpled smile when you are happy. Born under the charmed evening star, you do seem blessed with more than a fair share of loveliness and symmetry. Even excess pounds tend to be distributed evenly about your well-proportioned body.

But there are two sides to every story, as you should know, Libra, having just about invented the phrase yourself. Let's face it: Back here on earth, you are not always the picture of equanimity. When you are not being "nice" to the *n*th degree, you can be flighty, argumentative, judgmental, and downright moody. You are often indecisive and procrastinating, weighing and analyzing things to the point of tedium. Even your behavior alternates between balancing extremes. You are either a dedicated workaholic or the very personification of sloth. You are either a dispassionate, objective observer, or you are so overshadowed by your emotions you cannot see straight.

You are the one sign that is usually either very thin or pleasingly plump. Your scales dip and rise with some regularity as you vacillate between compulsive dieting and giving in to your love of comfort and fine food and drink. You would never let your weight get really out of hand, however; you're too obsessed with beauty and balance to do that.

That is the wonderful thing about you inconsistent Libras. You never stay high-and-mighty or down-and-out too long. You are ever determined to bring the opposing forces of your personality into equilibrium, and the moments when you succeed actually are quite heavenly.

An eternal balancing act. That is quite a feat of nerves and will, Libra. All that juggling can be the cause of much anxiety. No wonder you sometimes find solace in food. You crave pacifying foods like ice cream, or anything sweet, soft, and creamy, and you are almost universally carbohydrate and dairy eaters. As a means of oral gratification, lots of you chew gum, your fingernails, bite pencils, straws, and Styrofoam cups, lick your lips, and even chain-smoke.

Seated at the dining room table, however, you are far more selective about what goes into your mouth. Generally speaking, you prefer foods that are light and airy, like the element that rules your sign, and prepared delicately and close to its natural state, not smothered in heavy sauces. What is the quickest way to kill a Libra's appetite? Serve you filet of sole, mashed potatoes, and cauliflower. The monochromatic theme is a foolproof turnoff. You have a highly evolved aesthetic sensibility which is reflected in everything you do. You consider yourself an expert in the art of fine dining and know the rules of etiquette as well as Emily Post. You expect your food to be served properly and attractively, too. Chablis wine poured into a paper cup does not even merit drinking; you would rather sip water from a crystal goblet. You always require cleanliness, order, and a touch of elegance in your surroundings but especially when you eat. You have no stomach for garishness, ugliness, or squalor, which in constant or excessive doses can make you refined and sensitive Libras sick, physically and emotionally.

Of course, love is the food of your soul, Venus-ruled Libra. You are the sign of partnerships and relationships, and nothing quite upsets your delicate balance like heartbreak or rocky romance. Many of you believe there can be no true serenity in your life at all until you have found your "other half." One thing is for certain: The state of your love life usually is a pretty good indication of the direction in which the scales are tipping in any given week. Lost love usually results in weight loss, as does budding romance. However, the longer you are without a relationship, or trapped in an incompatible one, the higher the scales climb.

Then again . . . some of you Libras will argue that you are independent souls who get along quite well without a mate, thank you. And on your own, you do make a good show in public of appearing happy, not to mention flirtatious and irresistibly sexy. (Of course, the world rarely sees you out of sorts, because you tend to be reclusive when depressed.) Your need to be with people eventually draws you back into circulation, however, and given the choice, you usually opt to throw yourself head over heels into a relationship, sometimes to the point of subservience. Your desire to be comfortable sometimes expresses itself as a need to be taken care of, even pampered, like royalty, or like a child. You also like to please others and can be overly accommodating or excessively doting. But your nature cannot abide imbalance, and when caught in any one-sided relationship, you often compensate for the difference by overeating.

Love, leisure, luxury: That's all it takes to make for one content and well-adjusted Libra. You don't so much love money for its own sake, or as a symbol of power, but for the comforts, pleasures, and things it can buy. Some of you are social climbers and status seekers, but all of you simply feel at peace when you are surrounded by beautiful things. You invariably prefer quality to quantity and won't tolerate imitations. Your jewelry will be gold and diamonds, or you will have none. You prefer to own just three or four outfits from the best couturier than a closet full of ready-to-wear clothing. When you travel—which you love to do in style—it is to the chic vacation in-spots of the world, or you would just as soon stay home.

Home for you cultivated Libras is usually in or near a city. Although you love the tranquility and natural splendor of the countryside and the soul-soothing effects of the seashore, you experience withdrawal symptoms if deprived of cultural activities for too long. Your genuine fascination with artistic endeavors is one of the few things besides love that distracts you from food. Many of you have season subscriptions to the theater, ballet, symphony, or opera, and memberships to fine arts museums and libraries. Libras are often devotees of the international art scene and enjoy gallery-hopping in search of up-and-coming talent. Some of you are serious collectors, while others just like to see and be seen at trendy openings. You are usually book lovers, and many of you have a wonderful way with words. Even in everyday speech, you tend to use language with great precision, eloquence and, of course, logic. Some of you parlay this gift of gab into profitable careers in law and politics; many pursue vocations in the literary field.

People-watching is another urban pastime Libras love. Nothing pleases you more than a cup of cappuccino, a rich Italian pastry, and a front-row seat at a sidewalk café, where you can relax and enjoy the parade of beautiful people—nothing more than marching in it, that is. Whether it is on the Champs Elysées, Fifth Avenue, or Rodeo Drive, you love to spend long, lingering hours promenading and window-shopping on the world's most famous boulevards. It makes you feel as splendid as the idle rich, even if you cannot afford to buy a thing.

Of course, even on a beer budget, frivolous Libra, you will usually manage to find a way to indulge your champagne tastes—particularly when it comes to real champagne. But watch your alcohol intake: Too much alcohol consumption also leads to cravings for starches and sweets—your diet downfall. You have an insatiable sweet tooth, Libra, and hardly think twice about spending four or five dollars to buy a quarter-pound sample of imported bonbons. Why not? Some of those gourmet chocolates are as precious as rare works of art. Of course, you take equal delight in common penny candy. An old-fashioned sweet shop replete with soda fountain and glass jars of licorice sticks, gumdrops, and assorted caramels and nougats, offers its own kind of perfection to Libra. A few bucks here buys a choice of everything, so you irresolute creatures never even have to make up your minds.

If you make yourself ill finishing off that bag of goodies you just bought, Libra, you will compensate for the sugar overdose by consuming a "healthy" portion of protein. That is Libra's version of a "balanced" diet. Or, if you eat too much at your next meal, you will skip the following one or two. That is what you Libras call "balancing out the caloric intake." True, you will balance out, but in the long haul it is not at all a healthy way to eat. "Paying the piper" for your little indiscretions is a vicious cycle which creates a very erratic metabolism.

Logical Libra, you understand quite well that you are going to have to stabilize your eating patterns if you want to control your weight, but you often seem to lack the motivation to stick to a diet. You tend to like the easy life too much to put in the effort it takes to curtail your gastronomical desires. I know you can't be hurried during these indolent periods, my friend. You naturally require quiescent times to recharge your batteries. But afterward I know your energy will be flying higher than ever, and that is when I expect you to get down to business with your very own Libra Sun Sign Diet. It is designed to meet your unique nutritional needs and eating style. The colorful and tasty array of foods incorporated into your daily meal plans will be a feast for your refined eye and palate, and the diet is balanced to provide you with enough energy to keep those Libra batteries charged for the duration.

Find yourself a Libra friend to be your diet partner. You sociable creatures do function so much better in pairs. Now just think, Libra, there are no more decisions to be made. You have discovered the diet that will turn the scales once and for all.

Sexual Appetite

Libra, your natural elegance, warmth, and magnetism, spiced with just the right touch of flirtatiousness, combine to make you one deliciously tempting dish. Male or female, you are absolutely one of the most romantic, sentimental, idealistic, and charismatic lovers to grace this earth. Your own expectations of romance are so extraordinary, however, that Cupid himself seems at a loss to fulfill them. You Libras seek nothing less than beatitude in love, and you truly believe everyone should live happily ever after. The fact that few of us do does not daunt your faith. And you have put on many a pound awaiting Prince or Princess Charming to save you from grim solitude and carry you forth into matrimonial bliss.

Marriage is the ultimate goal of any Libra love relationship. You are known as the relationship-oriented member of the zodiac family, and a Libra out of love is a sorry sight indeed. You pine. You brood. Without a mate for counterbalance, your sense of self-worth plummets, and your insecurity sometimes causes you to enter into dependent relationships. On the other hand, your deep fear of doing just that—and losing yourself in a union—sometimes causes you to assume a staunch posture of independence, despite your obvious desire to be coupled.

It is curious how you otherwise dispassionately logical Libras, when it comes to love, become quite muddled in your thinking. It must be that bewitching influence of Venus. Your great romantic illusion is that fulfillment is something that comes from outside yourself—usually in the form of a mate, or, failing that, in the form of liquor and food—when the truth is that fulfillment is something generated from within. Your mistaken belief that the purpose of your life is to find your "other half" undermines your ability to find the harmonious union you seek.

What is the best diet advice I can give you love-struck Libras? First of all, make up your mind that the absence or presence of a lover will not hold sway over your scales. Learn to enjoy your time alone; that should not be difficult for someone whose talents and interests are as diverse as yours. And don't rely on others to give you the things that make you happy. Learn to buy yourself lilacs and roses. Above all, develop self-reliance and an unshakable sense of self-identity, which are no less important to the success of a marriage than they are to single life.

Strive for equality in your relationships. Both you and your partner must pull your own weight. You are cooperative by nature, fair Libra, and you are not interested in playing male/female roles strictly according to traditional lines anyway. You like to please and you also love to be pleased, but overdoing either in a relationship is sure to result in discord and discontent.

Libra's fundamental need for a strong, solid relationship and the stability and support of a partner is often forfeited to your desire for rapturous romance. Swept away by passion, you often leap into intimate relationships without first looking to see if your prospective lover is really up to the role. When the big letdown comes, you often cushion the fall with triple-scoop hot fudge sundaes and frozen cream pies. It would be a lot less bruising to the ego and less fattening besides for you to decide what your sexual needs are beforehand, then express your needs to each candidate so you are able to choose a partner who's willing and able to meet them should you become involved. That's right, Libra, I said *decide* and *choose.* Your uncanny ability to put yourself in someone else's shoes is not, alas, a talent the rest of the world shares. Don't expect your mate to know what you want if you don't name it. And don't expect your lover to be sexually aggressive only when *you* are in the mood. If that's what you need to make you happy, you have some serious rethinking to do.

You are appealing from the inside out, enchanting Libra, and generally speaking you are quite comfortable with your powerful sensuality. Even so, sex is usually a secondary consideration in your relationships, at least in their formative stages. You are certainly no prude—you are simply more interested in ideal love than in sex per se. You are most happy in a relationship when your lover is a friend and partner. You are great communicators and willing to put in the effort needed to make a romance work. Your belief in peace at any price, however, has been the justification both for your self-denigrating appeasement tactics and your stormy declarations of war. In the name of improving your relationships, some of you Libras engage in an unpleasant habit of comparing your mate to others, and your constant fault-finding compounded by your absolutely relentless pursuit of making your point, frequently lead to dissension—and then to the refrigerator door.

In the long run, your need for harmony does not allow you to remain in an antagonistic relationship. The moment you do not feel you are loved with the same capacity you love, you will retreat into your shell in frustration and despair. Likewise, if you suspect someone is vying for your place beside your lover, you will usually withdraw from the heat rather than compete for what is yours. You lack the killer instinct and are often all too willing to accept the consolation prize—usually an excuse to indulge your cravings for rich and creamy foods. On the other hand, you Libras can be fickle, too, and if you feel the sparks between you and your mate have died down and there are no more fireworks in sight, you won't sit around striking matches in hopes of reigniting the fire. You do know how to take control of your life when you want to.

Eating/Entertaining at Home

Libras love to be surrounded by people of all types and ages, and what better way to do it than entertaining at home. The combination of friends, fine food, and familiar surroundings strikes a perfect balance, and in that moment of symmetry you Libras absolutely radiate.

Charming, gracious, and convivial, you were born to play the role of host or hostess, and you take center stage every chance you get to throw a party. In preparation for a fete, you spare no detail, even if you have to stretch your budget. You spend hours going from one gourmet shop to the next, hunting down just the right mix of taste sensations to make up your lavish spread. Luxury items like pâtés, imported cheeses, exotic fresh fruits, and chocolate-covered strawberries are staples at Libra parties, as are the basic French breads and pasta salads.

If you are in a particularly energetic phase of your rest-and-activity cycle, you might whip up some of these delights from scratch. Probably, your orderly kitchen is well equipped to handle the task. If you are in a more quiescent period, however, you will tend to buy everything ready-made. And if you are feeling exceptionally lazy and frivolous, you may even have the affair catered—maids, waiters, bartenders—the works. That way you are completely free to mingle with your guests, and it's a welcome reprieve from the austerities of your diet, since talking to friends is the one activity that occupies your mouth with almost equal satisfaction as eating.

Quality and elegance are your main concerns. You love food prepared in small and bite-size servings. Canapés, hors d'oeuvres, and assorted quiches and pastries in miniature are perennial Libra favorites. Everything that is capable of sporting a toothpick will have one, to add color and balance to the presentation. You love to serve crudities on a silver tray—and don't anyone dare call those lovely rows of neatly sliced carrots, celery, broccoli, and peppers "vegetables." That would be as gauche as a Libra serving pretzels, chips, and onion dip.

Of course, your home is a study in beauty and refinement. Soft colors, soft music, and the soft touch of fresh flowers are standard features of your household. Your aesthetic flair is evident everywhere, from the tasteful furnishings to the elegant table settings: sterling silver, bone china, and crystal arranged in perfect symmetry on the finest linen tablecloth. The presentation of the meal itself is an art in which Libra excels. Every item of food has its own special serving implement, container, or dish. Bread will be wrapped in linen napkins in a silver basket, wine will be poured from a decanter, and dessert eaten from a parfait glass.

As for the food, generally speaking you Libras are not large meat eaters. You usually serve fare suited to the diet-conscious (light and low in cholesterol) because that is the way you delicate air signs prefer to eat. Dinner might start out with something like melon soup or fresh compote, and end with a large bowl of fresh grapes, and whatever comes between will be well balanced and delicious.

Now. That just about covers the basic Libra meal. So let's clear off the table and make some room for dessert. Lots of it. Dessert is your forte, and when you are not compulsively dieting, whipped cream is your middle name. Strawberry shortcake. Charlotte Russe. Cream pies. You can never serve just one dessert, partly because they all look so wonderful and you cannot decide which to choose, and partly because it's such a *sweet* way to end an evening and say goodbye to your friends. Besides, you love the applause, and this way are always prepared with an encore.

Let's face facts, my logical friend. All the chatting and low-calorie entrées in the world cannot compensate for the damage that can be wrought by one of Libra's famed last courses. After all, when your company goes home, who is left with half-eaten pies and unfinished cartons of ice cream? *You,* Libra. And that is usually when you begin your dangerous eat-and-starve method of balancing your caloric intake. Well, there is a healthier way to divide up the calories. Just split up the leftovers and send them home with your friends.

Food Shopping

Libra goes out to buy groceries for the pure pleasure of a shopping spree. The way some people haunt the back streets of Paris or the exotic markets of Fez, you get lost exploring supermarket aisles and excavating specialty shop shelves in search of your favorite foods. You shop with great care and deliberation. First stop is a tea and spice store for fresh dried herbs and ground coffee, then on to the old-fashioned bake shop for some Danish rings, rich butter cookies, and oven-fresh raisin pumpernickel rolls. The bioche and *pain au chocolat* you get direct from a local patisserie, and the prosciutto and fresh pasta you pick up at the quaint deli you discovered. The grains and all-natural salad dressing you buy at the health food store, and you will wait to pick up your produce until the farmer's market is open on Saturday. In the meantime, you can go to the supermarket to get your household items and a few packaged goods.

As long as the place is impeccably clean, you love to patronize small shops where you are on a first-name basis with the owners, who can recommend selections to you from their list of daily specials. Without their aid, you Libras face the imposing task of making up your own minds. You judge the quality, compare the prices, weigh the nutritional values, and consider several alternatives. You decide on a package of spinach ravioli, put it in your basket, walk a few steps, turn around and switch it for the cheese ravioli, put it in your basket, and repeat the process once again. You are not being wishy-washy. This is an important decision, and you thought you had weighed all the pros and cons when you realized at the checkout counter that, all things considered, ravioli wouldn't do at all. So you turned it in for a box of spaghetti. It's a process that would boggle the mind and try the patience of any other sign in the zodiac, but you Libras consider shopping *fun.*

Just as time is no object, neither is price. When you food-shop you are concerned with freshness, wholesomeness, and, above all, quality, and will pay the prices gourmet shops demand if they have the product you want. You may comparison-shop but you will never sacrifice appearance or taste for a few pennies' savings.

You also eschew additives and preservatives in food and absolutely abhor anything ersatz or artificial. You won't buy honey when you want sugar, carob when you want chocolate, or diet-brand colas when you want the real thing. Freeze-dried coffee is a kind of poison to you, whereas the coffee bean and the coffee mill are items you won't live without. And nothing would compel you to purchase "no-name" generic foods. To you it's inconceivable that a box so bland, so unattractive, could possibly contain something fit for human consumption.

You are much too discerning to be influenced in your food shopping by crass advertisements, although you will try a new product recommended by a friend or packaged so beautifully it simply catches your eye. You don't bother with specials or coupons, and though you often keep shopping lists, you rarely use them. You do have a frivolous habit of stocking up on foodstuffs because you buy many items just to avoid the decision of whether or not you actually need them. In this respect, one could say you are an impulse buyer—although you probably take a good two minutes to come to that "rash" conclusion.

Oddly enough, you are so entertained by shopping for food, you rarely think to sample your purchases. So what keeps you so enthralled? Imagining all the delicious ways you will consume the delights once you get them home. And that's the kind of food for thought that threatens to be fattening.

Social Dining

Social dining? Libra? Who else? What else? If you could spend your entire day hopping from café to café or pub to pub, socializing with a different friend in each place, you would do it. Sure, we all love the conviviality of café life, lingering over an espresso or a white wine spritzer as we chat. But you, Libra, are the unfortunate one who is slave to a merciless sweet tooth.

And no matter how interesting the latest installment in your buddy's soap-operatic love life, you just cannot keep your mind off those fruity, chocolaty, creamy desserts you saw in the display case when you came in. Between your vivid imagination and your lapses of self-discipline, it is inevitable that one of those irresistible little delicacies will end up on your plate.

Your fondness for this type of gastronomic experience is so extreme, you often choose to eat your meal in one restaurant and then go out to some little patisserie just to get your favorite dessert. That sort of extravagance characterizes Libra's style of dining out. You are utterly seduced by luxury and would love to bring back the days when one would not be seen tripping the light fantastic wearing anything less glamorous than black tie and tails or a sequined, beaded, bejeweled evening gown. For you, every dinner out on the town is an opportunity to dress up. And naturally you prefer to dine in elegant surroundings. White linen napkins and tablecloths, fresh flowers, candlelight, and the heavenly sound of two crystal champagne glasses clinking in a toast provide the perfect ambiance for you enchanting Libras to cast your spell. Actually, the very ultimate in luxurious dining for Libra isn't dinner at a four-star restaurant at all—it's champagne breakfast at a fine hotel with old-style European service. Now, that's the pampered life the way it should be.

Of course, you would not eat in any restaurant more than once that did not prepare and serve its food beautifully. Not that taste isn't important to you, too. But food that doesn't look appetizing will never find its way to Libra's lips. You agree with the Japanese who say, "we eat with our eyes," and you have a special fondness and respect for Japanese cooking, artistry, and display. And the soft-spoken, genteel, and dignified manner of Japanese service is balm to your delicate nerves. For their lightness and elegance of presentation, fine northern Italian food and French *nouvelle cuisine* also appeal to your palate. Salmon trout served with cucumber mousse and fruit salad with a sprig of fresh mint just sparkle on your plate, and a delicately prepared angel hair pasta primavera is like a little bit of heaven to the taste.

If the food or service is poor, you diplomatic creatures probably won't complain, or be the slightest bit rude, unless you are in one of your contrary moods; but you won't return to the restaurant either. On the other hand, you will be absolutely hooked on any eating establishment that ends a meal with such flourishes as serving complimentary mints and petit fours or presenting finger bowls to each diner plus a rose to each lady at the table.

With so much rich living, how can you possibly keep your weight in control, Libra? Well, you are fortunate to have a system of checks and balances built into your eating personality. First of all, you love to look great, and you devour compliments on your appearance with a gusto you never show when eating food. One comment on how lovely you look and you won't need another bite of food all evening. In addition, you well-mannered Libras consider it an impropriety to stuff yourself in public. Finally, you do have an instinctual sense of when it's time to return to simpler gastronomic living. After a few too many nights of dining debauchery, you will search out the cleanest-looking health food restaurant in town for a well-rounded, nutritious, and low-calorie meal. Your biggest social dining problem actually doesn't strike until you get home to your own kitchen and decide you owe yourself a reward for your "good behavior" at the restaurant. The truth is, many of your overweight Libras are actually closet eaters.

Special-Occasion Dining

There are two varieties of special occasions that tend to sabotage Libra's diet. The most frequent kind is the once-a-year extravaganza, which never comes only once a year in Libra's life because your many friends send you a constant stream of invitations to weddings, holidays, anniversary parties, and honorary dinners. And social Libra cannot resist the chance for a change of tempo, to get out of your house and dress up to the hilt.

The problem at these gala events is that after you have had the first two or three glasses of champagne, you begin to lose count of everything else you put in your mouth. Back comes your friendly waiter, this time insisting you should try an hors d'oeuvre. And you are quite polite and accept each invitation to taste just one, eating each with the speed and daintiness that etiquette demands. But don't kid yourself, Libra. Lots of dainty bites add up to one big "pigout." The average cocktail party lasts about two hours, and one hors d'oeuvre now and then adds up. When you have reached ten you have reached *ten.* Not a few. *Count* them.

If your diet somehow survives the potential ravages of the cocktail party, you will probably meet your Waterloo when you get to the buffet table. You just cannot choose between all those tempting selections and are bound to sample everything before the occasion is over. These events do seem calculated to be your ruination, Libra. But don't feel that your only alternative is to give up the party life you love so much. You can stick with your diet and still be the belle or beau of the ball if you simply take some preventive measures at the outset. First, tell your host or hostess about your predicament so everyone understands they are not to *"insist* you *must try one."* With that charming Libra voice that could melt an iceberg, I am not concerned anyone will feel insulted by your request. So much for pushy waiters. Now, Libra, you need some cocktail-hour diet savvy. Begin by drinking a full glass of water before you have your first drink and an additional glass of water before each subsequent drink. Alcohol dehydrates you, and the water acts to speed up the assimilation of alcohol by your body, thereby preventing the compulsive eating that usually accompanies liquor consumption. As for the hors d'oeuvres, choose them for their nutritional value—high protein, low sugar, and low carbohydrate. Deviled eggs, steak tidbits, and a taste of cheese should suffice.

Planned vacations and cruises are a less frequent type of special occasion but an equally dangerous one to the success of your diet. Your love of style and comfort usually demands that you travel first class, and who can resist the royal way in which hotels, airlines and cruise ships pamper their highest-paying customers? Certainly not you, Libra. If you plan to fly while dieting, you are better off going economy class. It is not just cheaper; it will get you where you want to go for far less cost in calories, too. Prior to flight time, try to avoid those airline club lounges as well. Mingling with the beautiful people, you find it too easy to indulge in a few high-calorie drinks. If you can't resist the party, then muster up your self-control, flash the bartender one of your dazzling smiles, and order soda water with a twist of lime. No one else has to know what you are—or aren't—drinking.

At all costs, Libra, you should avoid taking any cruises during your diet period, unless your ship is a floating spa. Since the days of the *Titanic,* ocean liners have been designed with one purpose in mind: to pamper, entertain, and feed the passengers as if there were no tomorrow. And as long as you are on the ship, there is no place to go to escape this orgy. To paraphrase an old expression, "a diet, like the good captain, always goes down with the ship." Do your body-beautiful a favor, Libra, and keep it safe on dry land.

Your Health

Libra, you must have harmony and balance in your life or you are likely to get sick. And you really do need your "beauty sleep." While you have a good constitution, rest and relaxation are of utmost importance to maintain health, especially when you are overworked. You are particularly vulnerable to colds and flu when your resistance is down, and you are also somewhat susceptible to migraine headaches and eye problems. Nervous tension is just about impossible for you Librans to endure. It often manifests itself in high blood pressure, acne, allergies, and susceptibility to viral and bacterial infections.

Libra rules the kidneys, pelvis, renal arteries, outer and upper parts of the liver, adrenal glands and adrenal cortex, lower lumbar region of the back and equilibrium of the lower back. Few of you get through life without suffering the pain of an occasional bladder or urinary infection. Many of you also suffer the pain of lower back incapacity and/or herniated or slipped discs. Very often your only means of relief is a chiropractor or physical therapist. However, you usually respond well to treatment due to your diligence.

Beware of excessive alcohol consumption, Libra, because it can cause severe damage to your most vulnerable areas—the kidney, bladder, and adrenal cortex. When the adrenal cortex is affected, hormone production is diminished and addiction results. Keep a check on your consumption of junk foods and sugar products, too, because you also have a proclivity towards diabetes and hypoglycemia, which should not be ignored.

Every sun sign has a tendency to have some diseases more than others. Possible problems for Libra include:

Abscesses	Pelvis
Adrenal glands (cortex)	Pyelitis
Atrophy	Renal arteries
Bladder infections	Skin diseases
Diabetes	Slipped, herniated discs
Disease of the liver	Spleen (as it is related to the
Disorders of the bladder	blood and lymphatic systems)
Eczema	Syphilis
Gravel in the bladder	Toxins in the blood
Injuries to the lower back	Uremia
Kidney	

Sodium phosphate is the Libra cell salt. Cell salts are naturally occurring minerals that are normal constituents of the body cells. They are found in trace amounts in foods, and plants, animals, and human beings require these compounds for proper nutrition. And, like vitamins, cell salts get used up. Sodium phosphate is the acid neutralizer cell salt, and homeopathic doctors often use this cell salt in the treatment of gout, ulcers, kidney stones, and acid stomach. Its primary function is preventing excess alkalinity or acidity in the bloodstream, thereby stabilizing the acid-base balance. This acid-base balance must be maintained for the body cells to function properly. With a deficiency of sodium phosphate, salt is formed by uric acid and is deposited around joints and tissues, causing swelling, stiffness, and other rheumatic symptoms. Sodium phosphate is also necessary for the function of the kidneys and the elimination of wastes, including the excretion of urine, which Libra rules. A diet that includes foods rich in sodium phosphate should help to avoid problems in these sensitive areas while aiding in the overall maintenance of good health.

It is also important that your lifetime maintenance eating program be rich in magnesium foods. Research has shown that magnesium has been helpful in the prevention of kidney stones. (See list included in your maintenance food chapter.)

Some additional health tips for my Libra friends:

Drink lots of unsweetened cranberry juice. It is low in calories and has excellent therapeutic benefits for bladder infections (a constant Libra complaint).

If you have been eating poorly and feel that your body needs an internal cleansing day, I would suggest a one-day watermelon fast. The fibers of the melon act like little brushes to clean the intestines. It is a natural cleanser that also helps to clean the liver and detoxify the body. And the natural fruit sugar in the watermelon will give you the necessary energy, so you do not feel at all tired. On this day, you may only have water, tea, herbal tea, or black coffee as a beverage.

Libra Daily Nutritional Supplements

- One general multivitamin with minerals
- 400 mg vitamin E
- 1,500 mg vitamin C
- 600–800 mg Os-Cal (calcium carbonate from oyster shells)

Libra, you can often get away with extra poundage because your weight is proportionately distributed. You always look in balance and your face is pretty, or handsome, despite some plumpness. However, a healthy Libra is a *balanced* Libra, and any diet—be it high-carbohydrate/low-calorie or low-carbohydrate/high-calorie—is not going to set well with you unless it is balanced, too.

Remember, Libra . . .

This diet is especially prepared to address your sun sign and *should not be interchanged with any other Sun Sign Diet.* It is important that you follow it exactly as it appears, for optimum weight loss and assimilation of nutrients. If you do, you will find you no longer have high and low dips in your energy cycle, your cravings for starches and sugars will be reduced, and you will diet effortlessly. Before starting your Libra diet, carefully read "General Diet and Maintenance Guidelines for All Sun Signs," found at the beginning of this book. Remember, drink 8 glasses of water daily. *Go for it.*

The Seven-Day
Libra Reducing Diet

I know what you are thinking, Libra . . . if the diet does not include some sweets and dairy products, and an occasional "hot and spicy" dish, you will never be able to stick to it. On the other hand, you really have to lose weight; you hate not looking great, and so, after all, with much deliberation, decide you will have a go at it.

You made the right decision, Libra. Your Seven-Day Libra Reducing Diet has been designed to meet all your nutritional requirements and to incorporate high-energy foods that are easily digested, quickly assimilated and as natural as possible. It provides the balance of proteins, carbohydrates, and fats your body demands on a daily basis. I know that many of you Libras eat very light breakfasts, or no breakfast at all. However, it is important that you do not choose to skip meals. If this is your tendency, *make sure you at least include the fruit portion of your breakfast or lunch.* Your body requires the natural fructose, and you will find that by eating it you actually lose more weight.

You should feel extremely "in tune" and "in balance" with your body for the duration of your diet. The inclusion of foods rich in vitamins C and E, magnesium, niacin, and iron will prevent the usual nervousness and lethargy Libra feels when dieting, and the specific foods and food combinations will counteract your sugar and carbohydrate cravings and produce maximum weight loss with a minimum amount of discomfort.

Watercress is a food you will encounter frequently on your Seven-Day Reducing Diet. For thousands of years, astrologers have associated watercress with your sun sign, primarily because it is a very powerful liver cleanser as well as an energizer. Unfortunately, most Libras "never touch the stuff" and are missing an important nutrient for your constitution. After you eat approximately one-half bunch of this green leafy vegetable, you will feel an instantaneous lift, dear Libra. But go slowly. If you feel a headache coming on, it is a good sign that your body is ridding itself of accumulated toxins, which indicates your need for watercress even more. However, moderation is the key, and you should not eat any more than is already indicated in your diet plan.

The Libra Sun Sign Diet also incorporates apricots into many meals because they have the highest iron content of any fruit. The almonds and tofu are high-quality, easily digestible sources of protein, and the grapes, which are rich in silicon, create a calming, balancing influence while satisfying your sweet tooth.

Please note the asterisked (*) foods which are on your daily diet plan. I have noted the vitamin and mineral content of these foods and the major reason for their inclusion in your program. Refer to the section "Notes to Libra Seven-Day Reducing Diet."

To further speed up your weight loss and suppress your appetite, you may choose to try a diet aid known in the United States as Glucomannan. It is extracted from the Japanese konjac root, a tuber that is very high in fiber. A final monograph on its effectiveness has not yet been established by the FDA, as it has no history of use in the United States before 1958; however, the konjac root has been cultivated and eaten in Asia for over a thousand years.

Glucomannan contributes to a decrease in cholesterol and triglyceride levels, and aids in maintaining low-density lipoprotein levels. It acts as a dietary fiber to increase viscosity and moisture content of food as it is digested, so that it forms a smooth, soft mass that moves easily through the intestinal tract. Digestion is slowed, so normal blood sugar levels are maintained after a meal. Two capsules taken three times a day may cut your appetite in half!

Eat what is scheduled for each day. (If you do not want something, leave it out, but do not substitute.) You may repeat this diet as often as necessary to achieve your desired weight loss. And to make sure there are no excuses whatsoever, I have included a binge day.

Your binge day is only to be used when you feel you will otherwise "blow your diet." It is designed so you can feel you have indulged without any impinging sense of guilt. Just make sure that you do not use it more than four times a month. (See binge day section.)

Stop procrastinating, Libra. This diet works. Now put it into action.

DAY ONE

BREAKFAST
>3 kiwi fruit*
>
>1 Tbsp. peanut butter*

LUNCH
>*All Fresh Fruit*
>an assorted fresh fruit plate (up to 3 cups of any fruit you wish)*
>
>black coffee,* tea, or water
>
>*Absolutely nothing else.*

DINNER
>8 oz. bowl of brown long-grain rice*
>>*or*
>
>1 baked potato* served with 2 tsp. diet margarine and herbs
>
>6–10 broccoli spears with lemon juice or 2 tsp. Parmesan cheese
>
>1 sliced tomato seasoned with basil
>
>iced tea, herbal tea, or no-sodium Perrier

EVENING SNACK
>3 fresh apricots (if unobtainable, substitute dried, unsulphured apricots)*
>
>tea or herbal tea
>
>*Remember, drink 8 glasses of water every day.*

DAY TWO

BREAKFAST

Cantaloupe Calcium Shake

½ cantaloupe mixed with 1 packet vanilla Alba 77 skim-milk drink and 3 ice cubes. Beat in blender.

LUNCH

1 toasted pumpernickel bagel with 1 oz. smoked salmon and 1 Tbsp. cream cheese, topped with 10 pistachio nuts*

sliced whole tomato

iced tea

or

Libra Strawberry Tofu

Make one package of strawberry D-Zerta diet gelatin according to package directions. When firm, place in blender with 8 oz. tofu.* Put in refrigerator for 2 hours. Top with 1–2 Tbsp. Cool Whip dessert topping. Serve with 1 whole sliced orange. Fantastic—and so filled with protein, it's too good to be true. (May be substituted for any lunch.)

MIDAFTERNOON SNACK

herbal or plain tea

DINNER

4 oz. dry red wine (optional)

4–6 oz. veal piccatta, veal chop, or veal scallopine, sautéed in white wine or lemon juice

large tossed salad or arugula, watercress*, lettuce, and spinach, seasoned with 2 Tbsp. lemon juice and kelp, or Pritikin no-oil salad dressing.

20 green grapes* frozen in freezer
(Put in the freezer the day before. When the natural fructose of grapes is frozen, it becomes extremely sweet and tastes like ice cream. Devour slowly.)

Remember, drink 8 glasses of water every day.

DAY THREE

BREAKFAST

¼ cup skim-milk ricotta cheese or cottage cheese

4–5 dried apricots mixed and put on a slice of rye toast

LUNCH

3½ oz. canned or fresh Chinook salmon*

salad of spinach, watercress, parsley, lettuce, and 2 Tbsp. Pritikin no-oil salad dressing

MIDAFTERNOON SNACK

1 Frozfruit fruit pop (any flavor except coconut or banana)

DINNER

Chinese-style Easy Tofu à la Libra

8 oz. cake of tofu

8 oz. can of bamboo shoots

1 cup fresh mushrooms

½ cup small snow peas

Stir-fry the above in Kikkoman reduced-sodium soy sauce. Add garlic and ginger,* kelp, and parsley.

salad of watercress, fresh spinach, and string beans, seasoned with Pritikin no-oil salad dressing

or

1 cup Libra Watercress Soup*

2-egg asparagus* omelet made with 1 tsp. butter or margarine, topped with 1 oz. Swiss cheese

strawberry D-Zerta diet gelatin

1 cup fresh strawberries

tea

Remember, drink 8 glasses of water every day.

DAY FOUR

BREAKFAST

> 1 oz. (¼ cup) Grape Nuts cereal
>
> ⅔ cup skim milk
>
> ½ cup fresh strawberries

LUNCH

> ### Libra Power Fruit Salad
>
> ½ papaya,* ½ mango, 3 apricots, 4–6 almonds,* topped with ¼ cup plain yogurt, farmer cheese, or skim-milk ricotta cheese.
>
> 2 breadsticks

or

> ### Minted Cantaloupe Soup*
>
> 2 cups cantaloupe
>
> 1½ cups chopped mint
>
> 3 Tbsp. plain yogurt
>
> ¼ cup dry white wine
>
> Blend, chill, and serve with salad or arugula and parsley.
>
> 2 breadsticks

DINNER

> ¼–½ broiled, baked, or barbecued chicken*
>
> 1 cup cauliflower* topped with 2 Tbsp. grated Parmesan cheese
>
> large salad of watercress, mushrooms, and sliced tomato, topped with basil, served with 2 Tbsp. Pritikin no-oil salad dressing
>
> 1 35-calorie Jell-O frozen pudding pop
>
> tea
>
> *Remember, drink 8 glasses of water every day.*

DAY FIVE

BREAKFAST

hard-boiled egg or 6 almonds

½ papaya

tea

LUNCH

Turkey Apple Cheese Salad*

3 oz. turkey breast served with alfalfa sprouts, chopped apple, 3–4 walnuts.

1 oz. Edam or Gouda cheese

1 can Yoo-Hoo diet chocolate drink

DINNER

Chinese wonton soup

6 oz. stir-fried chicken and broccoli with ginger

½ cup steamed rice

1 fortune cookie

Chinese tea

or

Pasta Treat

8 oz. pasta (use vegetable or durum wheat pasta),* sprinkled with 2 Tbsp. grated Romano or Parmesan cheese, topped with 2 Tbsp. skim-milk ricotta cheese.

1 cup steamed broccoli* with lemon juice and pepper

salad of watercress and tomato, with 2 Tbsp. Pritikin no-oil salad dressing

Remember, drink 8 glasses of water every day.

DAY SIX

BREAKFAST
>   1 toasted English muffin
>
>   2 oz. cottage cheese

LUNCH
>   same as Day One (fresh fruit plate)

DINNER
>   4 oz. white wine (optional)
>
>   4–5 oz. chicken livers* sautéed in white wine with herbs and 1 small onion
>
>   ½ cup steamed carrots
>
>   1 cup fresh strawberries with 1 Tbsp. Cool Whip dessert topping
>
> or
>
>   1–2 lb. broiled or steamed lobster*
>
>   1 serving broccoli
>
>   1 small mixed salad with vinegar and 1 tsp. oil
>
>   1 cup fresh strawberries with 1 Tbsp. Cool Whip dessert topping
>
>   *Remember, drink 8 glasses of water every day.*

DAY SEVEN

BREAKFAST

2 oranges, *or* 1 cup blueberries,* *or* ½ cantaloupe, *or* ½ fresh pineapple,* *or* 1 large banana

tea, black coffee, or water

Nothing but water until lunch.

LUNCH

large tomato stuffed with lump crabmeat, *or* solid tuna, *or* sliced chicken *or* 2 hard-boiled eggs

MIDAFTERNOON SNACK

herbal tea with honey

DINNER

4–6 oz. flounder or filet of sole* (broiled with lemon juice, no butter)

1 cup fresh or frozen asparagus

1 cup sliced cucumber, parsley, and watercress, with

1 Tbsp. yogurt sprinkled with basil for salad dressing

EVENING SNACK

as much D-Zerta diet gelatin as you like, any flavor

Remember, drink 8 glasses of water every day.

Notes to Libra Seven-Day Reducing Diet

Libra Diet Notes—Day One

This is a very low-calorie alkaline food day, including high-enzyme fruits and vegetables with all your necessary food requirements.

* Kiwi fruit and peanut butter is an excellent blend of carbohydrate, protein, and fat, and a delicate balance between alkalinity and acidity. Kiwis are rich in vitamin C.

* Fruit salad enzyme action serves to speed up the metabolism and makes for easy absorption of nutrients. Make sure you do not have any milk in your coffee, because it will slow down the entire process.

* Brown long grain rice is an excellent source of B vitamins and iodine. Rice also contains easily assimilated protein.

* Potatoes have one of the highest nutrient content of all vegetables. They are rich in vitamins A and B, and protein. Potatoes also contain alkaline salts, which aid in neutralizing acid waste and help cleanse the body by eliminating toxins, such as uric acid.

* Apricots are the best source of iron in the fruit kingdom. And Libras need iron.

Libra Diet Notes—Day Two

* Pistachio nuts are an excellent source of vitamin E and a Libra's favorite.

* Tofu is an excellent alkaline vegetable protein that is easily digested and easily absorbed into the bloodstream for quick energy without lethargy—a nearly perfect food for Libras. Combined with no-calorie Jell-O, it satisfies the need for something sweet but nutritiously low-calorie. You may substitute this for any lunch in your diet program.

* Red wine, believe it or not, does supply iron. Good for Libra women three or four days before menstruation.

* Veal is low-calorie, rich in phosphorus, and easily digested.

* Watercress is the natural food astrologically delegated to Libra. It is nature's diuretic, and rich in minerals, chlorine, sulfur, and calcium. Half a bunch of watercress gives you the same amount of calcium as a glass of milk.

* Grapes are an alkaline fruit. When frozen, the grapes' natural sugars are brought to the surface, and they taste like ice cream. A great way to fool your Libra taste buds.

Libra Diet Notes—Day Three

* Salmon is an excellent low-cholesterol and high-level protein food that is extremely high in vitamins A, B, and E.

* Ginger is a natural penicillin, which fights poisoning and bacterial infections.

* Libra Watercress Soup—a powerful internal cleanser that acts particularly on the liver. It is easily assimilated and delicious.

Libra Watercress Soup

½ bunch watercress
1 cup plain yogurt
1 envelope low-sodium onion bouillon
Put everything in the blender and purée. Makes 1 cup.

* Asparagus is an excellent diuretic food that contains the enzyme asparagine and helps to break up accumulated fat in the cells.

Libra Diet Notes—Day Four

* In Libra Power Fruit Salad, papaya contains the digestive juice papain, which has a soothing effect on the intestinal tract and is rich in vitamins A, B, and C. Almonds are rich in iron, potassium, and manganese.
* Minted Cantaloupe Soup is rich in vitamin C—and is fun.
* Chicken is chock full of almost every vitamin in your Libra Maintenance Diet and an excellent source of protein.
* Cauliflower is a nonstarch vegetable that is highly alkaline, containing vitamins A, B-1, and C.

Libra Diet Notes—Day Five

* Turkey, apple, cheese, walnuts, and alfalfa sprouts are rich sources of proteins, carbohydrates, and fats.
* Pasta is a tasty and available carbohydrate to satisfy those starch cravings. Use only vegetable or durum wheat pasta.
* Broccoli is also rich in calcium and a must when milk or milk products are not included in your menu.

Libra Diet Notes—Day Six

* Chicken livers are one of the best sources of vitamin B-12. They are also rich in pantothenic acid, and vitamins B, B-6, C, D, and lecithin.
* Lobster—simply a love of sensual Libras.

Libra Diet Notes—Day Seven

* Blueberries are rich in vitamin C and folic acid. Libra, you must replenish folic acid if you have been drinking liquor and sweet liqueurs.
* Pineapple is rich in bromelin, which helps break down protein and has excellent diuretic properties.
* Flounder or filet of sole is a low-calorie, low-cholesterol, rich source of B vitamins . . . excellent for your nerves, Libra. It is the perfect light meal before you repeat Day One of your reducing diet.

Step on the scale tomorrow. You will be very proud of yourself.

LIBRA TOTAL BINGE DAY

Even with best of intentions, Libra, there are times when you feel you must tip the scales and deviate from your diet, lest you lose your mind. For this reason, I have included a binge day. Use in moderation and read the following guidelines:

Before You Binge

1. Drink water.
2. Drink water.
3. Drink water.
4. Rest.
5. Brush your teeth and rinse with your favorite mouthwash.
6. Chew sugarless gum for 20 minutes.

You may find that the desire to binge has passed. However, if you are still suffering from intense food frustration, follow these basic binge rules:

Rule One

Under no circumstances should you ever binge before completing Day Five of your reducing diet. This will ensure a maximum weight loss with a minimum of food frustration.

Rule Two

If, for example, you binge on the sixth day of your diet, resume your diet the following day (Day Seven) with the menus for Day Six. If you binge for just one meal, such as lunch on Day Six, resume your reducing diet with dinner of Day Six of your reducing diet.

Rule Three

Bingeing is for when you get that creepy, anxious sensation, when you feel like pulling out your hair—strand by strand—and you cannot endure dieting for even one more moment. Before you do something you'll regret, give yourself a binge day. It's hoped that this will not be necessary more than four times a month.

Rule Four

After you have lost your first 10 pounds, you may vary your binge day with the binge day of the sun sign opposite yours, which is Aries.

Remember, an occasional binge day—when necessary—will allow you to indulge without guilt and still lose weight. Here, Libra, is your binge day menu.

Binge Day Menu

BREAKFAST
> 3 kiwis with 1 Tbsp. peanut butter
>
> 1 whole mango and 1 slice rye toast with butter
>
> *or*
>
> ½ cup granola cereal, 1 tsp. raisins, ¾ cup skim milk
>
> coffee with milk

MIDMORNING SNACK (optional)
> 20 Paul's Peanuts (no oil, no salt)

LUNCH
> 1 slice regular mushroom pizza
>
> ⅔ cup Tofutti frozen dessert or ½ cup ice cream
>
> *or*
>
> 4 oz. sangria (optional)
>
> 1 Mexican taco
>
> ½ cup Spanish rice
>
> *or*
>
> 4 oz. dry red wine (optional)
>
> 1 cup pasta mixed with broccoli and pimientos, seasoned with garlic, herbs, and 2 Tbsp. any reduced-calorie salad dressing

MIDAFTERNOON SNACK
> 1 natural Frozfruit fruit pop

DINNER
> 4 oz. dry red or white wine (optional)
>
> chef's salad with 2 Tbsp. blue cheese dressing
>
> 1 dinner roll with 1 tsp. butter
>
> *or*
>
> 4 oz. dry red wine (optional)
>
> 6–8 oz. broiled or baked bay scallops, shrimp, crabmeat, or crab claws (no butter, use lemon juice)
>
> 1 baked potato with 1 Tbsp. sour cream and chives
>
> small mixed salad with reduced-calorie salad dressing
>
> 10–15 natural or frozen grapes

Maintaining Your Ideal Weight

Libra Maintenance Foods for Optimum Health

When you have achieved your desired weight goal you should follow a maintenance diet rich in the specific nutrients that you, Libra, need each and every day.

Vitamin A

Vitamin A is necessary for healthy skin, eyes, and hair (Libras are very coiffure-conscious). It protects the tissue and linings of the digestive tract, kidneys, and bladder. Vitamin A also prompts the secretion of gastric juices necessary for protein digestion. Vitamin A in large doses can be toxic and should not be taken arbitrarily in vitamin form. It is far healthier to eat vitamin A-rich foods as listed below.

FOODS RICH IN VITAMIN A

Apricots	Honeydew melon
Bananas	Mangoes
Beets	Oranges
Broccoli	Parsley
Broiled liver	Peaches
Cantaloupe	Red chili peppers
Carrots	Salmon
Chicken liver	Squash
Egg yolk	Yams

Niacin (Vitamin B-3)

Niacin is essential to the metabolism of fats, proteins, and carbohydrates. Niacin in the body can be depleted by excessive sugar and carbohydrate intake, typical to Libra. In addition, niacin helps reduce cholesterol levels in the blood as well as promote weight reduction because of its ability to elevate and stabilize blood sugar levels. Libras, who are prone to hypoglycemia, should eat a niacin-rich diet for this reason, too. It has been proven effective in alcoholism treatment, and recent studies show it has some results in the treatment of acne, too.

FOODS RICH IN NIACIN

Alfalfa

Apricots

Avocados

Beef

Brown rice

Chicken (white meat)

Corn

Dried dates

Green peas

Halibut

Lentils

Liver

Mushrooms

Peanuts

Peas

Potatoes

Rice

Salmon

Tuna

Vitamin C

Vitamin C plays an important role in bolstering the body's ability to resist infection. It aids in the formation of collagen, a substance that constitutes about 35 to 40 percent of the body's protein and fortifies cells, keeping them in their natural formations and enabling them to resist any invading bacteria. Additionally, vitamin C is essential to the production of bacteria-fighting white blood cells and thus reduces the risk of enlarged tonsils and swollen glands in Libras, who are predisposed to these infections. By the same token, vitamin C minimizes Libra's risk of bladder and urinary tract infections by maintaining a healthy acid-alkaline balance in the urine.

FOODS RICH IN VITAMIN C

Alfalfa

Almonds

Apples

Apricots

Asparagus

Bananas

Beets

Blueberries

Broccoli
Brussels sprouts
Cantaloupe
Celery
Chicken
Cranberries
Currants
Grapefruit
Green peppers
Lemons
Oranges

Orange juice
Paprika
Parsley
Peaches
Pineapple
Skim milk
Strawberries
Tangerines
Tomatoes
Watercress

Vitamin E

Vitamin E is known as the anti-aging vitamin because it improves and maintains the health of cells in the body, especially those of the skin. Libra is susceptible to skin diseases, particularly eczema and acne. Vitamin E prevents radiation in the atmosphere from doing damage to cells, which would otherwise cause premature aging and aggravate skin disorders. Vitamin E is also an important detoxifying agent for the symptomatology of varicose veins. A deficiency in vitamin E could damage the kidneys, a sensitive area for Libra.

FOODS RICH IN VITAMIN E

Apples
Asparagus
Avocados
Apricots
Broccoli
Cabbage
Cheese
Chicken
Dried beans
Eggs
Egg yolk
Green beans

Mushrooms
Onions
Parsley
Peanut butter
Red wines
Salmon
Sardines
Shrimp
Spinach
Sunflower seeds
Sweet potatoes

Magnesium

Magnesium is one of the minerals essential to the body. It is necessary to maintain a proper balance of calcium and phosphorus. In addition, it has been found to be the single most effective ingredient in promoting good bone structure. A deficiency causes a disturbance of the calcification of the bone and can often lead to weakened or disintegrated disks in the lower back. Magnesium is important to a healthy nervous system as well. It not only helps to carry messages from the brain to the muscles, but is a natural tranquilizer—good for soothing and calming you anxious Libras.

Recent research shows that a deficiency of magnesium can cause kidney stones. (Remember, Libra, your sign rules the kidneys, and this could prove to be a sensitive area for you.) An adequate daily supply of foods rich in magnesium is often enough to prevent kidney stone formation.

FOODS RICH IN MAGNESIUM

Cabbage	Peaches
Carob	Pears
Cauliflower	Plums
Cherries	Radishes
Corn	Sesame seeds
Cucumbers	Spinach
Figs	Watercress

Sample Maintenance Menu

When you reach your desired goal, please follow the maintenance eating hints found in "General Diet and Maintenance Guidelines for All Sun Signs" at the beginning of this book for proper calculations of caloric intake.

I'm including a sample maintenance menu based on your sun sign for optimal Libra maintenance. When you create your own diet for yourself, try to choose many of the foods you eat from your Libra Maintenance Foods lists.

2,000 Calories Per Day

BREAKFAST	CALORIES
1 mango, *or* 1 cup strawberries	135–145
2 oz. Special K cereal	111
1 Tbsp. raisins	90
½ cup skim milk	43
coffee	0
	379–389

MIDMORNING SNACK
 1 oz. sesame seeds   167

LUNCH
  4 oz. white wine (optional)   83
  2-egg broccoli omelette with 1 tsp. margarine 300
  1 dinner roll with 1 tsp. butter   113
  garden salad with 2 tsp. low-calorie dressing 100

              596

MIDAFTERNOON SNACK
 1 cup grapes   114

DINNER
  baked halibut with lemon   214
  ½ cup steamed spinach   45
  1 baked potato with 2 Tbsp. sour cream and chives 191
  1 baked apple sweetened with sugar substitute 120

              570

  TOTAL DAILY CALORIES   1,992

  Remember, drink 8 glasses of water every day.

Restaurant Eating
The Libra Way

Perhaps you have seen the following dishes on restaurant menus. Both the dishes and the types of restaurants chosen will appeal to your Libra palate and satisfy your nutritional needs. Note that all of the recommended dishes contain the nutrients specified in your Libra Maintenance Foods lists.

In all menus, one appetizer plus one entrée equals approximately 600–700 calories.

Japanese Restaurant

APPETIZERS

Sliced mackerel in a bed of lettuce and scallions

Smoked salmon and raw beef with hot mustard, arranged like a flower

ENTRÉES

Fresh salmon grilled in teriyaki sauce

Sashimi—assorted filets of finely sliced raw fish, served with a dash of seasoning and soy sauce

Sliced prime rib with vegetables, seasoned with sesame sauce

Casserole of naturally raised tender chicken and fresh vegetables

Continental American

APPETIZERS
> Crudities
>
> Sliced tomatoes with mozzarella

ENTRÉES
> Crabmeat and asparagus tips salad
>
> Grilled baby chicken diablo
>
> Prime Western loin of lamb filet
>
> Smoked chicken and shrimp salad

French Nouvelle Cuisine

APPETIZERS
> Snails prepared in white wine, shallots, and garlic
>
> Seafood *pâté* served with fresh vegetables

ENTRÉES
> Escallop of salmon, lightly grilled
>
> Sautéed breast of chicken with mushrooms
>
> Veal chop in tarragon sauce
>
> Steamed bass with champagne

Seafood Restaurant

APPETIZERS
> Marinated bay scallops
>
> Fresh garden salad

ENTRÉES
> Fresh lump crabmeat sautéed with julienne ham
>
> Steamed California salmon or trout
>
> Fresh shrimp with crabmeat and avocado
>
> Grilled Dover sole with lime and chives

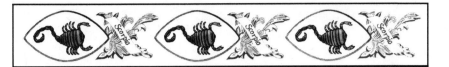

SCORPIO

October 24–November 22

The Scorpio
Personality

"I want, what I want, when I want it."

kay, Scorpio. Now that you want to lose the weight you have gained, you will surely be compulsive about it, as you are about everything. All or nothing, black or white, everything in the extreme—there is no room for gray areas in your life. You are always on the move and, compatible with your "all or nothing" nature, you never just do something halfway. Because of your extreme compulsiveness, when you decide to diet, you will diet.

Let's use that intensity so basic to your nature and concentrate on the good feelings you will have when you are in control of your weight. You, Scorpio, are very resourceful, motivated, powerful, and have the ability to release energy through psychic powers. A Scorpio needs proof of validity when doing something new, whether it be a diet or anything else in your life, so you will probe into all facets of how and why something works. You are relentless in your pursuits. You are especially aggressive when it comes to doing research and will look long and hard for the perfect diet. You are a "show me, prove it to me" person. Well, Scorpio, intuitively you will know this is the diet for you.

Your interest in psychology has taught you that a diet will not work for you in the long run if it does not address your unique life-style and behavior. You are not only forward thinking, avant-garde, and ahead of your time, you are smooth, different, unique, and often misunderstood. You are also sexy, sensuous, amorous, and passionate. And your passion is not only for sex, but often for knowledge. You read *Prevention* magazine, and *The*

Herbalist Almanac, subscribe to do-it-yourself books, and take self-improvement courses. You have read *Psycho-Cybernetics, The Power of Positive Thinking,* and *The Cosmic Laws of Energy.* Your search for knowledge in this area is unparalleled.

By this time, Scorpio, you have tried so many forms of therapy in the dieting process that you could write your own book. I suspect that you have been to a diet doctor, because pills offer a painless, magical way of losing weight fast and you want results yesterday. You may have tried hypnosis—although it really was a last resort and did not make you comfortable because you could not stand being under someone else's control. You have probably frequented a fasting resort, one or two spas, and all the Jack La Lanne's in your neighborhood.

Scorpios often spend their lives in the yo-yo syndrome of dieting—bingeing, then starving—going from one extreme to another. For this reason, you are often comfortable fasting or staying on mono-diets (which are quite repetitive and boring and encourage you to eat 14 grapefruit a day for 14 days). Part of the masochistic side of you tends to come to the surface in the dieting process, because you are so very hard on yourself.

If someone tells you something is impossible to do, your energies will quickly be ignited, ready to take on the challenge. Need I tell you, Scorpio, you must learn to practice moderation in all things; emotional extremism is as detrimental to your good health as is physical intemperance. Because Scorpios are famous for being compulsive and obsessive, when you feel your shape is not up to par or that you are losing the battle of the bulge, you will tighten your reins and, until the situation is under control, your diet will become a number one priority.

Scorpio is a complex sign, and Scorpios are often hard to understand. Just accept what you are. You can be provocative, but will be sure to be subtle about it. Sometimes you are a great pretender—calm, cool, detached on the outside, even when you are in turmoil on the inside. Scorpios cloak themselves in mystery and tend to keep lots of secrets. You are easily upset by the smallest slight and often think no one understands your feelings. And you will go to extremes to prove a point, no matter how long it takes or how much effort is required. Have you ever noticed, when you mention that you are a Scorpio some people's eyebrows raise up a bit? Perhaps they have heard that yours is a powerful sun sign, that you are extremely honest, that you tell it like it is. Obviously because of your upfront, honest approach to life, your friends are either friends for an entire lifetime, or they exit in the first half-hour after making your acquaintance. However, if someone is lucky enough to have you for a friend, they know that you will always be there for them. Your claim to fame is that when the chips are down and everyone else falls apart and leaves the scene, you can be counted on.

Scorpios are very serious about life. Friendship to you is very serious business. Often Scorpios were loners as children, and while you still seek your solitude, you take comfort in having a good friend. But as every Scorpio knows, it is only necessary to have one good friend; quality is far more important than quantity. When you receive support, or a kindness from another human being, you will return it tenfold.

You always operate in high gear—you walk quickly, think quickly, speak quickly, act quickly, and, of course, eat quickly. You feel compelled to burn the candle at both ends. There is no other way you can exist. You have a desire to do everything too fast, often exhausting yourself. But don't worry, Scorpio. Once you are exhausted enough, you will take time to relax.

Regardless of gender, you tend to overdo it when it comes to food, wine, and sex. You like food that comes in easy-to-open packages because it's quicker to get to. You love to wear comfortable clothing and shoes that you can kick off. For easy access—and speed—you'd love to have Velcro fasteners on all your clothing. And, because you are so intense and energetic, you'll wear out your partner before you even begin to tire. Oh yes, Scorpio, you are the passionate sign of the zodiac.

Sexual Appetite

Scorpios require a lot of sex. It is as important to you as food. In fact, to a Scorpio, sex is like food. If sexually deprived or frustrated, you will not feel satisfied and will raid the icebox to satisfy that empty feeling. If rejected in the lovemaking process, a Scorpio will eat anything in sight. Some Scorpios have been known to eat frozen pizza while it's still frozen. "Love me, love my moods, and love my changes of moods. But don't reject me."

Scorpio is a water sign, and water is the element that does not respond to words as well as to actions. You, Scorpio, want to devour your mate, physically and mentally. You may feel so passionate about love that you will not feel satisfied unless your lovemaking registers a 9.0 on the Richter scale. If you do not "feel" that this has happened, all the verbal communication in the world will seem to be a denial of your self-expression. Here, "feeling" is believing.

Scorpio, you sometimes feel you don't really deserve love and may say, "Love me because I'm bad; don't love me because I am nice." You like to maintain an air of mystery in your sexual life. You want depth in a sexual union. To keep your sexual appetite whetted, sex has to be a nurturing process that allows you to examine what is at the root of your emotions.

To fulfill your sexual appetite your mate would have to be a psychic. "You didn't read my mind" is usually one of Scorpio's unspoken sexual complaints. Communication here is essential. Your mate cannot read your mind, but he or she can respond to straight talk. This lack of communication contributes to timing problems, often experienced between you Scorpios and your mates. Matching your sexual rhythm to your partner's is quite important, so tell your partner what's happening, and what's not. By doing so, you'll increase the odds that your tension-building releases will coincide and neither of you will feel the frustration of being out of sync.

You love to conquer and to be conquered. You sometimes even consider sex a game—a game of intrigue, mystery, calisthenics, and creativity. But you have a strong sense of fidelity. Your weight will fluctuate according to your fluctuating love life. You are usually in control of your weight when you are in love and will tend to put on extra weight when looking for love or if your fall out of love. Any slight to the heart can send your weight soaring.

And, Scorpio, I have to tell you that your most orgasmic zone is your *G* spot. It is located between the *E* zone on the left and the *O* zone on the right. When you discover it, you will note it looks like this . . . *EGO.*

You have read Masters & Johnson, *The Joy of Sex,* and *More Joy of Sex,* but your own approach to sexual communication is much more basic. You subtle and sexy creatures give your messages with a look or a gesture or even a thought. You don't *talk* about sex. You just do it.

You want quality sex as much as you want quality carpeting. You may have dabbled in kinky sex or group sex, but only out of sheer curiosity— not out of any real sexual desire. Such experiences could never provide the deep and intense sexual union you need. You must never forget that you Scorpios are ruled by Pluto, the planet of birth and regeneration. You long to go to the absolute heights of love, and if it is not worth the conquest, you are just as capable of destroying what you have created. You often act in haste, then repent at leisure.

More than any other sun sign, you, Scorpio, truly feel that sex is dessert. That's precisely why you have enrolled in courses like "massage for couples," or "shiatsu," in an attempt to please and titillate the body even more. The Scorpio sexual appetite is extreme. There are days you are insatiable, and, if not fed, you will probably console yourself with chocolate-covered ice cream bonbons—and feel mighty guilty afterward. And then there are the days *and even weeks,* when you are totally preoccupied with a project, and sex is the furthest thing from your mind. It is very similar to your eating —binge today, starve tomorrow. Many of you have declared celibacy during a time in your life when you were preparing for some incredible feat. And many of you have explored the spiritual teachings of the great masters of zen and yoga who believe that only when your sexual desires are tucked neatly away in your top drawer can you possibly reach a higher plateau of serenity, known as "nirvana."

You see the pattern, my Scorpio friend? It's that all or nothing approach surfacing once again. Now that you have a better understanding of how you subconsciously allow your love life to wreak havoc on your eating behavior, find ways to alter your destructive habits. Remember the slogan, "Reach for your mate, instead of your plate." And if there is no mate about, don't fret: You are most ingenious and creative when it comes to solving this type of problem.

To experience more satisfaction, try giving more of yourself to the world. The more you give, the more you will get in return. Involve yourself in more meditative and spiritual pursuits. Learn to focus your strong passions on another, more universal type of love, and just keep concentrating on the heavenly body waiting to be yours.

Eating/Entertaining at Home

Although you Scorpios live fast-paced lives, you are real homebodies. You consider your home a sacred place, a total refuge from the outside world. Your home may display a skillful blend of traditional elegance and sleek contemporary comfort, accented with unusual and beautiful artifacts and accessories. It will bear the distinctive hallmark of your personality. It is at home that this often tense sun sign prefers to relax and recuperate from living life in the fast lane.

You love to entertain because you do it so well. Scorpio men and women are good cooks. You can whip up a storm of culinary delights that would impress the editors of *Gourmet* magazine. Or you can throw together some instant creation and serve it to company that evening. You don't find it necessary to test a recipe beforehand because you have an innate sense of how a dish will taste. And you know that it will be good. You regard cooking as what it really is . . . chemistry. You are fascinated by the way a specific process leads to a specific result, and probably have the very latest kitchen equipment on hand to guarantee that your experiments turn out just right.

You want your dinner to be memorable, unusual, dramatic, and mysterious. Your hors d'oeuvres—perhaps champagne, cheddar cheese, and caviar on pumpernickel rounds, or spinach crepes wrapped in phyllo pastry—always provide a tempting sampler of your superb culinary skills, and your guests are never disappointed by the parade of unique dishes that follow. You are tickled pink when guests say, "Oh my, what is this? I have never had it before and it is so delicious." Of course, you have chosen to serve a cold fruit soup in the winter, prepared from mangos, papayas, and coconuts (out of season), and topped with lichee nuts.

True to your excessive Scorpio nature, you will serve your intimate dinner party for four with enough food to feed the foreign legion, but you will serve it with flair, elegance, and charm enough for a royal family. The background music will be soft and romantic and the lighting soft but spectacular. And the dinner table will be set with linens in festive and coordinated colors, and inside each tall wine glass, a matching napkin drooping the corners to look like flower petals. Your centerpiece is often a beautiful array of fresh-cut flowers combined with slender candles, or an abundant display of fresh fruit surrounded by clusters of grapes and nuts and, oh yes, nutcrackers.

The conversation at your dinner table, Scorpio, might sound strange to other people. Whether you are debunking the old method of eyelid surgery or promoting the new therapy for disintegrated spinal disks, you will not miss the opportunity to educate your guests with your latest medical and health information or other esoterica.

Often your family and friends don't get to try out new dishes unless company's coming, because that is when you Scorpios shine. And your family understands your need for such motivation. You are extremely protective of your loved ones and work hard to create nutritionally balanced, nourishing meals. And, Scorpio, you are very possessive and strive to preserve all of your possessions—jams, jellies, your lover, your spouse, your leather boots . . . and your body. As in everything you do, you try to be perfect in your role as nurturer. You were the first to put sunflower seeds on the table and to introduce health foods into your daily diet.

You do enjoy making others happy, and you also enjoy challenging yourself to the impossible. So, I know you won't have any problem keeping to your own diet while you watch your friends and family enjoy the delicious spread you have served them.

Food Shopping

Scorpio, you are not particularly fond of shopping for food. Indeed, you consider it a colossal waste of time. Not surprisingly, when you are compelled to go, you will charge down the supermarket lanes as though activated by jet-propulsion rockets. To cut your shopping time in half, you often buy double loads of groceries on one trip. Your trick is to push one shopping cart filled to overflowing ahead of you while pulling a rapidly filling cart behind.

Two places you *will* spend time at are the produce section—feeling the fruits and vegetables for ripeness before you select them—and the dairy section, opening container tops to check for freshness. You also read labels. In fact, you Scorpios were reading them before FDA was a household word. Long before it was fashionable, you reduced your meat consumption, feeling that somehow beef was a second-rate protein. It was after coming to this realization that much of your eating habits changed, as well as your grocery purchases.

Disciples of Adelle Davis and Carlton Fredericks, you Scorpios often prefer to shop in health food stores where you know the food is not adulterated. For years, you have suspected white sugar, flour, and salt to be man's biggest diet enemy. And most of you are convinced that the ingestion, or lack of ingestion, of certain food groups will ultimately be linked to the rising incidence of cancer.

In true Scorpio fashion, you simply cannot stand to be "taken" or cheated. However, if a product passes your rigorous inspection, you will be the first in your neighborhood to try a new item that appears on the supermarket shelves and to share it with your friends. You have taken the time to learn the tricks of the supermarket trade, and you know how to ferret out the real bargains from the hypes as well as how to tell the genuinely healthy and natural foods from ersatz nutriments. As a result, you probably have the best self-taught nutritional background of any sun sign, although you are often known to be a better teacher than follower of your own advice.

Scorpio, it is especially important that you not go food shopping when you are hungry. You have little patience for shopping to begin with, and after racing up and down those aisles, you are likely to arrive at the checkout counter with two missing slices of cheese and a half-consumed can of soda. Of course, nothing is more exasperating to you than waiting on a long checkout line, and you may reach even deeper into your shopping cart in search of a pacifying goody, unless you find some interesting magazine to distract you. And you often bag your own groceries out of sheer frustration of watching an inefficient cashier. At times like those, you will vow to restrain your buying impulses next time around and use the express lane. Or, better still, you promise yourself to call and have your food delivered.

Social Dining

Scorpios love to eat in restaurants that are off the beaten path—undiscovered, secluded, intimate, but gastronomically superb. An old Victorian mansion with elaborate dining rooms, windows almost as high as the ceilings, and wood burning in the fireplace, or an inn tucked away on a mountaintop or on an island cove simply catches your fancy—and the ever-present aroma of warm bread emanating from the kitchen promises that a truly fresh apple pie will be served for dessert.

When you tire of the intimacy of the quiet little table in the corner, however, you will seek out the establishment sporting neon lights, blaring music, and massive, oversize seats for a noisy Yuppie cast of thousands. There is no middle of the road for you Scorpios.

You love Italian cuisine. Prosciutto and melon, smoked salmon, and air-dried beef, or *bresaola,* as any paisano calls it, are among your favorite dishes. When you can't get away to sit at a café on the shores of the Mediterranean, you might console yourself by finding a restaurant that serves *bronzino,* as Mediterranean rockfish is known. You water signs are always nuts for seafood and love any restaurant that overlooks a harbor or shore. There you can be sure the fish your waiter just served you was alive and swimming just a few hours before. You love to pick your own live lobster fresh from a tank, and if you have ordered a large one, you do not expect to be served a crustacean that looks little enough to have been caught with a mosquito net.

You do look for quality in the food you consume, especially in its manner of presentation and service, but Wedgwood china and crystal candlesticks do not compensate for two endive leaves and a meager portion of meat on your plate. The light look and taste of French *nouvelle cuisine* is not a Scorpio's cup of tea.

But rich foods or *spicy* foods . . . well, that is another story. Is there a Szechuan chef who exists who can make a "hot and spicy" soup pungent enough for Scorpio's tastes? Your eyes may tear and your cheeks may flush, but you will love every drop and morsel of such an exotic—but traditional —specialty. Any fire you can quench with a glass of cool wine, whatever vintage, pleases you the most, and the rules of red or white be damned. You would never be subject to an old winemaker's principles, although you do know your wines and you are well aware of all the fine amenities—like a taste of sorbet between courses—that make a memorable meal.

Even for the finest restaurant, you will rarely wait in line, and you hate to be kept waiting when you are hungry. When you sit down to your table, you expect to be served *pronto.* At the very least, you Scorpios reason, you should be brought your bread and water, which is even served to prison inmates.

Should you dine at some world-renowned restaurant during one of your dedicated dieting periods, I know you controlled Scorpios will maintain an almost martyr-like stoicism that far exceeds the capabilities of most of us mortals. If a dessert cart loaded with strawberry soufflé, chocolate rum mousse, and zabaglione passed by you, you would ignore it. If a slice of the greatest New York cheesecake were planted right in front of your eyes, you would just stare right back. Not a morsel would touch your lips. When you make up your mind to diet, you are absolutely unshakable.

True to your secretive natures, you Scorpios often don't let anyone know you are even dieting at all. You will devise little ways of cutting calories, such as ordering a club soda with a lime twist, trimming all the fat from your meat, or eating just a bite of your baked potato. But about other things you are anything but discreet. In fact, you are more than outspoken. If you have enjoyed a satisfying repast, you will be effusive in your praise. You will genuinely compliment all who served you, extending your praises to the chef and maître d' and anyone who will listen.

And if the food or service is poor? Everyone is sure to hear about that, too, especially your unfortunate waiter. If he is unwitting enough to hand you your check with a smile and cheerfully ask how you enjoyed your meal, he will receive a stinging reply that is anything but cryptic. "As a matter of fact," you will say in your most precise and controlled voice, "it was the lousiest meal I have ever had, and you have some nerve passing this off as food."

Well, I just hope you didn't blow your diet *eating* it, my friend.

Special-Occasion Dining

You just remembered that you have a special function to attend tomorrow, and you are already wondering—and worrying—how you will stay on your diet. You don't really want to sabbotage your successful dieting pattern at this time, but you don't really want to let anyone know that you are on a diet either. Well, you could just use that special occasion as a wonderful excuse to go on a binge. Here you are again, Scorpio, caught up in extremes.

Whatever you decide, you don't need to jeopardize the ultimate weight goal you have set for yourself. There are ways you can stick to your diet at special occasions without anyone being the wiser. Bring your own food with you in a serving bowl, but bring enough for the entire clan. Then, everyone will think how very considerate you were to cook up this special dish for all to eat. Or, if you want to partake of the gourmet goodies served by your host, you can just ask for small servings, nibble at the food, and perhaps even hide a piece of the Chicken Cordon Bleu in your paper napkin. And, voila, everyone, including your host, will think you have cleaned your plate.

Even if you choose to use this occasion as an excuse to go off your diet, you do not have to blow it for good. On the day of the occasion eat only that one special meal and on the following day eat only two meals (breakfast and lunch, breakfast and dinner, or lunch and dinner). While you will probably neutralize your overindulgence by fasting in this way, I do not recommend this method of balancing out your caloric intake as a way of life. But once in a while to save you Scorpios from your all-or-nothing diet extremes, it is worth a try. Just get right back on your Scorpio Sun Sign Diet, pronto, and you will still be in control of your weight loss.

Of course, nothing lures Scorpio off a routine like traveling, which you consider to be one of your most special delights. When you are exploring the globe, you are learning, searching, discovering—so how can you resist sampling the foods? I know one Scorpio, for example, who won't be a day in Paris without a cup of *café au lait* at a bistro, although home in New York she wouldn't think of drinking the stuff. When you see a Spanish street vendor or hear the dulcet tones of an Italian waiter singing, *"Mangia, mangia,"* you Scorpios are likely to throw caution to the wind, no matter how straight a diet course you have been sailing the year through.

At the other extreme, you are the classic "food stowaway," and many a customs clerk has stopped you for transporting cans of sardines and tuna, jars of mushrooms, and boxes of raisins over a foreign border. Wherever you go, you don't leave home without your most prized possessions— artificial sweeteners, immersion heaters, bouillon cubes, tea bags, and instant coffee. Some of you clever Scorpios view your travel time away from the confines of your kitchen refrigerator as a welcome escape from gluttonous habits. Upon your return from a two-week escapade abroad, you are likely to present yourself Monday morning at the office a surprising fifteen pounds lighter.

Oh Scorpio, will the rest of the world ever understand you?

Your Health

The Scorpio health picture is typical of your nature. You can destroy your body with excesses, melancholy, or hard work. You look upon eating as an oral sexual experience, protective and indulgent . . . and, as you know, often self-destructive. Need I tell you, Scorpio, you must learn to practice moderation in all things. Unchecked emotions can manifest in a pattern I call "angry eating." If you fall into this category you are the November sign that stands in front of the refrigerator, opens the door, and plugs anything into your mouth in an attempt to calm yourself down. Temporarily, your anger is relieved from the tranquilizing effect of the food. Your brain is now busy telling your body to digest the calories rather than allowing it to deal with your heated feelings of anger.

Scorpio, my friend, you have two important lessons to learn if you wish to control your weight forever. The first one is to truly work on your low frustration tolerance, so that anger does not enter your life as quickly. The second is to learn that your life can work smoothly even if you give control over to someone else. Here is your opportunity. If you do not try to control what you eat . . . you will be a winner at the game of losing. Just this once, allow me to be in control.

It is very important, due to the tension you often experience, that the acid/alkaline pH of your body be kept as balanced as possible. Chinese medicine would refer to this as the universal yin/yang principle.

Scorpio rules destruction and elimination, and controls the red pigmentation in the blood. Your sun sign also rules the uterus, prostate gland, testicles, penis, vulva, reproductive organs, nasal bone, pubic bone, lower lumbar vertebrae, colon, and rectum.

Diseases to which Scorpios are subject include:

Acute fever	Prostatic strictures
Blood diseases	Ruptures
Fistulas	Ulcers
Hemorrhoids	Urethral strictures
Infections and diseases of the	Vaginal infections
reproductive system	Venereal disease
Ovarian cysts	

The Scorpio diet must be rich in foods that contain high amounts of vitamin B-complex, vitamins C and E, zinc, folic acid, potassium, phosphorus, and selenium. Illness may be caused by a buildup of toxic waste materials, so you should promote elimination. For optimum health, be sure to include foods that add bulk, such as salads and bran, in your diet. Periodic fasting and/or occasional use of a mild herbal laxative may enhance your feeling of well-being.

You also require a lot of vitamin B-12 in your diet. Insufficient B-12 results in anemia because of insufficient iron in the system. In addition to causing anemia, B-12 deficiency prevents the production of sex hormones and can cause underdevelopment of breasts and sex organs. The established requirement for Scorpios is 2 to 4 micrograms per day. Absorption of B-12 is inhibited by excessive amounts of mucus in the small intestine, often caused by allergy to dairy products.

Calcium sulfate is the Scorpio cell salt. Cell salts are naturally occurring minerals that are normal constituents of the body cells. They are found in trace amounts in foods, and plants, animals, and human beings require these compounds for proper nutrition. And, like vitamins, cell salts get used up. Calcium sulfate is an important constituent in the cells of all connective tissue and is absolutely essential to the healing process. Calcium sulfate prevents gastric juices from dissolving the stomach lining, and a deficiency of this cell salt usually causes stomach problems. Since it is also important in forming the reproductive hormones, lack of it affects the ovaries, testes, and prostate gland. Whenever something has to be eliminated from the body, calcium sulfate is reported to be effective.

FOODS RICH IN CALCIUM SULFATE

Asparagus	Kale
Black cherries	Leeks
Cauliflower	Mustard greens
Coconut	Onions
Figs	Prunes
Garlic	

Scorpios should avoid diets rich in saturated fats and should follow a diet generally high in protein, including plenty of lean meat, seafood, eggs, poultry, nuts, and soy products. In addition, your diet should include fresh fruit and vegetables, asparagus, figs, coconuts, and prunes.

Often, Scorpios prefer hot and spicy foods and hot beverages. In fact, almost all your food has to really stimulate your tongue and taste buds. With your intense personality, your nervous system is often in a state of flight.

Scorpio Daily Nutritional Supplements

- Super B-complex multivitamins
- One general multivitamin with minerals
- 400 mg vitamin E
- 2,000 mg vitamin C
- 25 mg zinc (recommended for adults only)

Remember, Scorpio . . .

This diet is uniquely prepared to address your sun sign and *should not be interchanged with any other Sun Sign Diet.* It is important that you follow the diet exactly as it appears, for optimum weight loss and assimilation. Before starting your Scorpio diet, carefully read "General Diet and Maintenance Guidelines for All Sun Signs," at the beginning of this book. Remember, drink 8 glasses of water daily.

You will never have to be a member of the yo-yo team again, dear Scorpio, because this diet has been prepared to meet your biological, chemical, nutritional, and behavioral needs.

Good luck and *go for it.*

The Scorpio
Two-Week
Reducing Diet

This diet has been designed to meet the Scorpio nutritional needs, while taking into consideration the Scorpio life-style. It is a high-protein, low-carbohydrate diet well suited for the high-energy Scorpio. It also has a straightforward, no-nonsense approach to dieting, one that explains, step by step, the reason each food item is incorporated in your diet plan.

The first day of your diet is programmed for a potassium-rich liquid fast that will flush all of the toxins out of your body and eliminate water weight. This day will act to normalize and balance your body's acid/alkaline pH factor. By nature of your zodiac sign, you Scorpio tend to retain water easily in your cells. For this reason, your daily diet includes quality potassium-rich foods for their excellent diuretic qualities. They will help flush out the sodium from your body, which is so often the cause of edema. The inclusion of high-fiber foods in your diet will help alleviate Scorpio's usual constipation problems.

You will find the use of apple-cider vinegar (2 teaspoons in an 8-ounce-glass of water) is an excellent diet aid. It will help tame your robust appetite for starchy bread products. The potassium/phosphorus balance in the apple-cider vinegar will definitely help cut down your appetite. Have it with meals and perhaps once midday for optimal effect.

To further speed up your weight loss and suppress your appetite, you may try a diet aid known in the United States as Glucomannan. It is extracted from the Japanese konjac root, a tuber that is very high in fiber. A final monograph on its effectiveness has not yet been established by the

FDA, as it has no history of use in the United States before 1958; however, the konjac root has been cultivated and eaten in Asia for over a thousand years.

Glucomannan contributes to a decrease in cholesterol and triglyceride levels, and aids in maintaining low-density lipoprotein levels. It acts as a dietary fiber to increase viscosity and moisture content of food as it is digested, so that it forms a smooth, soft mass that moves easily through the intestinal tract. Digestion is slowed, so normal blood sugar levels are maintained after a meal. Two capsules taken three times a day may cut your appetite in half!

Please note the asterisk (*) that appears after certain foods listed in your diet. I have noted the vitamin and mineral content of such foods, and the reason for their inclusion in your diet. You will find an in-depth discussion of each day's menu at the end of your Scorpio Reducing Diet, in the section "Notes to the Scorpio Two-Week Reducing Diet."

Do not mix your menus. Eat what is scheduled for that day. (If you do not want something leave it out, but do not substitute.) You may repeat the full Scorpio Two-Week Reducing Diet as often as necessary to achieve your desired weight loss.

I know underneath that superhero willpower, Scorpio, you are a mere mortal soul like the rest of us, and thus have included a Scorpio binge day. When you find yourself gnawing away at your fingernails and on the verge of pulling your hair out, use your binge day. But remember, no more than four times a month.

Your Scorpio diet coupled with your strong willpower and motivation are a sure bet for your success.

WEEK ONE

The first week of the Scorpio diet leaves few options. The first day is designed to balance your pH factor, which is probably disproportionate due to your style of living.

DAY ONE—ALL LIQUID DAY*

For the next 24 hours, you may not have any solid food, but you will indeed be having energized food in liquid form. Make your own soup, consisting entirely of fresh vegetables and water to balance acid and alkaline properly. Drink this throughout the day, hot or cold. An excellent way to start your diet, the soup will act as a natural diuretic. You are definitely one of the water-retainers of the Zodiac. For this reason, dieting or not, you must drink water throughout the day.

ON RISING

> 8 oz. water and 2 tsp. lemon juice
> 1 cup of tea

THROUGHOUT DAY

> ### Scorpio Vegetable Soup
> 10 cups water
> 6 fresh whole tomatoes
> 1 head cabbage, cut up
> 1 head lettuce, cut up
> 2 large onions
> 2 zucchini
> 6 carrots
> 2 bunches parsley
> 4--5 stalks celery
> Combine the above ingredients in a large pot. Bring to a boil and simmer, covered, for about one hour. Let cool and put entire contents through blender or food processor until liquid. Drink throughout the day.
>
> D-Zerta diet gelatin—as much as you want
>
> *Remember, drink 8 glasses of water every day.*

DAY TWO*

The second day is an all-protein day which will rid your body of excess water and sugar.

BREAKFAST
>   2 hard-boiled eggs

>   *or*

>   3 oz. tuna fish, (water-pack only)

>   *or*

>   6 oz. tofu

LUNCH
>   4–5 oz. lean meat, chicken, fish or veal

>   *or*

>   8 oz. tofu

MIDAFTERNOON SNACK
>   1 hard-boiled egg (if hungry)

DINNER
>   satisfying amounts of broiled, baked, or steamed chicken, fish

>   *or*

>   veal (baked in tomato juice)

EVENING SNACK
>   2 oz. cottage cheese (optional)

>   black coffee, tea, or no-sodium diet soda (limit, 2 cans)

>   *Remember, drink 8 glasses of water every day.*

DAY THREE

The third day the pH factor in your body will again be balanced. You must use only fresh fruit*. The enzyme bromelin in the pineapple will act as a catalyst and break up the fat composition. It will also start the metabolic burning system, and once again act as a diuretic. The sunflower seeds in the evening will fill your calcium needs, *but must not be included* if you are on "watermelon for the day."

ENTIRE DAY
> 2 whole fresh pineapples*

or

7 whole grapefruit

or

7 whole oranges

or

6 papayas

EVENING SNACK
> 1 oz. unsalted fresh sunflower seeds*

or

ENTIRE DAY
> as much watermelon as you would like all day long
>
> black coffee, tea, or water—no diet soda

An excellent cleanser for toxic Scorpios—very sweet, satisfying, and yields a 2-pound weight loss. *But absolutely nothing else must pass your lips.*

Remember, drink 8 glasses of water every day.

DAY FOUR

BREAKFAST

    3 kiwis* and hot tea with sugar substitute

or

1 cup fresh or ½ cup unsweetened or frozen strawberries

LUNCH

    ½ papaya* and ½ broiled or baked chicken

    no-sodium seltzer, tea with lime, or black coffee

DINNER

    ½ papaya and ½ broiled or baked chicken*

    3 kiwis

    D-Zerta diet gelatin

    no-sodium seltzer with lime

EVENING SNACK

    herbal tea

Remember, drink 8 glasses of water every day.

DAY FIVE

Day Five is a high-protein, low-carbohydrate day, packed with high-energy food. It is important that you have watercress and parsley where indicated. They are extremely important to the Scorpio diet. Eat at least ½ bunch watercress during the day (carry it with you when eating out and add it to your salad.

BREAKFAST
> 1 whole grapefruit or ½ pineapple
>
> coffee or tea (no milk or milk products*)

LUNCH
> 2 eggs (any style, cooked with 2 tsp. margarine)
>
> large plate of fresh asparagus (all you can eat), topped with 2 Tbsp. Parmesan cheese
>
> 2 oz. licorice

DINNER
> 4 oz. dry Chablis wine (optional)
>
> 6 oz. broiled, baked, or steamed fish (no butter—use lemon juice or ¼ cup Mexican salsa*)
>
> 2 cups watercress,* parsley, and raw spinach, seasoned with 2 Tbsp. Pritikin no-oil salad dressing
>
> no-sodium seltzer with a twist of lime

EVENING SNACK
> as much D-Zerta diet gelatin as you want
>
> *Remember, drink 8 glasses of water every day.*

DAY SIX

Another important day of pushing high-enzyme food and fiber. This will help counteract constipation; the potassium, silicon, and phosphorus content is abundant, and a Scorpio can never get enough of these. Try to drink a glass of water with each apple so that it fills you up more.

ENTIRE DAY
> a total of 8 apples for the day

EVENING SNACK (optional)
> 1 cup unsalted air-blown popcorn

or

> 2 Tbsp. unsalted sunflower seeds

BEVERAGE
> black coffee, tea, herbal tea, or water *only*

> *Remember, drink 8 glasses of water every day.*

DAY SEVEN

Another high-protein, low-carbohydrate, Scorpio-regenerating food day. If you do not have too much weight to lose, you may have a Bloody Mary with dinner.

BRUNCH*

> 2 eggs*
>
> 2 tsp. caviar and 1 oz. Nova lox
>
> sliced tomato
>
> 1 Wasa Crisp Bread

MIDDAY SNACK

> 1 whole grapefruit or orange

or

> 2 oz. licorice

or

> 1 Frozfruit fruit pop

DINNER

> 1 glass Chablis (optional)
>
> ½ chicken, baked, broiled, or boiled
>
> asparagus* (as much as you want)
>
> 1 cup watercress* and parsley, with 2 Tbsp. no-oil Pritikin salad dressing
>
> D-Zerta diet gelatin—any flavor, all you want
>
> *Remember, drink 8 glasses of water every day.*

You must be very proud of yourself. How much have you lost? Perhaps 5 pounds, maybe 6 or 7? Well, Scorpio, you should feel as though you are again in control.

On the next page, your reducing diet for Week Two begins. You will note that you have a few more options in your combinations. Now that you've done so well in Week One, it's time to put your creative talent to work, particularly at dinnertime.

WEEK TWO

Week Two is rather simple. You will note that at lunchtime I have included sardines, one of the most perfect foods for a Scorpio, supplying every needed vitamin and mineral and providing incredible staying power. Sardines will keep you from feeling hungry for hours. If you go to a restaurant and cannot order sardines, substitute salmon.

In Week Two, you may have 2 cans of diet soda, one on Day Five and one on Day Seven. But try to use no-sodium brands. (Regular diet soda has more salt in 1 can than there is in 4 ounces of steak.) If you have less than 10 pounds to lose, on Day Seven you may have a Bloody Mary or 1½ ounces of liqueur.

BREAKFAST CHOICES FOR WEEK TWO

Choose one: ½ grapefruit, ¼ fresh pineapple, 1 apple, ⅔ cantaloupe, 2 tangerines, 1 cup fresh strawberries*

and

5 almonds*

hot tea

or

1 slice pumpernickel bread with 1 tsp. pure apple butter (limit 3 times per week)

4 oz. unsweetened grapefruit juice

or

1 large banana*

café au lait (with 2 oz. milk)

LUNCH EVERY DAY

4 oz. white wine (optional)

huge salad, consisting of: lettuce, tomatoes, cucumbers, parsley, watercress, broccoli, cauliflower, and raw mushrooms

and

3½ oz. can of sardines in mustard sauce or oil (if packed in oil, drain and blot on paper towel); toss sardines on salad and serve with 1 Tbsp. horseradish

If you absolutely do not like sardines, you may substitute one of the following:

3½ oz. Chinook salmon*

3½ oz. Bismarck herring*

2 hard-boiled eggs

6–8 oz. tofu

4 oz. cottage cheese* (limit 3 times per week)

DINNER EVERY DAY

6 oz. broiled or baked chicken, fish, or liver

and

1 cup asparagus, cauliflower, or water-pack artichokes

and

2 cups of salad from ingredients listed above in lunch menu, with 2 Tbsp. Pritikin no-oil salad dressing

D-Zerta diet gelatin—all you want

EVENING SNACK

1 35-calorie Jell-O frozen pudding pop, strawberry

Remember, drink 8 glasses of water every day.

Notes to Scorpio Two-Week Reducing Diet—Week One

Scorpio Diet Notes—Day One

* This is an excellent way to break the vicious cycle of constant overeating. It will add alkaline properties to your already acid constitution (excellent remedy for acid stomach). After 24 hours you will have lost your craving for sugar. The Scorpio Vegetable Soup has been designed to feed your body the proper minerals and vitamins. It is rich in vitamin C; the 6 tomatoes yield a whopping 1466 mg of potassium, and the other vegetables are rich in vitamin C and folic acid. Expect to urinate a lot today.

Scorpio Diet Notes—Day Two

* Day Two is a low-carbohydrate, high-protein day, which Scorpios handle very well. Because you will not be eating any sugars or starches, you will rid the body of more excess water weight. (Scorpio's are never short on water.) It offers more than adequate protein, and is strong in the B vitamins, vitamin E, and zinc.

Scorpio Diet Notes—Day Three

* Fresh fruit is fortified with powerful enzymes that act to digest food, rid the body of accumulated toxins, and speed up your metabolism. Your body needs the carbohydrates and natural fructose. The order of active fruit-enzyme power is pineapple, papaya, grapefruit.
* Pineapple is rich in the enzyme bromelin, which works to break up accumulated fats in the cells, and chlorine, which has an invigorating effect upon the kidneys and liver.
* Sunflower seeds are rich in vitamin B-6, potassium, magnesium, calcium, fiber, and lecithin. Especially good for the brain and nerve tissues.

Scorpio Diet Notes—Day Four

By now, Scorpio, you are looking in the mirror and marveling at your incredible weight loss. Pretty fantastic, isn't it? Well, let's continue and accomplish your goal.

It is important not to allow your body to become used to one particular food, or one style of eating. Flipping from carbohydrates one day to protein the next does not allow your metabolic rate to become static. In other words, it is always changing your set point. (If you absolutely cannot have today's menu, you may repeat Day Two.

* Kiwis will supply you with quality fruit enzyme of vitamin A.
* Papaya contains the digestive juice papain, which has been used as treatment for ulcers. Papain has a soothing effect upon the digestive system, especially the stomach and intestinal tract. Papaya is also rich in vitamins C, B, and A.
* Just 3½ oz. of chicken (you are allowed much more) offers 243 grams of phosphorus. It is rich in vitamins B-2, B-3, B-6, B-12, folic acid, and calcium. What a bargain food for your Scorpio constitution.

Scorpio Diet Notes—Day Five

* Do not use any milk in your coffee or tea. Not even a smidgin, Scorpio. It stops the enzyme action of the breakfast fruit.
* The watercress programmed for your dinner meal has more calcium than a glass of milk.
* Mexican salsa is delicious over fish, and has a nice tangy taste that Scorpios love. It can be purchased in any health food store and some supermarkets, and is made from jalapeño peppers. Your programmed diet day is full of vitamins B, C, E, folic acid, selenium, and zinc.

Scorpio Diet Notes—Day Six

This is a day of total martyrdom. I know it won't be easy, but it will be well worth the results.

At this point your body needs an extra push of fiber (constipation slows down your system), and you need a good dose of phosphorus and magnesium. The apple represents the perfect balance of both minerals, is satisfying and filling, and has a high alkaline pH concentration.

Scorpio Diet Notes—Day Seven

* Breakfast and lunch are rich in vitamin B-2 (riboflavin). Vitamin B-2 functions as part of a group of enzymes that are involved in the breakdown and utilization of carbohydrates, proteins, and fats.

* If you choose to have your eggs hard-boiled, you will experience longer satiety value. It takes almost as much caloric energy to digest, as the egg yields, and each contains 6 grams of protein. A good source of vitamin E, folic acid, phosphorus, and iron.

* It is important that you have your salad of watercress and parsley. Both herbs are rich in calcium and vitamin C, and substitute your need for milk.

* Asparagus is an excellent diuretic food, containing vitamin B-1 (thiamin). It contains the enzyme asparagine, which helps to break up accumulated fats in the cells.

Okay, Scorpio—now you can see that you can lose weight and feel just great when a diet is based entirely on your sun sign needs. Because of your compulsive nature, many of you will be asking, "Can I return to Day One again?" You may return to Day One if you will only be staying on your diet for a month; if you need to diet longer, you will find that you will still lose a lot of weight the second week (as long as you do not change *one* thing) and that you will be able to stay with the diet as a comfortable way of life. The choice is up to you.

Notes to Scorpio Two-Week Reducing Diet—Week Two

You will note that I emphasize large salads or raw foods. Raw foods are rich in enzymes—those miracle workers that serve to extract vitamins and minerals from foods and produce healthier Scorpios. You should become aware of the power of health in raw fruits and vegetables. Remember the key to good health is not what you eat, but what you assimilate. The best assimilation takes place with foods that are close to nature.

* Salmon is an excellent low-cholesterol, high-level-protein food that is

extremely rich in vitamins A, B, and E. Horseradish is an excellent blood cleanser.

* Bismarck herring allots 20 grams of protein per serving and is rich in vitamins B-2, B-3, B-12, D, phosphorus, calcium, and potassium.

* Please note that all your calcium requirements per day are met with any of the above choices of protein.

* Cottage cheese or skim-milk ricotta are good sources of calcium. (Limit to 3 times per week.)

* Strawberries act as a blood purifier, are rich in vitamin C, and have excellent enzyme power, which helps to break down fat cells.

* Almonds are a superb nonanimal protein, rich in iron potassium, manganese, and phosphorus.

* Bananas are a good source of vitamin B, yielding 370 mg of potassium, 8 mg of calcium, and 33 mg of magnesium. You may freeze them, and they will taste like banana ice cream. If you choose banana, do not include the almonds.

Now examine your heavenly body. You may repeat your Scorpio Sun Sign Diet until you achieve your desired weight loss.

SCORPIO TOTAL BINGE DAY

Scorpio, with all the extremes in your life, you sometimes need to let go. I have given you that option with a binge day. Now remember, Scorpio, you have a tendency to go overboard, so be careful!

Before You Binge

1. Drink water.
2. Drink water.
3. Drink water.
4. Rest.
5. Brush your teeth and rinse with your favorite mouthwash.
6. Chew sugarless gum for 20 minutes.

You may find that the desire to binge has passed. However, if you are still suffering from intense food frustration, follow these basic binge rules:

Rule One

Under no circumstances should you ever binge before completing Day Five of your Scorpio Reducing Diet. This will ensure a maximum weight loss with a minimum of food frustration.

Rule Two

If, for example, you binge on the sixth day of your diet, resume your diet the following day (Day Seven) with the menu for Day Six. If you binge for just one meal, such as lunch on Day Six, resume your reducing diet with dinner of Day Six of your reducing diet.

Rule Three

Bingeing is for when you get that creepy, anxious feeling, when you feel like pulling out your hair—strand by strand—and you cannot endure dieting for even one more moment. Before you climb the walls, give yourself a binge day. It's hoped that this will not be necessary more than four times a month.

Rule Four

After you have lost your first 10 pounds, you may vary your binge day with the binge day of the sun sign opposite yours, which is Taurus.

Remember, an occasional binge day—when necessary—will still allow you to lose weight (without guilt). Here, Scorpio, is your binge day menu.

Binge Day Menu

BREAKFAST

1 bagel with diet butter or 1 Tbsp. cream cheese

1 oz. smoked salmon

café au lait

or

2 scrambled eggs with 1 Tbsp. caviar (optional)

café au lait

LUNCH

4 oz. white or red dry wine (optional)

1 slice pizza with mushrooms

½ cup any flavor sherbet or Tofutti frozen dessert

or

1 cup linguine, macaroni, or spaghetti with garlic, basil, and oregano

1 Tbsp. oil mixed with ¼ cup tomato juice

MIDAFTERNOON SNACK

1 strawberry or cantaloupe Frozfruit fruit pop

DINNER

4 oz. white wine (optional)

1–2 lb. steamed or broiled lobster (no butter)

large tossed salad with lemon juice

1 sliced tomato with basil

or

6–8 oz. any broiled or baked fish of your choice

large serving of broccoli

½ baked potato with 1 Tbsp. sour cream and chives

Remember, drink 8 glasses of water every day.

Maintaining Your Ideal Weight

Scorpio Maintenance Foods for Optimum Health

Whe you have achieved your desired weight goal you should follow a maintenance diet rich in the specific nutrients that you, Scorpio, need each and every day.

Vitamin B-12

Vitamin B-12 is necessary for normal metabolism of nerve tissue involved in protein, fat, and carbohydrate conversion. Vitamin B-12 helps prevent anemia by regenerating red blood cells, which are ruled by Scorpio. It helps increase energy, improve memory and balance, and maintain a healthy nervous system. B-12 has often been considered the nerve vitamin, so important to the hyper Scorpio. It also aids in the production of DNA and RNA, the body's genetic material.

FOODS RICH IN VITAMIN B-12

Alfalfa sprouts	Dairy products
American cheese	Eggs
Beef	Green peas
Bran	Herring
Chicken	Liver
Chicken livers	Milk
Cottage cheese	Muscle meats

297

Pickled foods	Skim milk
Prunes	Soy bean products
Raw oysters	Swiss cheese
Sardines	Trout
Shellfish	Yogurt

Vitamin C

Excessive stress, cigarette smoking, and drinking uses up the necessary vitamin C in your body. Vitamin C helps heal wounds, burns, and ulcers, and aids in the prevention of common colds by strengthening the immune system. It also acts as nature's natural laxative. Scorpios tend to have problems with constipation and can eliminate this problem by incorporating more vitamin C foods in their diet.

FOODS RICH IN VITAMIN C

Alfalfa	Currants
Almonds	Green Peppers
Apples	Grapefruit
Asparagus	Lemons
Bananas	Oranges
Beets	Orange juice
Blueberries	Paprika
Broccoli	Parsley
Brussels sprouts	Pineapple
Cantaloupe	Skim milk
Carrots	Strawberries
Celery	Tomatoes
Chicken	Watercress
Cranberries	

Vitamin E

Vitamin E is considered the sex vitamin. It increases sexual potency and virility, and acts as an anti-aging vitamin. Vitamin E is an antioxidant; it has the ability to unite with oxygen and prevent it from being converted into toxic peroxides. This leaves the red blood cells filled with a greater supply of oxygen which the blood carries to all organs of the body. It stimulates urine excretion and helps to lower blood pressure. Vitamin E supports the proper functioning of the pituitary and adrenal hormones. Scorpio, this is one of your more important vitamins. It is even more successful when combined with selenium.

FOODS RICH IN VITAMIN E

Apples	Mushrooms
Asparagus	Parsley
Avocados	Peanut butter
Broccoli	Salmon
Cabbage	Sardines
Carrots	Shrimp
Cheese	Spinach
Chicken	Sunflower seeds
Eggs	Sweet potatoes
Halibut	Turkey
Liver	Wheat germ
Milk	

Selenium

Selenium works with vitamin E to make it more efficient. Males have a stronger need for selenium since half their body's supply is concentrated in the testicles and seminal ducts.

FOODS RICH IN SELENIUM

Eggs	Garlic

Zinc

Zinc is an essential mineral involved in the synthesis of proteins and in enzyme action. Remember, Scorpios need a high-protein diet. Zinc in conjunction with vitamin C really helps to strengthen your immune system. Zinc has recently been found to be an effective treatment in both male and female infertility (no wonder, since Scorpio rules the reproductive organs). And zinc is the most important mineral in eliminating prostate problems.

FOODS RICH IN ZINC

Chopped meat	Milk
Eggs	Pumpkin
Lamb	Wheat germ

Folic Acid

Folic acid is essential in producing the necessary quantity and adequate size of red blood cells necessary for proper liver function. If you drink too much wine or liquor, folic acid must be replaced daily. Most important, folic acid is also interrelated with endocrine gland function, a vital part of the Scorpio reproductive system.

FOODS RICH IN FOLIC ACID

Asparagus	Kidney
Avocado	Lamb
Beet greens	Lima beans
Broccoli	Liver
Brown rice	Peanuts
Chard	Potatoes
Cottage cheese	Smoked ham
Endive	Spinach
Green leafy vegetables	Turnips
Kale	

Potassium

Potassium keeps the body fluids properly balanced and helps attract nutrients from the blood stream into the cells. It activates many enzymes and is essential for muscle contraction. Much stress is put on the muscles of the Scorpio physique because Scorpios have a tendency to keep their body tense. As mentioned earlier, Scorpios have a problem (especially women) with water retention. You will find that incorporating potassium-rich foods in your diet will eliminate this edema. And the diuretic action of potassium foods often reduces common allergies.

FOODS RICH IN POTASSIUM

Almonds	Potatoes
Asparagus	Prunes
Bananas	Salmon
Beets	Sardines
Broccoli	Sesame seeds
Buttermilk	Skim milk
Cantaloupe	Strawberries
Coconut	Sunflower seeds
Green leafy vegetables	Tuna
Lemons	Turkey

Phosphorus

Phosphorus works in combination with calcium and is usually present in most foods. It is essential for healthy kidney functioning and for the transference of nerve impulses. Remember that the excretory system is ruled by Scorpio. Phosphorus should always be balanced with a ratio of 2.5:1, calcium to phosphorus.

FOODS RICH IN PHOSPHORUS

Almonds	Liver
Apples	Milk
Avocados	Mushrooms
Beef	Nuts
Beef liver	Parsley
Beets	Pumpkin seeds
Cherries	Rice
Chicken	Salmon
Corn	Scallops
Egg yolks	Spinach
Grapefruit	Tuna
Halibut	Veal
Lima beans	

Scorpio Sample Maintenance Menu

When you reach your desired goal, please follow the maintenance eating hints found in "General Diet and Maintenance Guidelines for All Sun Signs" at the beginning of this book for proper calculations of caloric intake.

I'm including a sample maintenance menu based on your sun sign for optimal Scorpio maintenance. When you create your own menus for yourself, try to choose many of the foods you eat from your Scorpio Maintenance Foods lists.

2,000 Calories Per Day

ON RISING	CALORIES
1 glass warm water with 2 Tbsp. lemon juice sweetened with 2 packets of sugar substitute	14

BREAKFAST

8 oz. skim milk beat in blender with	80
1 banana, and	80
2 Tbsp. raw wheat germ	56
1 Wasa Crisp Bread	35
black coffee or tea (no milk)	0
	251

LUNCH

3¾ oz. sockeye salmon	190
¼ cup potato salad	100
alfalfa sprouts, lettuce, tomato	75
¼ cup coleslaw	77
1 slice pumpernickel or black bread	79
no-sodium diet soda, black coffee, or tea	0
	521

MIDAFTERNOON SNACK

1 whole orange or apple	80

DINNER

1 glass Chianti wine (optional)	75
5–6 oz. sirloin steak	575
½ cup Jerusalem artichoke (cubed)	75
1 sliced fresh tomato	27
salad of lettuce, spinach, watercress, cucumber	150
1 Tbsp. blue cheese dressing	68
	970

EVENING SNACK

1 cup fresh strawberries	45
½ cup sherbet	120
	165

TOTAL DAILY CALORIES	2,005

Remember, drink 8 glasses of water every day.

Restaurant Eating the Scorpio Way

Perhaps you have seen the following dishes on restaurant menus. Maybe you have ordered them, and maybe not. Included here are dishes chosen to specifically appeal to the Scorpio palate. Note that all of the recommended dishes contain the nutrients especially important for you and which are included in your Scorpio Maintenance Foods lists. In all cases, one appetizer plus one entrée equals approximately 500–600 calories.

French Restaurant

APPETIZERS

Artichokes in vinaigrette dressing

Steamed mussels with white wine and shallots

ENTRÉES

Steak with peppercorns, flamed

Loin of lamb with fresh mint

Chicken braised in champagne with mushrooms

Filet of salmon with herbs

Italian Restaurant

APPETIZERS

Italian ham with melon

Clams on the half shell

ENTRÉES

Veal sautéed with fresh baby artichokes

Boneless chicken in wine

Shrimp broiled with anchovies and caper sauce

Mignonettes of beef

Japanese Restaurant

APPETIZERS

Vegetables or fish with vinegar sauce

Soy bean soup

ENTRÉES

Casserole of meat, fish, and vegetables, cooked at the table

Smoked salmon and raw beef with hot mustard sauce

Sukiyaki

Chicken boiled and seasoned with seaweed, horseradish, and exotic vegetables

American Restaurant

APPETIZERS

Shrimp or crabmeat salad

Assorted fresh fruit

ENTRÉES

Filet of sole almondine

Lobster with light wine sauce

Rack of lamb au jus

Steak tartare

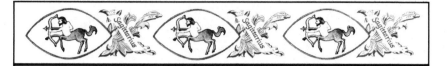

SAGITTARIUS

November 23–December 21

The Sagittarius Personality

"A moment on my lips, forever on my hips."

Enthusiastic, jovial Sagittarius, whatever you do in life, you do with gusto. You work hard, you play hard; but the single-mindedness of your activity never weighs down your buoyant disposition. Your capacity for making the best of every circumstance, for the sheer enjoyment of the moment, is unrivaled. You have an indomitable spirit and an unshakable belief that "good will out."

Cynics would say you have your head in the clouds. They are just jealous because nothing seems to worry you—not even the fact that too much good living may add pounds to the waistline. They may try to poke a hole in your balloon with pointed remarks about how pleasantly plump you look these days. But your inevitably light-hearted retort—"I'm not overweight, I'm just too short"—is likely to leave your detractors deflated.

Lucky for you, Sagittarius, that many people born under your star are not very heavy. Your on-the-go life-style prevents the extra pounds from accumulating too easily. But those of you who do put on weight often have a hard time taking it off. You step on a scale infrequently, and when you do, you take your weight fluctuations in stride. You may become philosophical about it, like my mother, who had a classic Sagittarian rationalization if someone mentioned she had gained some weight: "No I haven't," she would say. "They are cutting the garments smaller this year."

Those of you who admit to a few extra pounds tend to be blithely optimistic that tomorrow you will simply lose them. You can picture the new, thinner you already. How might this weight-loss miracle occur? You

307

visionary Sagittarians cannot be bothered with such minor details. When you do go on a diet, you will be extremely open about the fact. But generally speaking you are too concerned with having a good time to pay much attention to your food consumption and its effects.

Food, friendship, and fun. Those are the three essential ingredients of dining pleasure for Sagittarius. You truly enjoy the social aspect of eating— being with friends, or meeting new ones, and the opportunity to share your philosophies of life, your heartfelt humor, and an occasional good joke. You are frequently the dinner guest of others, because people seem to enjoy your refreshing candor and your famous wit, which is known to be as charming and clumsy as a puppy.

It is rare to see you upbeat, offbeat Sagittarians depressed about anything, even your weight. Your overeating is rarely emotionally triggered. You simply like to eat too much as a way of life. You clean your plate at mealtimes with the same purposeful abandon with which you live. You consume your share of ice cream and chocolate (fresh-dipped strawberries are your favorite), but you are not really noshers. Snack foods are mere tinder for the Sagittarian fires, which require some hefty logs to keep burning.

Naturally athletic, you like to get the "right start" to your active day. You will eat a breakfast of champions, a lunch fit for an Olympic gold medalist, and a dinner suited for a marathon runner on the eve of a big race. Complex carbohydrates and grains really satisfy your need for hearty fare. Some of you super-Sagittarians are able to polish off a heaping portion of lamb chops and mashed potatoes, then happily help yourself to seconds and thirds.

Your appetite is never so robust, expansive Sagittarius, as when you are traveling or enjoying the great outdoors. Horseback riding down the Grand Canyon, bicycling through Europe, or mountain climbing in the Andes, you thrive on adventure, the more far-flung the better. Nothing gives you the visceral experience of another culture like the taste of its native cuisine. When you cannot get away from home, however, a jaunt to a local Ukrainian restaurant or a foray into Thai gourmet cooking will satisfy the Sagittarian wanderlust.

By the same token, your thirst for fresh air and wide open spaces can be quenched, temporarily at least, just by sitting on a patch of green lawn. You love the sight, sound, and smell of meat sizzling on a backyard barbecue, and you love the taste of anything cooked over charcoal. A picnic in the countryside also tickles your soul. You will pack a basket full with bread and cheese, and a little *eau de vie* of course, and hike until you find a spot to spread your blanket. You won't cancel the excursion if the sun hides behind a cloud or if the wildflowers you had hoped to pick along the way are only weeds. You will eat anywhere outdoors—in a haystack or a swamp, in the fog or drizzle—to escape the routine of the kitchen table.

Sagittarius, you alone among the signs of the zodiac truly know how to turn the world into your playground and all life into a special occasion. Your unique outlook makes a glorious design for living, although it can kill a diet if you let it. The answer is not to alter your perspective or change your modus vivendi. You do not have to curb your appetite for African safaris and rare taste treats of "rhino au gratin"; just get right back to your diet the moment you step on home shores. When the time comes once again, it should not be so hard to say no to a second slice of ordinary roast beef or a humdrum baked potato. Simply close your big eyes and call up those stores of Sagittarian willpower. Don't forget your sense of humor, either: A little dose of it can go a long way to console your disappointed desire. Just say: "A moment on my lips, forever on my hips," and we do know about the Sagittarius hips.

According to astrology, your sign rules the hips and thighs, and those of you who lead more sedentary lives will find that extra calories tend to settle where you sit. Fortunately, many of you do have a natural love of exercise and sport, because getting rid of those saddle bags takes a goodly amount of running, walking, racquetball playing, or leg lifts—not to mention self-control of your eating, my fun-loving friend. Yes, I know that the thought of a diet is like a wet blanket on your fiery soul. You dislike restrictions of any kind on your life-style and ideas, and your generous nature is unpracticed to saying *no* to anybody, least of all to yourself. Just lunching with a dieter is enough to make you strain at the bit. Hard-boiled eggs and cottage cheese, or grapefruit and water-pack tuna, simply isn't your idea of a meal, and you have little tolerance for neurotic types who constantly watch what they eat. Life is too short to spend it counting calories, is your philosophy, impatient Sagittarius. And you are likely to apprise your companion of this opinion without ceremony, as you notoriously blunt and oblivious creatures are known to do. Of course, you will probably follow that offhanded slight with one of your ingenuously charming smiles and admit to your offended friend that you are planning to start your own diet tomorrow (*mañana* is your favorite word). As a sign of your sincerity, you order a tuna salad sandwich with french fries and tell the waiter to hold the extra mayo.

Your irrepressible good humor and outgoing personality are what get you—and your friends—through the worst days, Sagittarius, and I know they are just the qualities that will ultimately see you through your diet. You also have a strong sense of self-worth, and that is a basic ingredient to success in any endeavor. But let's speak frankly here my outspoken friend. Although you like to think of yourself as a free spirit, someone who acts on impulse and lives strictly for the moment, underneath that bravado you are not such a reckless soul. You are actually goal-directed, even idealistic, and you are fundamentally interested in self-improvement. There is a rather philosophical side to you concerned with moral and ethical principles, with law and tradition. Granted, your relationship to these values is inclined to be iconoclastic; but deep, deep down, you truth-seeking Sagittarians are a bedrock of conservatism. While you like to *feel* you are free to break any boundary, you do not always choose to do so.

All these qualities add up to a very sturdy individual with enough energy and self-control to do anything you put your mind to. Add to these attributes the legendary Sagittarian luck, and it is no wonder you are perusing this book right now. Chances are, you stumbled upon *The Sun Sign Diet* just at the very moment you absolutely decided to get your weight under control.

Well, you really have had a stroke of good fortune because the Sagittarius diet is designed to meet your unique nutritional needs and psychological makeup. And you won't have to sacrifice your natural vitality, or even your fun. I guarantee you will find enough variety and tasty, hearty food on your diet menus to satisfy even your lusty palate.

I know you love to gamble, Sagittarius, and I hate to disappoint you but your Sun Sign Diet is a sure bet. Just follow it as directed, and you can't lose anything but excess pounds.

Sexual Appetite

Sagittarius the archer, your astrological symbol is the Centaur, a mythical monster with the head, trunk and arms of a man, and a horse's body and legs. Half human, half beast, you are at once the soul of reason and the embodiment of animal appetites—altogether a fascinating creature, though somewhat difficult to domesticate. Anyone wishing to try should understand from the outset that both forces—intellectual and sensual, spiritual and physical—demand balanced expression in your life and relationships. Without other channels available, you unbridled Sagittarians inevitably turn to overeating as an outlet for your excess energy.

For a happy union, your partner must be your friend foremost, and then your consort. To keep up with you, he or she will also have to be equal parts playmate and teammate, romantic and adventurer, metaphysicist and jock. Your approach to sex is lighthearted and spontaneous. You like it to be fun, active, and very physical, of course—a bit like sports. Sex with Sagittarius must be exciting, inspired, and creative. You yourself are quite a skilled tease, and your lover likewise will have much more fun breaking you in by dangling sweet carrots just out of reach under your nose than by constantly feeding you sugar cubes. While you are not overemotional in love, you are warm and attentive and also enjoy the opportunity for intimate conversation that comes in the afterglow of lovemaking.

Just jogging around the bed can get so *booorrring,* however. You do not like to feel obligated to make love, and you do require a variety of physical outlets, Sagittarius. Ennui has been the downfall of many a diet, and you would do well to ponder the fact that you sometimes confuse your own natural restlessness with boredom. You tend to be most content in a relationship when sex is something great you do with your lover as a break from skiing, skydiving, windsurfing, and sailing. For your Sagittarian nature boys and girls, just about nothing beats a box of chocolate donuts like sharing the great outdoors with someone you love—unless, perhaps, getting your tight-muscled body massaged by your mate once you are back inside.

Open, honest communication, free of judgments, is an important part of your sexual needs, too. In love, you have galvanic responses. You are very affectionate and deeply vulnerable—and sometimes very volatile. You are also a sucker for flattery. You think intelligence is a very sexy quality and love to be appreciated for your own. If you feel it is absolutely true, you enjoy any compliment to the effect that your body is sexy, too.

You yourself have a rather quirky, sometimes blundering style of communication. You tend to say whatever comes to your mind without much thought, a technique that can be disarming as often as it is charming. One thing that can be said for certain, what one sees in the archer is what one gets. There is little pretentiousness in you, Sagittarians.

Compatibility on all levels is essential to you and unfortunately very difficult to find. You can be a person of great extremes, demanding communication, attention, closeness one moment, freedom, space, individual expression the next. It is not unlike you to take a leisurely stroll with your lover, then suddenly gallop off, your bow and arrow aimed at some nameless target, leaving your bewildered mate in a cloud of dust behind you. There are not many individuals in this world flexible enough to wait around until you return to the stable, or perceptive enough to know you Sagittarians always will. Of course, with those thoroughbred legs of yours, you are well equipped to enjoy a good chase, footloose Sagittarius. Flirting is as delicious to you as cream-filled candies, and as natural as breathing. But you are not adulterous: You are basically a moral character and quite trustworthy once the knot has been tied. And woe to the mate that questions your integrity.

You Sagittarians are among the most friendly, gregarious creatures in the zodiac. Friendships take a high priority in your life, and your spouse had better be prepared to share you with your many fans. Left alone in a public place you will innocently befriend a stranger in a matter of minutes, and never even think there could be ill effects when your mate returns to find you. Obviously, a possessive, clinging, or jealous lover could never understand your freedom-loving spirit; the Sagittarian who ever gets hitched up to one of these types will be one busted bronco indeed. And all the hot-fudge haystacks in the world won't undo the damage to your trampled soul.

True love, when you find it, is very sacred to you, romantic Sagittarius. I know you are willing to work long and hard for the survival of a relationship. Just be careful you do not stay in a bad match simply out of loyalty or principle. Remember, you will not find the way out of an unhealthy or unsatisfying emotional entanglement looking into your refrigerator, Sagittarius. Do some real soul-searching to discover the source of your frustration. Then go straight to your mate and tell-it-like-it-is, as only you archers know how. Even extra pounds cannot weigh down your expansive spirit for long. Your sunny attitude gives you power to turn a stale relationship into a growing one. And a growing relationship can keep Sagittarius so busy, you won't even think of food.

Entertaining/Eating at Home

The Sagittarian host or hostess loves to entertain. You like to think of your home as your stage, a place where you can really let the showman in you come out—and there is plenty of ham on those Sagittarian bones. You really do like to see your friends have a good time when they visit, and they do make such an appreciative, if captive audience for your culinary extravaganzas.

Ordinarily you don't care much for impromptu visits by friends. For expected company however, you are capable of cooking up a storm. You keep a file box of recipes you have gathered from friends, family secrets that have been handed down for generations, and others charmed away from chefs you have met around the world. Generous to a fault and often extravagant, you spare no expense in preparing a meal for invited guests and will hire household help if your budget allows it. Then you can be blissfully free—in true Sagittarian style—to enjoy your own cooking and company.

For a person who spends so much time on the road, you actually put a great deal of care into your home. It is generally open and spacious, or at least designed to give the appearance of being so. You can't tolerate cramped quarters for long, although some of you manage to thrive quite happily amidst the clutter of carved antiques, oriental rugs, exotic sculptures, and other treasures you have collected on your global travels or picked up at auctions and flea markets, which you love to haunt. It is no coincidence that such Sagittarian homes resemble museums of antiquity.

You are natural curators and will gladly give your company a guided tour of your collections if they show the slightest interest, or even if they don't. Your possessions are not just for show, however. Your company will be seated at an elegantly appointed dinner table set with beautiful handmade linens retrieved from some attic trunk, imported bone china, and heirloom crystal and serving pieces.

Whether you serve a cuisine with an international flavor or down-home cooking that could have come straight from Grandma's oven, your guests will enjoy a tasty, well-orchestrated meal served graciously and gracefully by their sociable Sagittarian host. You are always the life of a party, funny Sagittarius, especially your own. Any guest at your table will feel comfortable, well taken care of, and most definitely well fed.

Alas, my friend, you do love to pile food on a plate and watch your guests consume it with zeal. You really do not like people dieting in your house; as mentioned, calorie-counters cramp your carefree style. The fact is your own libertine spirit is quite infectious, and around you, your reducing friends may have a difficult time remembering why they had even *tried* to decline the extra serving of potatoes. Caught up in that boundless Sagittarian energy, the most conservative individual has been known to throw caution to the wind.

Do have some sympathy for your guests, good-willed Sagittarius. Let them leave food on their plates if they want; then give the leftovers to your pet. Animal lovers all, you Sagittarians are bound to have at least one hungry little beast around your house.

Besides, it wouldn't hurt you either to do the same with the extra food on your plate.

Food Shopping

Only Sagittarius could turn something as mundane as grocery shopping into a form of recreation. The sprawling, ultramodern supermarket sets something free in you, and you have been known to push your basket down the aisles practicing your latest break-dance moves to the music broadcast over the store loudspeakers. You stretch and bend to the beat as you reach for items on the upper and lower shelves, incorporating your activity into an exercise routine. Or you brush up on your basketball game practice-shooting canned goods into your shopping cart. Doing two things at once is always twice the fun for energetic Sagittarius.

You get vicarious pleasure just going through the imported food section. The flavors of far-off lands captivate you, and you are carried away to Iberia just picking up a jar of Spanish artichokes. As you explore the shelves for new and exotic taste sensations, you discover an interesting looking item, a Portuguese number called Snails à la Farego. Sure you will give it a try. Another can lands in the basket. Later you spot a box of English biscuits, a jar of French preserves, and a container of that new *gelato*—you know, like the one you sampled in Venice. Or was that Sorrento? Again high-priced, high-calorie items go into the cart. But who's counting? Not you, extravagant Sagittarius.

You don't watch the clock when you shop either. You often spend hours in the supermarket, but only a small fraction of the time directly engaged in selecting groceries. In between combing the aisles for a bar of soap (after eight years shopping in the same store, you still don't know where anything is) and chatting with your good friends Charlie the deli man, Tracy the store manager, and the nice old gentleman who needed help choosing a box of spaghetti, you just don't have much attention to pay small details like the fine print on food labels, comparison-pricing, or tracking down coupon items. You buy almost strictly on impulse, motivated by Madison Avenue catchwords like *naturally good, new, enriched,* and *value-packed.* Convenience foods are a staple in the diet of busy Sagittarius, and you tend to go through the frozen foods section, in particular, as if you were playing "supermarket sweetstakes," unable to resist any item that promises to save you time in the kitchen. You also can't resist buying a few "fun" foods, especially the kind you can eat on the run.

Obviously, your spontaneous shopping methods do not allow much time for checking grocery lists. That you do when you get home and unpack your many bags. I wouldn't be surprised if you forgot the butter and eggs, Sagittarius. However, I would be amazed if you left out that package of chocolates you were eyeing on Aisle 3 and that bag of thick-sliced potato chips you checked out on Aisle 8.

I know shopping is such fun when you do it your way, Sagittarius, but you are going to have to be slightly more systematic for the duration of your reducing diet. You will make your whole life easier by planning and purchasing the list of groceries you need at the start of each week. It will save you time in your busy schedule and allow you to stick to your diet effortlessly.

Social Dining

Dining out with Sagittarius is an adventure in eating. Your favorite type of restaurant defies categorization. Ideally it serves foreign fare, of course, perhaps Chinese, Indian, or Japanese. But there is a little bit of Christopher Columbus in your bones, and you always enjoy a menu that offers a journey into the unknown. If you stumble upon a tasty treasure, you will make a return trip with shiploads of friends to share the experience.

Good old American cuisine also suits your versatile palate, as long as it is served in somewhat exotic surroundings. A seaside shanty with New England charm, a mountain inn replete with working fireplace, anything folksy appeals to your easygoing style. Forward-looking Sagittarian also enjoys joining the trendy crowd at the latest fashionable establishment. Eating baby ribs barbecued on a mesquite grill amidst neon lights, art deco, and multilevel dining rooms is an acceptable alternative to dinner in the local Little Italy.

Your busy work and travel schedules often make it difficult for people to pin you down to a dinner date. You frequently cancel at the last minute or show up late to the restaurant.

You tend to use the unpredictability of your engagements as an excuse to break your diet. You feel you cannot pass up the opportunity to indulge when the waiter puts that basket on the table filled with assorted crunch truffles, loaves of fresh stone-ground breads, and homemade muffins. It is the house specialty, after all, and Lord knows when you might have another chance at this place. Besides, it is so much more *fun* to eat. You'll probably want to make a toast to it, and order another round of spirits for the table.

Undoubtedly, you have promised yourself, "to start my diet tomorrow for sure." Well, did you forget tomorrow's luncheon invitation to the newest continental restaurant in town, my procrastinating friend? Why not put down your glass of wine right now and try spreading the good cheer with a little sparkling water and lime instead. It's as bubbly as the best champagne without any of the empty calories, and really just as much fun. Then, if you feel the uncontrollable urge to splurge, pay the check. If you want to be reckless, leave your typically generous tip. Ask for your leftovers in a doggie bag (and make sure you feed them to the doggie) and charge out the restaurant door.

Believe it or not, that super-duper, once-in-a-lifetime specialty you pass up *will* be available to you on this earth at some later date.

Just *not* tomorrow, okay?

Special-Occasion Dining

Active, outgoing, and openhearted, you have friends in every corner of the globe, not to mention around every corner of the city, and they like to keep you on the move from dawn to dusk with endless honorary breakfasts, luncheons, and dinners, casual get-togethers, and formal soirées. Beside your membership on the wildlife conservation committee, the world peace association, and the cultural activities board, you also have a year-round schedule of fundraising parties and cocktail hours to attend. It really is tough to stick to a diet with so much good food available to you all the time.

Holiday occasions are the real test of Sagittarian mettle. You just cannot say no to those tempting specialty foods Aunt Gertrude bakes this one season out of the whole year. Well, my self-indulgent friend, *try.* Turning down those goodies is the best gift you can give to yourself any holiday season. Nothing else in the world can give you that sense of pride you will feel when you step on the scale at the holiday's end and haven't gained an ounce.

The trouble is, impulsive Sagittarius, that you never need a special day on the calendar as an excuse to make an occasion, anyway. Sagittarians are ready at a moment's notice for an outing. You love to spend lazy afternoons picnicking by an old water mill, rowboating on a duck pond, or strolling down a country lane. You enjoy a day at the races, the horse show, or the Derby—all things equestrian interest the archer. You love outdoor sports in most any shape or form—a friendly softball game, a serious tennis match —and the activity keeps your mind and hands off food. The danger strikes when you join the crowds in the grandstands to watch your favorite home team play. For Sagittarius, rooting at a ball game is almost as much fun as playing one—*more* fun if you consider all the hot dogs and beer, popcorn and ice cream you can eat between cheers.

A camping trip is one of your all-time favorite occasions. Sleeping under a moonlit sky is as near to heaven as Sagittarius can get on earth, just about. And nothing beats eating by a campfire, especially if the meal is trout you fished from the brook yourself.

Just remember, Sag, one self-indulgent day does not put an end to your dreams for a thinner you. You can enjoy a special occasion—the camaraderie of friends and the pleasure of physical activity or mental stimulation —without helping yourself to all that fattening food. If you must indulge, save some crumbs off your plate for the wildlife. I know you love to feed your feathered, finned, and four-legged friends, and better they should eat the calories than you.

Your Health

Sagittarius, your innate compulsion to be and feel fit coupled with your unlimited optimism makes you one of the healthier signs. You are not the type to worry or belabor your problems, and even when you are sick, it is hard to keep you in bed.

Fresh air, and plenty of it, is as vital to you and your health as water is to the fish. You are a natural athlete, and truly need to be both physically and mentally active. However, in your penchant for nonstop activity, you sometimes lose sight of your own limitations. As inherently strong as your constitution is, it is not invulnerable to disease, and you do get sick when you wear down your resistance. And you have suffered more than one accident in your life, due to your restless exuberance. On the other hand, if cooped up, or deprived of exercise and fresh air, you tend to lose your optimistic outlook, and illness often results.

Moderation is obviously the key to maintaining your health. It is especially true of your diet. You tend to put on weight by overindulging at mealtime and on special occasions, not because you eat between meals. Your love of rich foods, meat, and good wine may be especially detrimental because you have a tendency to build up cholesterol and have liver problems. And remember, alcohol is loaded with empty calories. I know food and spirits warm your heart, but it is time you got a little more control over your overactive eating.

Your sign rules the liver, hips, thighs, the expiratory functions of the lungs, the pelvis, buttocks, sciatic nerve, gluteus muscles, arterial system, and especially the iliac arteries. You have a proclivity toward weakness or disease in these areas, and proper precautions should be taken to protect them.

Other health problems common to Sagittarians include:

Bronchitis	Nerve disorders
Diabetes	Paralysis of the limbs
Fractures	Pulmonary disease
Hemorrhoids	Wounds through falling, cutting, or
Hypoglycemia	sports
Lung troubles	

These problems may or may not manifest during your lifetime.

The Sagittarian diet should be rich in choline, biotin, lecithin, inositol, and vitamins C, B-6, and K. Vitamins C and B-6 are needed to protect your circulatory system, and deficiencies could be conducive to pulmonary diseases. Both vitamin B-6 and biotin assist in reducing high levels of cholesterol. Vitamin B-6 is also necessary for healthy muscles; a deficiency is likely to produce weakness.

Inositol, choline, biotin, and vitamin K are important for healthy metabolism and proper fat distribution. Lecithin helps to burn up excess fat and prevents the formation of cholesterol as well.

Silica is the Sagittarius cell salt. Cell salts are naturally occurring minerals that are normal constituents of the body cells. They are found in trace amounts in foods, and plants, animals, and human beings require these compounds for proper nutrition. And like vitamins, cell salts get used up.

Silica is flint or quartz, and when seen under a microscope, its particles are sharply pointed. Its shape leads some to call it "nature's knife," or "nature's surgeon." Silica is mainly concerned with the body's waste-removal system. Silica forces wastes, such as pus from pimples and boils, to rise to the surface of the skin where it can be excreted through the pores. Once wastes have been eliminated, silica further works as a healing agent at the site of the eruption.

An essential constituent of the connective tissues of the brain, the sheaths which cover the nerves, and the lens of the eye, silica is also necessary for healthy vision and a healthy nervous system, as well as healthy muscles— all sensitive areas for Sagittarius. A lack of this cell salt can cause cataracts, nervous disorders, bad memory, and an inability to connect one's thoughts. Silica also helps to maintain hair's healthy luster and to prevent bones, teeth, and fingernails from becoming brittle.

FOODS RICH IN SILICA

Brown rice	Parsnips
Cherries	Prunes
Figs	Sage
Fruit skins	Strawberries
Marjoram	Vegetables

I know your nervous system is in high gear and you need lots of outlets for your excess energy. But you can't just dance the pounds away. Your philosophical attitude ("Well, that's the way it is") will not impress the scale either. I am not suggesting you do anything as extreme as a total fast, but I am not beyond making an appeal to your religious and spiritual nature: Even the Bible recognizes the health benefits of periodic or partial abstinence from food. Face the truth. The best thing for you to do for yourself is to go through a period of serious dieting. I know you will succeed because more than any other sign in the zodiac, your optimism and positive attitude will carry you through.

Sagittarius Daily Nutritional Supplements

- Super B-complex multivitamin with zinc
- 2,000 mg vitamin C
- 400 mg vitamin E

Remember, Sagittarius...

This diet is especially prepared to address your sun sign and *should not be interchanged with any other Sun Sign Diet.* It is important that you follow the diet exactly as it appears, for optimum weight loss and assimilation. Before starting your Sagittarius diet, carefully read "General Diet and Maintenance Guidelines for All Sun Signs," found at the beginning of this book. Remember, drink 8 glasses of water daily.

You will never have to be a member of the yo-yo team again, dear Sagittarius, because this diet has been prepared to meet your biological, chemical, nutritional, and behavioral needs.

Good luck, and *go for it.*

The Sagittarius
Seven-Day
Reducing Diet

Y ou are not usually given to overweight, Sagittarius, and when you do
get fat it is simply from too much eating. You don't like to deny yourself
anything. You are in love with life, and dieting spoils the fun. Take heart,
dear friend, I wouldn't think of ruining your good times. The Sagittarius
Reducing Diet will allow you to achieve maximum weight loss with the
minimum of discomfort.

Look at the following diet as a new adventure in your life. It is a little
unorthodox, designed for your style of living, body chemistry, and metabolic makeup. It enlists foods to counteract your sugar and carbohydrate
cravings and allows you to eat somewhat impulsively, so you feel just a
little reckless—as if you are not really dieting at all.

Knowing how you hate to be enslaved to your kitchen, I have been
especially careful to include in your diet frozen and convenience foods.
They will make your life easier by freeing you from cooking. However, if
you wish to prepare everything from scratch, you will find directions listed,
too. And knowing how you hate to be a party-pooper, Sagittarius, I have
even included some wine and champagne, so you need not put a damper
on your social life.

To further speed up your weight loss and suppress your appetite, you
may choose to try a diet aid known in the United States as Glucomannan. It
is extracted from the Japanese konjac root, a tuber that is very high in fiber.
A final monograph on its effectiveness has not yet been established by the
FDA, as it has no history of use in the United States before 1958; however,

the konjac root has been cultivated and eaten in Asia for over a thousand years.

Glucomannan contributes to a decrease in cholesterol and triglyceride levels, and aids in maintaining low-density lipoprotein levels. It acts as a dietary fiber to increase viscosity and moisture content of food as it is digested, so that it forms a smooth, soft mass that moves easily through the intestinal tract. Digestion is slowed, so normal blood sugar levels are maintained after a meal. Two capsules taken three times a day may cut your appetite in half!

In addition, to help tame your appetite for starchy bread products, I suggest the use of 2 teaspoons of apple-cider vinegar in an 8-ounce glass of water with all your meals. The high content of potassium and phosphorus will help to suppress your appetite. If you wish, you may drink a glass in the middle of the day for a quick pick-me-up.

Please notice the asterisks (*) that appear after certain foods listed in your diet. I have noted the vitamin and mineral content of the food and the major reason for its inclusion in your program. Refer to the section "Notes to Sagittarius Seven-Day Reducing Diet."

Eat what is scheduled for that day; if you do not want something leave it out, but do not substitute. You may repeat this diet as often as necessary to achieve your desired weight loss. And to make sure there are no excuses whatsoever, I have included a binge day, which appears at the end of your reducing diet with proper instructions.

Your binge day is only to be used when you feel you will "blow it." It is designed so you can feel you have indulged without any impinging sense of guilt. Just make sure that you do not use it more than four times a month.

You win almost every gamble you take, Sag. You simply were born under a lucky star. That's probably why you picked up this book and are holding it right now. As fortune would have it, here is your very special diet that will guarantee success if you follow it as prescribed. Be as honest with yourself as you are with everyone else, and take the plunge with a twinkle in your eye.

DAY ONE

BREAKFAST

1 small banana* and 5 almonds*

coffee with a little milk

LUNCH

6 oz. tomato juice

2-egg mushroom, spinach, or broccoli omelette, sprinkled with marjoram*

DINNER

8 oz. frozen Celentano Lasagne* (any supermarket)

salad consisting of: 2 cups watercress,* parsley,* lettuce, spinach, and radishes, 2–3 Tbsp. Pritikin no-oil salad dressing

1 cup fresh strawberries marinated in wine

EVENING SNACK

D-Zerta diet gelatin candy*

NOTE: In place of Celentano Lasagne you may use 1 cup of durum wheat pasta and serve with ¼ cup Aunt Millie's natural tomato sauce and 2 Tbsp. Parmesan cheese.

Remember, drink 8 glasses of water every day.

DAY TWO

BREAKFAST

1 slice raisin toast with 2 oz. cottage cheese

LUNCH

2 all-beef frankfurters* (no roll)

sauerkraut*—as much as you want, but no relish

1 light beer or Diet Coke

DINNER

¼–½ baked, broiled, or barbecued chicken* (no skin); prepare with ¼–½ cup Mexican hot salsa or use ½ cup tomato juice

2 cups (well-packed) salad, consisting of 1 sliced green pepper,* ½ bunch watercress and parsley, 1 whole tomato with basil, fresh spinach leaves, and radishes, 2–3 Tbsp. Pritikin no-oil salad dressing

EVENING SNACK

1 strawberry or raspberry Frozfruit fruit pop

or

D-Zerta diet gelatin candy with 1 Tbsp. Cool Whip dessert topping

Remember, drink 8 glasses of water every day.

DAY THREE

BREAKFAST
>   1 cup Golden Wheat Lites
>   1 cup skim milk

LUNCH
>   8 oz. tomato juice
>
>   3 oz. water-pack tuna* or salmon*
>
>   *or*
>
>   1 vanilla Danny-in-a-Cup frozen yogurt
>
>   1 cup fresh strawberries
>
>   iced tea, black coffee, no-sodium seltzer, or no-sodium diet soda

DINNER
>   ½ grapefruit or 1 glass white Chablis wine
>
>   Mrs. Paul's Fish Dijon with Asparagus
>
>   *or*
>
>   Mrs. Paul's Shrimp Primavera with Fettucine Pasta*
>
>   Bird's Eye chinese-style stir-fry vegetables with seasoning (⅔ box)
>
>   1 can Yoo-Hoo diet chocolate drink

Remember, drink 8 glasses of water every day.

NOTE: You may substitute 4 oz. broiled or baked filet of sole or shrimp (no butter) for Mrs. Paul's entrées.

DAY FOUR

BREAKFAST

½ cup All-Bran Flakes*

2 tsp. raisins and 1 tsp. sunflower seeds*

¾ cup skim milk

LUNCH

4 oz. dry white wine (optional)

4 oz. any fresh fish, prepared without butter (use lemon juice or white wine)

2 cups tossed salad consisting of alfalfa sprouts, lettuce, spinach, mushrooms, and watercress, seasoned with 2 Tbsp. lemon juice or Pritikin no-oil salad dressing

DINNER

6 oz. veal steak, cube or cutlet, sautéed in white wine

½ cup steamed brown or white rice

1 sliced whole tomato with basil and oregano

SNACK

2 cups air-flow unsalted popcorn

Remember, drink 8 glasses of water every day.

DAY FIVE

BREAKFAST

4 oz. unsweetened grapefruit juice or ½ grapefruit

2 eggs prepared to any style with 1 tsp. diet margarine

black coffee, tea, water (no milk)

LUNCH

¼ lb. cold roast beef (purchase at deli)

1 sliced whole tomato (sprinkled with marjoram)

salad of lettuce, cucumber, watercress, and parsley, with 2 Tbsp. Pritikin no-oil salad dressing or lemon juice and garlic pepper

no-sodium diet soda, iced tea, or black coffee

DINNER

¼ lb. cold roast beef

9 oz. fresh or frozen asparagus* sprinkled with 2 Tbsp. Parmesan cheese

1 cup fresh strawberries (add 1 packet Equal sweetener) or ½ cup unsweetened frozen strawberries

EVENING SNACK

all the D-Zerta diet gelatin *or* candy you want (no Cool Whip today)

Remember, drink 8 glasses of water every day.

DAY SIX

BREAKFAST

> 4 oz. unsweetened prune juice*
>
> 1 slice raisin bread with 1 Tbsp. apple butter

LUNCH

> fresh fruit salad*—3 cups, absolutely nothing else
>
> black coffee, tea, or no-sodium diet soda (no milk)

DINNER

> 2 broiled lean lamb chops* or 6 oz. lean minute steak or London broil
>
> 6–8 broccoli* spears with garlic pepper
>
> ½ cup cooked carrots
>
> D-Zerta diet gelatin candy with 1 Tbsp. Cool Whip dessert topping

EVENING SNACK

> D-Zerta diet gelatin or candy
>
> *Remember, drink 8 glasses of water every day.*

DAY SEVEN

BRUNCH

6 oz. dry champagne or Bloody Mary (optional)*

2-egg omelette (prepared with 1 tsp. diet margarine) and 2 Tbsp. red or black caviar*

½ toasted bagel

or

6 oz. dry champagne or dry white wine (optional)* or grapefruit juice

2-egg frozen waffles with 2 Tbsp. diet maple syrup, topped with 2 Tbsp. Cool Whip dessert topping

MIDAFTERNOON SNACK

1 Frozfruit fruit pop

DINNER

6 oz. cold roast turkey with salad of 1 whole apple, 6 almonds, and alfalfa sprouts, seasoned with 2 Tbsp. reduced-calorie mayonnaise (May substitute chicken for turkey.)

or

4 oz. wine spritzer (optional)

4–6 oz. any broiled or baked fish, prepared without butter

or

1–2 lb. lobster, prepared without butter

fresh or frozen, lightly steamed asparagus, seasoned with lemon

juice and pepper and Parmesan cheese to taste

1 35-calorie Jell-O frozen pudding pop

Remember, drink 8 glasses of water every day.

Notes to Sagittarius Seven-Day Reducing Diet

Sagittarius Diet Notes—Day One

* Banana is rich in your needed vitamins B-6, K, and biotin.
* Almonds are a source of vitamin C, biotin, and lecithin. This will get you off to a good start.
* Marjoram is a spice rich in the Sagittarius cell salt silica.
* Celentano Lasagne is a calorie-controlled carbohydrate meal that won't even let you know you are dieting.
* Watercress and parsley are fine sources of calcium and must be included for proper health whenever indicated.
* D-Zerta diet gelatin candy has the staying power of gelatin protein and when prepared in the following manner is extremely filling and sweet. You may have anytime during the day when you are hungry.

D-Zerta Diet Gelatin Candy

Use 2 packages of any flavor D-Zerta diet gelatin and mix *with only* 2 cups of hot water. Consistency will be thick. When hardened, cut in bite-sized pieces and eat like candy.

Sagittarius Diet Notes—Day Two

* Sauerkraut has excellent enzyme qualities as a result of the fermentation process. It will aid in the digestion of the beef protein and should be eaten together. You can have as much as 1 cup sauerkraut if you wish.
* Chicken is rich in vitamin B-6, folic acid, inositol, choline, and biotin. Green peppers are rich in vitamin C.

Sagittarius Diet Notes—Day Three

* Tuna and salmon are rich in the B vitamins and the tomato juice is a good source of vitamin C.
* Danny frozen yogurt may be sinfully delicious, but it is also a good source of vitamin B-12 and enriches the intestinal flora. It should help your cry for "ice cream."
* Mrs. Paul's Fish Dijon with Asparagus or Shrimp Primavera with Fettucine Pasta meet your nutritional requirements under strict calorie control. (You may substitute 4 oz. baked or broiled filet of sole or shrimp for Mrs. Paul's light seafood entrées.)

Sagittarius Diet Notes—Day Four

* Bran Flakes and sunflower seeds are both excellent laxative foods. Sunflower seeds are rich in lecithin, zinc, inositol, and biotin, and important in the Sagittarius diet.

* Veal is a fine low-calorie choice of protein for you because it is resplendent with the B vitamins.

Sagittarius Diet Notes—Day Five

This is a low-carbohydrate, high-protein day for you, Sag, designed to get your metabolism burning and eliminate any excess water. Do not have any milk in your coffee today.

* Asparagus is an excellent diuretic food. It also contains the enzyme asparagine, which helps to break up accumulated fats in the cells.

Sagittarius Diet Notes—Day Six

* Prune juice is rich in vitamin B-6 and the Sagittarius cell salt, silica.

* Fresh fruit salad is power packed with enzymes that will help to break down fat, speed up your metabolism, and give you quick energy. Do not have any milk products.

* Lamb chop is a good source of choline, biotin, zinc, and inositol. Your Sagittarius constitution demands this fare.

* Broccoli is a good source of calcium and vitamin K.

Sagittarius Diet Notes—Day Seven

* Caviar is a terrific source of inositol and makes you feel very special.

* Dry Champagne, Bloody Mary, and white wine are optional, and if not served with brunch, then may be served with dinner.

* Turkey and lobster could be your mainstay diet foods. They give you energy because they are sources, once again, of your specifically needed vitamins. Who said dieting can't be fun?

TOTAL SAGITTARIUS BINGE DAY

When you feel that you simply cannot stay on your diet one more day . . . lest you lose your sanity, your sense of humor, and direction, you have the option to use your binge day. But follow the following rules precisely.

Before You Binge

1. Drink water.
2. Drink water.
3. Drink water.
4. Rest.
5. Brush your teeth and rinse with your favorite mouthwash.
6. Chew sugarless gum for 20 minutes.

You may find that the desire to binge has passed. However, if you are still suffering from intense food frustration, follow these basic binge rules:

Rule One

Under no circumstances should you ever binge before completing Day Five of your reducing diet. This will ensure a maximum weight loss with a minimum of food frustration.

Rule Two

If, for example, you binge on the sixth day of your diet, resume your diet the following day (Day Seven) with the menu for Day Six. If you binge for just one meal, such as lunch on Day Six, resume your reducing diet with dinner on Day Six of your reducing diet.

Rule Three

Bingeing is for when you get that creepy, anxious feeling, when you feel like pulling out your hair—strand by strand—and you cannot endure dieting for even one more moment. Before you climb the walls, give yourself a binge day. It's hoped that this will not be necessary more than four times a month.

Rule Four

After you have lost your first 10 pounds, you may vary your binge day with the binge day of the sun sign opposite yours, which is Gemini.

Remember, an occasional binge day—when necessary—will still allow you to lose weight (without guilt). Here, Sagittarius, is your binge day menu.

Binge Day Menu

BREAKFAST

6 oz. apple juice

2 Aunt Jemima blueberry waffles with 2 tsp. Featherweight diet maple syrup

2 strips bacon

coffee with 1 Tbsp. Cool Whip dessert topping

LUNCH

1 slice pizza

10 french fries

½ cup vanilla ice milk

no-sodium diet soda or Perrier with an orange twist

MIDAFTERNOON SNACK

2 gingersnap cookies

DINNER

4 oz. glass dry white wine (optional)

4 oz. veal scallopine with ½ can artichokes (or ½ 9 oz. frozen package)

1 medium-sized baked potato with 1 Tbsp. sour cream and chives

Bird's Eye french-style long grain rice, french-style green beans, diced onions, wild rice, and mushrooms

EVENING SNACK

1 cup air-blown popcorn with 1 tsp. diet margarine dripped on top

Remember, drink 8 glasses of water every day.

Maintaining Your Ideal Weight

Sagittarius Maintenance Foods for Optimum Health

When you have achieved your desired weight goal you should follow a maintenance diet rich in the specific nutrients that you, Sagittarius, need each and every day.

Vitamin C

One of the more important functions that vitamin C performs is aiding in the formation of collagen. Collagen is a substance which makes up over 40 percent of the body's protein. It is absolutely crucial to the maintenance of strong, healthy bones, cartilage, and tendons, which Sagittarius must protect because you are prone to accidents and especially susceptible to fractures of the thighs and hips.

Vitamin C also helps to maintain the elasticity of capillaries, veins, and arteries, troublesome areas for Sagittarius who rules the iliac arteries and veins.

FOODS RICH IN VITAMIN C

Alfalfa	Beets
Almonds	Blueberries
Apples	Broccoli
Asparagus	Brussels sprouts
Bananas	Cantaloupe

333

Carrots
Celery
Chicken
Cranberries
Currants
Grapefruit
Green peppers
Lemons
Oranges

Orange juice
Paprika
Parsley
Pineapple
Skim milk
Strawberries
Tomatoes
Watercress

Vitamin B-6

Vitamin B-6, important for the maintenance of healthy muscle functioning, is a must for you, Sagittarius, because your sign rules the upper leg muscles. A deficiency of B-6 produces muscle weakness. Vitamin B-6 also aids in the distribution of water in the fatty tissues. Lack of vitamin B-6 can cause cholesterol deposits to collect in veins, a dangerous condition for Sagittarius, who is predisposed to pulmonary disease.

FOODS RICH IN VITAMIN B-6

Alfalfa sprouts
Avocados
Bananas
Beef liver
Brewer's yeast
Cabbage
Chicken (white meat)
Chicken liver
Egg yolk
Fish
Green peppers
Honey

Lamb
Lentils
Mackerel
Peanuts
Prunes
Salmon
Skim milk
Sunflower seeds
Tuna
Turkey
Wheat germ
Whole milk

Vitamin K

Vitamin K is crucial to normal blood clotting. It is needed to synthesize four of the five coagulation factors that cause blood to clot when there is internal hemorrhaging. Vitamin K also seems to be important in the metabolism of fat.

FOODS RICH IN VITAMIN K

Alfalfa	Corn
Asparagus	Eggs
Bananas	Green peas
Bran	Liver
Broccoli	Milk
Brussels sprouts	Mushrooms
Cabbage	Spinach
Camembert cheese	Strawberries
Carrots	Tomatoes
Cauliflower	Watercress
Cheddar cheese	Wheat germ

Inositol, Choline, and Biotin

Inositol aids in the oxidation of carbon dioxide. Along with choline, it plays an essential part in metabolism and fat distribution. The two also work together to synthesize lipids, such as lecithin. Biotin also takes part in the metabolism of lipids, carbohydrates, and proteins. Recent research shows biotin may reduce the incidence of high cholesterol, hypoglycemia, and diabetes, blood diseases to which Sagittarius is prone. Although all three of these vitamin-like substances are synthesized in the body, the amounts synthesized internally are insufficient and must be supplemented dietarily.

FOODS RICH IN INOSITOL

Alfalfa sprouts	Lamb
Apples	Lentils
Cantaloupe	Peanuts
Carrots	Rice
Cauliflower	Strawberries
Cheese	Sunflower seeds
Chicken	Tomatoes
Eggs	Veal
Grapefruit	Watermelon
Halibut	

FOODS RICH IN CHOLINE

Alfalfa sprouts	Beef
Apples	Carrots
Asparagus	Caviar

Eggs	Rice
Green beans	Spinach
Lamb	Trout
Liver	Veal
Milk products	Wheat germ

FOODS RICH IN BIOTIN

Alfalfa	Lamb
Almonds	Lentils
Avocado	Liver
Bananas	Peanuts
Beef	Rice
Cauliflower	Strawberries
Cheese	Sunflower seeds
Eggs	Tomatoes
Halibut	Veal
Heart	Watermelon
Kidney	

Lecithin

Lecithin, as stated above, is manufactured by inositol and choline combining. Its primary job is burning up excess fat. Lecithin also forms an important portion of brain and nervous tissue—about 17 percent of the brain consists of lecithin. Lecithin also helps prevent the formation of cholesterol, which could lead to pulmonary problems. The inclusion of foods rich in lecithin helps protect the Sagittarius sensitive circulatory system.

FOODS RICH IN LECITHIN

Almonds	Rice
Avocado	Sesame seeds
Barley	Tuna
Beef	Turkey
Chicken	Veal
Liver	Wheat
Milk	

Zinc

Zinc is an essential mineral involved in the synthesis of protein and in enzyme action. Remember, Sagittarius, you need a relatively high-protein diet. Zinc in conjunction with vitamin C really helps to strengthen your immune system.

If you are diabetic or a heavy drinker, you need higher intakes of zinc.

FOODS RICH IN ZINC

Beef	Onions
Eggs	Pumpkin seeds
Lamb	Soy beans
Milk	Sunflower seeds
Mushrooms	Wheat germ

Sagittarius Sample Maintenance Menu

When you reach your desired goal, please follow the maintenance eating hints found in the "General Diet and Maintenance Guidelines for All Sun Signs" at the beginning of this book for proper calculations of caloric intake.

I'm including a sample maintenance menu based on your sun sign for optimal Sagittarius maintenance. When you create your own menus for yourself, try to choose many of the foods you eat from your Sagittarius Maintenance Foods lists.

2,000 Calories Per Day

BREAKFAST

½ fresh grapefruit	37
2 slices Downyflake french toast	270
with 1 Tbsp. Featherweight syrup	17
3 links Morning Star breakfast sausages	114
coffee, tea	0
	——
	438

LUNCH

4 oz. wine (optional)	83
Fresh fruit salad	60

Shrimp and pasta salad:

½ cup shrimp (sautéed quickly in lemon)	80
½ cup noodles	108
diced tomato, mushrooms, green pepper, scallions	30
2 tsp. sesame oil	80
2-inch slice garlic bread	80

	521

MIDAFTERNOON SNACK

1 Danny-in-a-Cup frozen yogurt	180

DINNER

1 light beer (optional)	95

2 tacos:

2 tortilla shells stuffed with	134
⅗ oz. lean ground beef chuck	214
diced tomato, onion, green pepper	30
¼ cup grated cheddar cheese	113
topped with Ha Cha Cha sauce	10
½ avocado served with sliced tomato	153

	749

EVENING SNACK

2 cups Jolly Time microwave popcorn with natural butter flavor	110

TOTAL DAILY CALORIES	1,998

Remember, drink 8 glasses of water every day.

Restaurant Eating the Sagittarius Way

Perhaps you have seen the following dishes on restaurant menus. Both the dishes and the types of restaurants chosen will appeal to your Sagittarius palate and satisfy your nutritional needs. Your lust for foreign fare has not been forgotten. You love to travel, and if you can't get there by air, train or sea, you'll get there via food. With this menu you can explore Italy, France, and Mexico.

In all menus, one appetizer plus one entrée equals approximately 600–700 calories.

Italian Restaurant

APPETIZERS

Stuffed mushrooms

Sliced mozzarella and tomatoes

ENTRÉES

Eggplant stuffed with ricotta cheese, baked in a light tomato sauce

Veal, sage, and prosciutto on a bed of spinach

Durum wheat pasta and Italian vegetables*

Veal sautéed with tomato, mushrooms, and peppers

* If your choice, eliminate appetizer.

Mexican Restaurant

APPETIZERS

Tortilla with salsa (baked, not fried)

Nachos, baked

ENTRÉES

Chicken enchiladas

Red snapper, served with a vegetable and tomato sauce

Chicken or beef tacos (ask that the tortilla be baked, not fried)

Stuffed green peppers

French Restaurant

APPETIZERS

Artichoke in vinaigrette dressing

Baked snails in wine and garlic

ENTRÉES

Frogs legs sautéed in lemon

Fricassee of chicken in raspberry vinegar

Choucroute of fresh salmon with cabbage

Loin of lamb with fresh mint

American Restaurant

APPETIZERS

Fresh-cut fruit slices

Chopped chicken livers

ENTRÉES

Pasta and spinach salad with mussels

Veal stew

Barbecued veal chop

Rib-eye steak

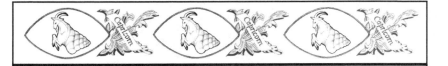

CAPRICORN

December 22–January 20

The Capricorn Personality

"He that is master of himself will soon be master of others."

If you are aware of and emphasize the positive personality traits with which you were born, this diet will work for you. You, Capricorn, are, most of the time, an excellent dieter, because there is a part of you that handles the rigors of self-denial quite well. You have a healthy respect for self-control. You are very disciplined, goal oriented, well-organized, have great determination and tremendous inner strength. You love and need a challenge. What a powerhouse of fine qualities to bring to this diet.

To the above you can add great willpower, tenacity, and perseverance; and you are very good at adhering to details. You are a cautious person. You consider yourself the master of your own destiny, and will search to find the perfect solution to everything. Not surprising, you usually do find it. Your strong convictions and your ability to overcome almost all obstacles certainly say, "Okay. I am ready to start dieting and I won't allow myself or anyone else to sabotage my plans."

Now that you are feeling pretty good about yourself, I know that you will take your dieting commitment seriously. You take all commitments seriously. You are not afraid to put in the effort it takes to stick with a diet because you believe that you get what you work for. You set lofty goals and you reach them. No matter how long you have to pursue something, the knowledge that you will ultimately succeed keeps you right on course. You are truly the sign that understands the adage, "knowledge is power."

One of the major causes of illness for Capricorn is your tendency to bottle up emotions—in fact, you sometimes give the impression of not having any. Capricorns will carefully conceal pain so no one knows you are suffering. Your innate sense of dignity and propriety inhibits you from expressing your innermost feelings. You like to keep a low profile and you really don't feel comfortable being with people who go overboard expressing their emotions. You have a tendency to be shy and, perhaps, more serious than your friends. You must work to develop a sense of compassion for your own weaknesses and those of others. And, most importantly Capricorn, you must learn to release your tensions, both physically and verbally.

Your career is one of the most important things in your life. You have a tendency to be a workaholic, and often expect other people to have the same ability and tendency. You are a hard taskmaster but never ask anyone to do something you would not do yourself. If you don't allow enough time to do a job perfectly, you'll come up with the perfect excuse—"But I didn't have enough time." The Capricorn personality does not thrive being pushed or threatened. You will respond to reason and a sense of duty. The best way to approach you is to appeal to your need to be needed.

You like to follow tried and true methods and often reflect on the past. You have an excellent memory for days gone by and remember the smallest details of events that happened long ago. You use life's experiences, rather than intuition, as guidelines for most decision making. But destiny somehow has a way of piling up the pounds, and though Capricorn is usually moderate in eating and drinking, even the most controlled Capricorn will at one point need to diet. However, that is a fact that you will not share with anyone. You will just diet—and won't talk about it. You are hypersensitive about weight gain because you feel it is a sign of weakness and loss of control. And to lose control is intolerable to you.

Capricorns are perfectionists and also demand perfection in their body. Your body represents a strong and firm foundation and you intend to take care of it for the rest of your life. This gives you a deep concern for the foods you consume and this is why you are probably opposed to eating foods with additives and preservatives.

Capricorns worry. You worry about your business, your family, your health, yesterday's news and tomorrow's IRS audit. You worry about social security and your pension plan, even if you are not due to collect it for twenty years. Under pressure you might throw caution to the wind. When your life becomes emotionally stressing, you become irritable, depressed, detached. At this point, if you decide to binge, it will be with ice cream, creamy malteds, pies, cakes, breads, and traditional foods like Momma used to make. You were born with a wisdom beyond your years, however, and you old goats are much too responsible and self-controlled to indulge very long in a devil-may-care diet.

Sexual Appetite

You are a tiger or tigress in the boardroom, but you are somewhat timid and modest in the bedroom. Capricorns are in need of a great deal of touching, holding, loving, and sex. And while you are not the most demonstrative sign of the zodiac, on a one-to-one basis you are quite smoldering, sexy Capricorn, capable of great sexual endurance. You Capricorns need to learn to show more of your sexual vulnerability. You need a little dose of immoral courage. And you need proof. You will devise little tests to prove that love is real. When you commit to a sexual relationship it must provide protection and security.

When the sexual revolution arrived along with the women's movement, for the first time it seemed possible that women could receive the same sexual gratification as men, with no strings attached. Capricorn women discovered lust and passion, and it was an important discovery; however, lust and passion only with nice men. Sometimes, Capricorn, you are torn between the right kind of person and the person who turns you on. Many a Capricorn has gained weight pondering this difficult choice.

Letting go sexually involves an opening up—both physically and emotionally. And that sort of opening up involves trust. It means saying, "I'm going to feel whatever I feel at a given moment. If I feel passionate, I'm not going to hold myself back." The ability to let go is no small task for you. However, once you do, you will emerge radiant and in touch with your sexuality.

Usually, Capricorn, you have a lot of patience with your mate because you are willing to struggle like a mountain goat to reach the top of the mountain. David Viscott, noted psychologist, must have had Capricorns in mind when he said:

> Relationships seldom die because they suddenly have no life left in them. They wither slowly, either because people do not understand how much or what kind of upkeep, time, work, love and caring they require or because people are too lazy or afraid to try. A relationship is a living thing. It needs and benefits from the same attention to detail that an artist lavishes on his art.

You Capricorns are extremely loyal sexual partners and demand the same loyalty from your mate. When sex is not readily available, or if you have been turned down by your partner, you may confuse sexual hunger with physical hunger. You go right to the refrigerator. And what do you eat? Bread, ice cream, or some other sweet. While satisfying your sweet tooth will temporarily make up for the feeling of rejection, you will pay for it in excess pounds in the long run.

If you become more aware of and learn to monitor this problem, you will find that you have a better handle on some of the subconscious patterns that make you eat for the sexually lean times. Plan ahead. Have other options readily available: Read a good book, exercise, jump rope, jog.

Most important, you must communicate your needs to your partner. Often, dear Capricorn, the problem is that you cannot or do not ask for sex as often as you would like it. That's your homework assignment; it will help keep you skinny.

Eating/Entertaining at Home

The Capricorn home says, "welcome." It bespeaks your love of comfort, earthiness, and tradition, and in it your dinner guests will always find a pleasant refuge. You eschew the decorated look for the personal touch, and whether your style is strictly of a period or passionately eclectic the effect will be undeniably soft and cushiony. Your furnishings tend to be classic, understated, accented by beautiful artifacts, oriental rugs, quality wood tables, unusual collectibles. Your own handicrafts are likely to be on display, probably near your favorite spot in the house, your wood-burning fireplace.

For you, entertaining at home is an opportunity to share the love, life, and friendship of your guests. You have the ability to throw a dinner party worthy of the award of excellence and still provide your company with a sense they are partaking in a simple, satisfying home-cooked meal. A damask tablecloth sets the stage of your formal dining room table, adorned with sterling silverware, individualized crystal salt and pepper shakers, fresh-cut flowers, and your favorite limited-edition china. (You are the type to turn over a plate just to make note of its origin.) You are thoroughbreds and entertain with an innate touch of class. You take great pains to organize the seating arrangements, and are very conscious of the likes and dislikes of your guests. (You are likely to keep such information catalogued, along with your recipes, on your home computer.) You love on such occasions to bring out your favorite vintage wine from your cabinet and present it to your guests with an introductory speech about its heritage that would impress the toughest critic.

As for the meal, you will choose from a repertoire of dishes based on award-winning recipes from Betty Crocker and *Good Housekeeping*, from your mother's favorite specialties, or from traditional holiday menus. You maintain a well-organized recipe box which enables you to adapt your meals to anyone's tastes without requiring extraordinary expense, and your butcher-block kitchen is designed for your practical methods of cooking.

Many of your childhood memories are intertwined with the aromas and flavors of long-ago meals. And you enjoy preparing hot chocolate or hearty franks and sauerkraut for your own family and friends because you feel you are enriching their own future memories of their time with you. You are definitely a family-oriented person who is quite traditional. Thanksgiving, Christmas, Passover—holiday celebrations with all the customary trimmings—are always celebrated in your home. Lots of Capricorns own pianos because you associate the solid massiveness of this instrument with stability, permanence, security. Besides, nothing pleases you more than to have your company sing along with some nostalgic tunes. You almost feel that it is your responsibility as a mother, father, daughter, son . . . or *Capricorn,* to make these holidays festive.

With food so symbolic of sentiment and love, you must work extra hard to stay with a diet, Capricorn. You often say to yourself, "How can I resist joining my loved ones for a midnight snack?" Well, just think about how often you have soothed your harried nerves with a tall glass of milk and a generous hunk of chocolate cake only to regret the calories later, and I know you realistic Capricorns will find the inner resolve to forego any future late-night parties around the kitchen table.

When all is said and done, you usually do not like fancy preparations if you are not entertaining, despite your superb culinary skills and the fact that it warms your heart to feed a friend. You consider it a waste of time to spend your life cooking and cleaning when there are more important things to be done—like working.

Food Shopping

Before you go food shopping you are sure to check to see what food items need to be replaced. No double guessing for you, Capricorn. You have a sophisticated (practically computerized) system for filing coupons. You have even thought about marketing your own food-shopping program. You often write your list according to the arrangement of the supermarket; or at the very least you have grouped items into categories, such as "dairy," "household," "frozen foods." This precision almost always guarantees that you will arrive home without forgotten purchases.

Because you often worry about the future and the unknown, you tend to plan ahead when it comes to buying groceries. You have enough food supplies tucked away in your cupboard, or freezer, to enable you to whip up a first-class meal, literally from soup to nuts, should the unexpected happen—uninvited company arriving at your door, a sudden earthquake, snowstorm, avalanche! Your motto, remembered since your childhood scouting days, still remains: Be prepared.

You know where to spend and where to save. You always bring back bottles and redeem cents-off coupons. If there is a "special," the Capricorn will buy it. If it is sold in bulk, you will surely purchase it. You are an incredible bargain hunter and will travel great distances to get the best discounts, then freeze and save the bargains you bought. You go through almost as much freezer paper and aluminum foil as toilet tissue. Your careful methods of food preparation do not always allow for shortcuts, however. Convenience products and TV Dinners have always been regarded as something less than substantial. Capricorns are frugal and resourceful. You will closely watch the cashier at the checkout counter as he or she rings up your merchandise, and you will not be too shy to request a recheck of the register because, "there is no way those few items could add up to so much." You are very loyal to neighborhood vendors, even so. You often create goodwill and as a result get just a little bit more service and price breaks than other patrons. You are food savvy, and your local grocers learn fast enough that no one can pull the wool over Capricorn's eyes. You have a collection of helpful shopping hints worthy of a professional home economist. Some food and diet wisdom my practical Capricorn friends have taught me:

- "Delicious" apples are the sweetest and the best.
- Contrary to Chiquita Banana, you can store them in the refrigerator when ripe—they last longer.
- Diet bread is often ordinary bread sliced thinner. Look for calories per ounce.
- Anything that is marked "dietetic" is immediately twice the price.

You hate to see food wasted, Capricorn. If an item is a day old or not looking too fresh, you will bring it to the attention of the supermarket manager and then request a discount. Tonight's dinner is sure to include the freshest and ripest groceries you bought this afternoon, and the week's menus will be carefully planned around the food on hand in your refrigerator. Of course, you always turn packages over to see the pull date before you purchase them. One of these days, some impossible package code like 6-7-1-2-1 will be cracked by a feisty Capricorn.

Social Dining

Think about your dinner last night, Capricorn. You were dining alone and, as always in your singular state, you ate very simply. You have been known to frequent the local delicatessen when the urge for a hot pastrami or corned beef sandwich becomes overwhelming. But your choice yesterday was a good old-fashioned cafeteria with steam tables, plenty of hot food, and inexpensive prices.

Now, *social* dining is altogether a horse of another color. Then you like to dine in fine restaurants. Admit it, Capricorn, there is a part of you that is a social climber, and especially in business you feel it is important to impress your clients with the choice of a superb restaurant, perhaps one in which the maître d' greets you by name. You enjoy transacting business where you might be noticed. Let us not forget, making the proper business deal means money to Capricorn, and money represents security in your life. You are smart enough to keep your alcohol consumption to a minimum because you would never want to lose control. Fortunately, this helps curb the temptation to stray from your diet on these endless "power" breakfasts, luncheons, dinners.

You do like to keep your life as predictable as possible. You often consult restaurant guides because you like to know what you are in for. When you find a restaurant you like, you will go back to it over and over again, even several times in the same week. You are never entirely comfortable choosing from a menu with no prices. And even at one of the finer dining establishments, you will send back your food if it has not been properly prepared: It has to be perfect!

When you are not closing some important business deal, you hard-driving Capricorns do know how to create romance. You are apt to choose a French bistro where the melodic chords of a violin and harp are heard in the background and the decor, the food and the people are *très* chic. But your personal preference on an evening out with friends might lead you to a hearty American dinner at a rustic old inn where potbellied stoves are burning and a potbellied chef reminds you of James Beard. You enjoy the country charm of wood paneling, richly colored upholstery, and overstuffed chairs. Underneath it all, you Capricorns are steak-and-potatoes types. Somehow, it is difficult to imagine you ordering consommé, even the jellied kind. Do you even know what color it is?

Special-Occasion Dining

Normally, you Capricorns are quite reserved and responsible, and that is why special occasions are so troublesome for you—just because they are special. You tend to give yourself license at these times to do what you wouldn't consider doing at any other, that is, let yourself go. You get surprisingly sentimental at such events as Christmas, your birthday, your mother's birthday, even your cat's birthday. But please beware. These feelings should not be interpreted as signals to digress from your diet. Should your cat's birthday take place during your ten-day diet, it is all right to celebrate, but choose wisely, eat small portions of whatever you wish. Do not worry about offending the host or hostess, and for goodness' sake remember: It is only one meal, not an excuse for a three-day feast.

Plan your own event if you are in the mood to attend one. You are generally so habitual in your behavior, that any activity out of the usual is something for you to look forward to, even if the occasion is unrelated to food. If it's a wedding, think of the occasion as time to dance. If it's a picnic, think of it as an opportunity to play a game of softball, volleyball, or horseshoes. Allow yourself to enjoy the pleasure of doing something different, and it will satisfy you just as much as overindulging in goodies.

I know I can depend on you Capricorns to take the necessary precautions to avoid blowing your diet completely when a tempting occasion arises. First of all, you can prepare by cutting down your food intake the day before a festivity, and also on the day following, in order to successfully continue your weight-loss program. You can also cook or bake something in advance to take along to the special occasion. You love to do things like that anyway, and that way you can guarantee all the ingredients in at least one dish are low-calorie. No guilt, no remorse, no cheating, no negative thoughts. Just forgive yourself this one special meal and just pick up your diet wherever you left off.

Your Health

As adults, Capricorns are known to have strong, healthy bodies, although as children your constitution is sometimes fragile and weak. Cramps and stomachaches often kept you home from school in your youth. Sensitive, worrisome Capricorn, your stomach is often the barometer of your emotions. Whenever you are in a stressful situation or undergoing emotional upheaval, your stomach starts to churn. It is a weakness you have learned to camouflage as you have gotten older, appearing calm and confident to the rest of the world. However, your cool exterior does not fool your digestive organs. Your constant drive for success and your ambitious, hardworking nature can wreak havoc on your nerves, and there are times you worry so much about your health that friends might have said you are a hypochondriac.

You should never eat when you are upset. Shoving food in your mouth to assuage nervous tension is not what your Capricorn body needs. You need to take a big breath, sit down, and relax. It is especially important that you develop some outside recreation hobby that is simply fun. It will serve to bring a little more balance in your otherwise hard-driving life. You know, Cap, you place too much emphasis on your career and station in life.

In medical astrology, Capricorn rules the patella, knees, joints, bones, epidermis, process of the gallbladder, and by reflex action the stomach.

Diseases to which Capricorns are subject, but which may or may not manifest themselves in your lifetime, include:

Allergies	Glaucoma
Arthritis and rheumatism	Hearing disorders
Curvature of the spine	Poor posture
Dental problems	Problems in the joints
Depression	Sciatica
Excess calcium deposits	Skin diseases (rashes, eczema)
Excess perspiration	Slipped disks
Frequent colds	Sluggish circulation
Gallbladder problems	Weak knees

Your ruling cell salt is calcium phosphate which helps to build strong bones and teeth. Cell salts are naturally occurring minerals that are normal constituents of the body cells. They are found in trace amounts in foods, and plants, animals, and human beings require these compounds for proper nutrition. And, like vitamins, cell salts get used up.

FOODS RICH IN CALCIUM PHOSPHATE

Almonds	Cucumbers
Asparagus	Egg yolk
Barley	Lean meats
Beans	Plums
Blueberries	Spinach
Cabbage	Strawberries
Celery	Whole wheat

The Capricorn diet must be high-protein, rich in foods that contain high amounts of vitamins A, all the B's, but especially riboflavin (B-2), C, D, E, calcium, lecithin, and fiber. Lack of these nutrients may cause gall stones, or burning sensation in the upper chest, pain beneath one or both shoulder blades, sharp chest pains, and an inability to catch your breath. Sometimes, you may experience trouble assimilating calcium, so you should be sure to include milk and milk products as often as possible. In addition, because of your sensitive stomach, it would be wise to avoid very cold or iced drinks. And don't worry so much.

Your Capricorn Reducing Diet has taken all of the above nutritional needs into account to guarantee you your weight will be lost and you will feel better than ever.

Capricorn Daily Nutritional Supplements

- One general multivitamin with minerals
- One multiple vitamin B-complex (B-100)
- 2,000 mg vitamin C with bioflavonoids
- 200 IU units vitamin E
- 600–800 mg Os-Cal (calcium carbonate from oyster shells)

Remember, Capricorn...

This diet is especially prepared to address your sun sign and *should not be interchanged with any other Sun Sign Diet.* It is important that you follow the diet exactly as it appears, for optimum weight loss and assimilation. Before starting your Capricorn diet, carefully read the "General Diet and Maintenance Guidelines for All Sun Signs" found at the beginning of this book. Remember, drink 8 glasses of water daily.

After you reach your desired weight, turn to the end of the chapter and you will find a long list of the maintenance foods you should incorporate in your diet of programmed Capricorn eating for the rest of your life. Remember, that these are the special foods that your body needs.

Make this a lifetime of eating with the stars.

The Capricorn Ten-Day Reducing Diet

Capricorn, this is a down-to-earth, realistic diet designed for your maximum weight loss and will allow you to gain control over your eating problems. You will find that the Capricorn Ten-Day Reducing Diet will meet the demands of your active life-style as well as your nutritional, chemical, and metabolic requirements for good health, putting you back in control of your eating behavior.

The first three days are supercharged with fruit, an important aid in the digestion and assimilation process. Fruits act as a catalyst, firing up your metabolic system to burn proteins and carbohydrates more efficiently. Days Five through Ten offer many options within the reducing day categories to allow you some freedom in planning your menus. I know I can count on your self-discipline and motivation to follow this precisely.

Your Sun Sign Diet even provides for your cravings for creamy comfort foods. You will find the day of bananas and milk totally satisfying while still allowing you to stay in control of your diet.

To further speed up your weight loss and suppress your appetite, you may choose to try a diet aid known in the United States as Glucomannan. It is extracted from the Japanese konjac root, a tuber that is very high in fiber. A final monograph on its effectiveness has not yet been established by the FDA, as it has no history of use in the United States before 1958; however, the konjac root has been cultivated and eaten in Asia for over a thousand years.

Glucomannan contributes to a decrease in cholesterol and triglyceride levels, and aids in maintaining low-density lipoprotein levels. It acts as a dietary fiber to increase viscosity and moisture content of food as it is digested, so that it forms a smooth, soft mass that moves easily through the intestinal tract. Digestion is slowed, so normal blood sugar levels are maintained after a meal. Two capsules taken three times a day may cut your appetite in half!

Please note the asterisked (*) items which appear after certain foods listed in your menu plan. You will find a detailed explanation of their vitamin and mineral content, and direct information as to why they are essential components of your successful diet regimen located in the section, "Notes to Capricorn Ten-Day Reducing Diet."

Follow the diet exactly as designed; do not mix your menus. Eat what is scheduled for that day. (If you do not want something, leave it out, but do not substitute.) This diet is nutritiously balanced so as to allow you to use it for the duration of your entire weight loss. Just repeat the ten menus to see results week after week.

Underneath that cool, disciplined façade of yours, Capricorn, you really are a mere mortal soul like the rest of us. With this in consideration, I have included a binge day for you too. When you begin to feel that you are really going to lose your cool—absolutely blow your top, use your Capricorn Total Binge Day. But remember, no more than four times a month.

This dynamic diet combined with your self-control and discipline, Capricorn, is your key to success.

Good luck, and *go for it.*

DAY ONE—ALL FRUIT DAY*

BREAKFAST
>1 apple or 1 whole grapefruit

LUNCH
>an assorted fresh fruit plate—up to 3 cups of any fruit you wish
>
>black coffee, tea, or water
>
>*Absolutely nothing else.*

MIDAFTERNOON SNACK
>1 whole grapefruit

DINNER
>an assorted fresh fruit plate—up to 3 cups of any fruit you wish
>
>black coffee,* tea, or water (no diet soda today*)
>
>*Absolutely nothing else.*
>
>*Remember, drink 8 glasses of water every day.*

DAY TWO—ALL BANANA AND MILK DAY*

BREAKFAST

> 1 banana and 8 oz. skim milk or buttermilk (put in blender with ice cubes, add sweetener)

LUNCH AND DINNER

> 4 bananas and 2 more glasses of skim milk or buttermilk, spaced throughout the day

> (You may freeze peeled bananas in aluminum foil. Freeze for at least 4 hours; may be left in freezer up to 4 days. They taste like ice cream.)

> *Remember, drink 8 glasses of water every day.*

DAY THREE—FRUIT AND PROTEIN DAY

BREAKFAST AND LUNCH

Choice of:

1 whole fresh pineapple*

4 whole papayas*

4–5 cups fresh strawberries*

DINNER

Choose satisfying portions* of:

baked or broiled chicken, turkey, filet of sole, flounder, lean meat, or veal chop

and

2 sliced tomatoes seasoned with basil and oregano

BEVERAGE

no-sodium seltzer, no-sodium Perrier, café espresso with a twist of lime, tea, Red Zinger, or an herbal tea of choice

Remember, drink 8 glasses of water every day.

DAY FOUR

BREAKFAST

4 oz. cranberry juice or orange juice

¼ cup bran buds or flakes*
1 cup skim milk

LUNCH

4 oz. sliced chicken, turkey, or cold roast beef

1 Wasa Crisp Bread

salad: lettuce, sliced tomato, fresh mushrooms, watercress, and parsley, seasoned with 2 Tbsp. Pritikin no-oil salad dressing or lemon juice and herbs

iced tea, hot tea, no-sodium club soda, diet soda, or seltzer

SNACK

10–15 pistachio nuts

DINNER

4 oz. glass white wine or champagne (optional)

6 oz. any broiled or baked fish in lemon juice, with 1 cup linguine* mixed with 2 Tbsp. Mexican salsa*

salad of watercress,* parsley,* arugula, and radishes

café espresso with lemon peel or your choice of beverage

or

Crabmeat and Artichoke Surprise

6 oz. fresh or frozen crabmeat (any supermarket)
9 oz. box frozen artichokes
Defrost both and mix artichokes with 8 black olives, ½ cup plain yogurt, 3 scallions, one bunch watercress.* Beat in blender and pour over crabmeat.

D-Zerta diet gelatin—as much as you want

Remember, drink 8 glasses of water every day.

DAYS FIVE THROUGH TEN

You have a choice of five breakfasts and five lunches. You may vary them, or eat the same one every day. The choice is yours. Each choice is combined to release the highest amount of energy and nutrition for you. You can eliminate but you cannot add or change the combinations given. Do not exceed programmed quantities if you wish to achieve maximum results.

BREAKFAST
> Choice of:
>
> 1 cup plain yogurt
>
> > *or*
>
> 4 oz. skim-milk ricotta cheese
>
> > *or*
>
> 4 oz. Light n' Lively cottage cheese,* sprinkled with 2 Tbsp. unsalted sunflower seeds*; sugar substitute, and cinnamon may be added if desired
>
> coffee with a little milk, tea, or herbal tea
>
> > *or*
>
> ### *Strawberry or Papaya Smash Drink**
> Blend 1 cup fresh strawberries or ⅔ cup unsugared frozen strawberries, or one whole papaya with a packet of vanilla Alba 77 skimmilk drink. Beat with 2 ice cubes until frothy.
>
> black coffee, tea, or herbal tea
>
> > *or*
>
> 1½ cups fresh blueberries* or 1 package unsweetened frozen blueberries
>
> black coffee, tea, or herbal tea (sugar substitute allowed, but absolutely no milk products with this breakfast)
>
> > *or*
>
> ### *Scrambled Egg, Cheese and Salsa*
> Scramble one egg in nonstick pan with 2 oz. skim-milk ricotta cheese* and 2 Tbsp. Mexican salsa. Delicious and nutritious.
>
> coffee with milk
>
> > *or*

1 toasted bagel with 1 tsp. cream cheese and diet jam (once per week)

4 oz. unsweetened grapefruit juice or ½ grapefruit

LUNCH

Choice of:

Apple Spinach Cheese Peanut Salad

Raw spinach leaves with 1 sliced apple, 3 oz. Light 'n Lively cottage cheese, 10 unsalted natural Paul's Peanuts (or 5 pecans), and 1 Tbsp. raisins.

café au lait, espresso, or iced tea

or

Pasta Delight with Apple* (once per week)

Eat one whole apple (ten minutes before pasta so that enzymes from apple will act to digest pasta more efficiently).

Pasta

1 cup durum wheat or whole wheat pasta cooked with garlic, pepper, oregano, herbs, and pimentos. Season with 1 tsp. diet margarine.

café espresso, black coffee with lemon peel, or no-sodium club soda with a twist of lime

or

Fresh Fruit Plate

Consisting of ½ cantaloupe, or ½ grapefruit, and ½ orange, ½ pear, ¼ pineapple, ½ apple, and 15 grapes. If eating at restaurant, you may order up to 2 cups absolutely fresh fruit salad.

black coffee, iced tea, hot tea, or herbal tea (absolutely no milk with this meal)

or

Baked Potato Feast*

1 very large baked potato served with ¼ cup plain yogurt and seasoned with dill, chives, scallions, garlic and thyme, served on a bed of lettuce and spinach leaves.

no-sodium diet soda or seltzer with a twist of lime, or hot tea

or

2 Hard-Boiled Eggs Salad

Slice 2 hard-boiled eggs* and serve with 1 whole sliced tomato seasoned with basil and oregano.

1 cup salad consisting of watercress,* spinach, and parsley seasoned with lemon juice and garlic pepper

no-sodium seltzer with a twist of lime or no-sodium diet soda

DINNER

1 cup Lipton Trim Soup (beef, tomato, chicken)

and

Large salad every day consisting of the following:

Broccoli*	Escarole
Cauliflower	Green pepper
Celery	Lettuce
Chinese cabbage	Mushrooms
Cucumber	Spinach
Endive	String beans
	Watercress

Use 2–3 Tbsp. Pritikin no-oil salad dressing, or lemon juice and garlic powder.

Choice of 4–6 oz. baked, broiled, or steamed (no butter, just lemon juice):

Bismarck herring (3½ oz.)*	Halibut
Canned Chinook salmon (4 oz.)	Lobster (1–1½ lb.)*
Chicken*	Pacific sardines (3½ oz.)*
Chicken livers	Red Snapper
Codfish	Salmon
Crabmeat	Shrimp
Filet of sole	Veal
Flounder	

and

Choice of 1 cup: cooked cauliflower, broccoli, spinach, asparagus,* or 1 whole fresh artichoke, served with warm lemon juice and garlic pepper and dill topped with 1 Tbsp. parmesan cheese.

unlimited amounts of D-Zerta diet gelatin or D-Zerta diet gelatin candy (see recipe Sagittarius Diet Notes—Day One) with 2 Tbsp. Cool Whip dessert topping *or*

1 35-calorie strawberry Jell-O frozen pudding pop

decaffeinated coffee, espresso coffee with a twist of lime, tea, rose hip herbal tea, or chamomile, no-sodium seltzer or Perrier

That's it! Repeat Day One to continue diet.

Remember, drink 8 glasses of water every day.

Notes to Capricorn Ten-Day Reducing Diet

Day One

* Fresh fruit is fortified with powerful enzymes which act to digest food, speed up your metabolism, and to rid the body of accumulated toxins. As the fruit begins to cleanse your system, you will notice a feeling of elevation, lightness, energy. The diuretic nature of many of the fruits will result in increased urination today.

* No milk allowed today. If you choose to have coffee for your beverage, it is absolutely imperative that you do not consume even the smallest bit of milk. Milk products will stop the enzyme action of the fruit and you will prevent a good weight loss.

* No diet soda today. The chemicals, additives, and preservatives in diet soda similarly inhibit the enzyme action of the fruit.

Day Two

I am sure that you are pleased with your weight loss this morning, Capricorn, and you will find the same results with today's menu.

* The calcium-rich skim milk or buttermilk combined with a banana (supplying 370 mg of potassium, 33 mg of magnesium, vitamin C and B-6) fills your vitamin requirements. In addition, the above vitamin combination is especially calming to the nerves, a usual Capricorn complaint. You may space your lunch and dinner any way you wish. You will hardly even feel like you are dieting.

Day Three

The fruit and protein combination has been designed for ultimate weight loss but high energy output.

* Once again, your breakfast and lunch is packed with live enzyme fruit. You have a choice of either pineapple, papaya, or strawberries. Pineapple is rich in chlorine, has an invigorating effect upon an overworked liver,

has natural diuretic properties, and it is one of the highest enzyme fruits. Papaya, rich in vitamins C, B, and A, and the enzyme digestive juice "papain," has a soothing effect on the stomach and intestinal tract. Fresh strawberries, are vitamin C-rich and another good choice for you. Do not mix your fruits. Whichever fruit you choose, you must have it at both breakfast and lunch.

* I have not listed a specific amount of protein for your dinner menu; by now, your body is ready to tell you when you have had enough. If you choose to have coffee for a beverage, it must not contain any milk.

Day Four

* Constipation and Capricorn seem to be synonymous. Bran buds or flakes for breakfast today.

* Lunch and dinner are high-riboflavin menus. Remember riboflavin functions as part of a group of enzymes that are involved in the breakdown and utilization of carbohydrates, proteins, and fats.

* Today you have a choice of two dinners. Many of you are looking for linguine or spaghetti at this point in your diet regimen. However, make sure that you use durum wheat linguine or spaghetti.

* Mexican salsa is made of chili peppers which are extremely rich in vitamins A and C. They are good for the digestive and circulatory system.

* It is important that you have your salad of watercress and parsley. Both herbs are rich in calcium and vitamin C and substitute your need for milk.

Days Five through Ten

I can always count on my Capricorn friends for staying well within the guidelines and rules of any diet and for this reason give you the option to make your choices from your programmed meals.

All the breakfast and lunches have been designed for optimum weight loss, while meeting all your Capricorn nutritional requirements. If you do not want to eat everything programmed for a particular meal, leave it out. Make no substitutions.

You will experience a wonderful feeling of well-being as the pounds just melt off.

Some Food Facts You Will Want to Know for Reducing Days Five through Ten

* Blueberries, an excellent enzyme fruit, help to break down fat cells.

* Potatoes are very rich in potassium. It's satiating power will keep the hunger pangs away.

* Asparagus is an excellent diuretic food, containing vitamin B-1 (thia-

min). It also contains the enzyme asparagine, which helps to break up accumulated fats in the cells.

* Sunflower seeds are rich in B-6, potassium, magnesium, calcium, fiber, and lecithin. Especially good for the brain and nerve tissues.

* Hard-boiled eggs have long satiety value, and take almost as much caloric energy to digest as the egg yields. Each egg contains 6 grams of protein. A good source of vitamins A, B-2, D, E, folic acid, phosphorus, and iron.

* Just 3½ oz. broccoli, rich in vitamin A and all the Bs, has 267 mg of potassium and 1.5 mg of fiber.

* 3½ oz. cottage cheese is rich in riboflavin as well as other B vitamins and calcium.

* Chicken is a good source of vitamins B-2, B-3, B-6, B-12, and folic acid.

* 3½ oz. of watercress has 606 mg of potassium, 50 mg of folic acid, and is chock full of vitamins A, B-2, C, as well as fiber.

* Bismarck herring yields 20 grams of protein per serving and is rich in vitamins B-2, B-3, B-6, B-12, and D, phosphorus, calcium, and potassium.

* Sardines supply you with vitamins B-2, B-3, B-12, D, iron, magnesium, potassium, and 525 mg of calcium (that's twice the amount in an 8 oz. glass of milk).

* 3½ oz. cooked lobster meat has 128 grams of protein and only 95 calories.

CAPRICORN TOTAL BINGE DAY

Capricorn, there are times when you need to let go. I have given you that option with a binge day. Now remember, Capricorn, you have a tendency to go overboard, so be careful.

Before You Binge

1. Drink water.
2. Drink water.
3. Drink water.
4. Rest.
5. Brush your teeth and rinse with your favorite mouthwash.
6. Chew sugarless gum for 20 minutes.

You may find that the desire to binge has passed. However, if you are still suffering from intense food frustration, follow these basic binge rules:

Rule Number One

Under no circumstances should you ever binge before completing Day Six of your reducing diet. This will ensure a maximum weight loss with a minimum of food frustration.

Rule Number Two

If, for example, you binge on the sixth day of your diet, resume your diet the following day (Day Seven) with the menu for Day Six. If you binge for just one meal, such as lunch on Day Six, resume your reducing diet with dinner on Day Six of your reducing diet.

Rule Number Three

Bingeing is for when you get that creepy, anxious feeling, when you feel like pulling out your hair—strand by strand—and you cannot endure dieting for even one more moment. Before you climb the walls, give yourself a binge day. It's hoped that this will not be necessary more than four times a month.

Rule Number Four

After you have lost your first 10 pounds, you may vary your binge day with the binge day of the sun sign opposite yours, which is Cancer.

Remember, an occasional binge day—when necessary—will still allow you to lose weight (without guilt). Here, Capricorn, is your binge day menu.

Binge Day Menu

BREAKFAST

½ cantaloupe or ½ orange or 4 oz. orange juice and 1 English muffin or bagel with 1 tablespoon peanut butter and diet jam

café au lait (2 oz. regular milk)

or

½ cantaloupe or ½ orange or 4 oz. orange juice and 1 Aunt Jemima blueberry waffle with 2 Tbsp. diet maple syrup and 1 Tbsp. Cool Whip dessert topping

café au lait (2 oz. regular milk)

LUNCH

1 frankfurter with sauerkraut and mustard on roll

½ cup vanilla, chocolate, strawberry, or coffee ice cream

no-sodium diet soda

or

1 serving Sara Lee cheesecake with 1 cup fresh or frozen strawberries

café au lait (2 oz. regular milk)

or

1 slice pizza with mushrooms

½ cup Tofutti

no-sodium diet soda

DINNER

1 light beer or 4 oz. white wine or sangria (optional)

6 oz. hamburger or ½ barbecued chicken and 10 french fries and large tossed salad with 2 Tbsp. salad dressing of your choice

SNACK

Yoo-Hoo diet chocolate drink with 1 tsp. Cool Whip dessert topping

Maintaining Your Ideal Weight

Capricorn Maintenance Foods for Optimum Health

W hen you have achieved your desired weight goal you should follow a maintenance diet rich in the specific nutrients that you, Capricorn, need each and every day.

Calcium

There is more calcium in the body than any other mineral, and almost all of the body's calcium is found in the bones and teeth. Because 20 percent of an adult's bone calcium has to be replaced every year (due to new bone cell formation, and because old cells break down), it is vital that you replenish your supply of calcium. Capricorn rules over the bones in your body and Capricorns tend to have back problems more than any other sun sign. The proper amount of calcium will help prevent fragile and brittle bones, arthritis, atherosclerosis, leg cramps, acne, and nail problems.

Calcium aids your nervous system, alleviates insomnia, and prevents rickets. In addition, calcium assists the blood clotting process and helps regulate the balance of alkali to acid in the blood. When calcium is combined with magnesium the ratio should be 2:1, twice as much calcium as magnesium. For adults, 800–1200 mg of calcium is the RDA.

Vitamin A

You need vitamin A, Capricorn, to help maintain clear, bright healthy eyes and skin. In fact, vitamin A plays a significant part in protecting your skin from premature aging as well as acne. It is absolutely essential for protein metabolism in the liver where approximately 85 percent of the body's vitamin A is stored. Vitamins A and E play an important part in protecting your lung tissue. However, taking supplementary vitamin A pills can be toxic, and unless advised by your physician should be avoided. Vitamin A should be derived from the following food sources.

FOODS RICH IN VITAMIN A
(Think of yellow and orange-colored fruits and vegetables)

Bananas	Oranges
Beets	Parsley
Broccoli	Peaches
Broiled liver	Potatoes
Cantaloupe	Red chili peppers
Carrots	Salmon
Chicken liver	Squash
Egg yolk	Yams
Mangos	

The B Vitamin Group

The more you worry, the more depressed you become and the more you need a healthy supply of foods rich in vitamin B. I have yet to meet a group of greater "worriers" than Capricorns. The B-complex group maintains muscle tone in the gastrointestinal tract, and aids in the general functioning of the nervous system. A diet supplying sufficient B vitamins makes for a healthy gallbladder.

One very important member of the B-complex group for the Capricorn constitution is vitamin B-2, or riboflavin.

Vitamin B-2 (Riboflavin)

Riboflavin functions as part of a group of enzymes that are involved in the breakdown and utilization of carbohydrates, fats, and protein, and regulates the delicate sodium-potassium balance in the body. Most recently, studies have linked a deficiency of riboflavin with anemia and hypoglycemia (low blood sugar). Stomach cramps, ear infections, and cracks at the corners of your mouth are indications that your riboflavin intake may be too low.

Capricorn, you require more riboflavin foods in your diet than any other sun sign because you do have a proclivity toward problems involving the eyes, such as conjunctivitis, glaucoma, night blindness, cataracts, impaired vision, and eye fatigue. You will note that your Capricorn Reducing Diet is chock full of riboflavin foods.

In combination with vitamin A, riboflavin maintains the health of the mucous membranes throughout the body and especially protects the skin. Oily skin, itching, scaling of the scalp, dermatitis, and even acne should have you questioning your riboflavin intake.

FOODS RICH IN RIBOFLAVIN

All dairy products	Milk
Apples	Papaya
Beef	Parsley
Blueberries	Peanuts
Broccoli	Salmon
Celery	Soybean products
Cottage cheese	Spinach
Dark-green leafy vegetables	Strawberries
Dried apricots	Tomatoes
Eggs	Veal
Lecithin granules	Watercress
Liver	Yogurt
Mangos	

Vitamin C

Vitamin C is one of the vitamins the body cannot manufacture for itself, or store from day to day. This is true for every sign, but for you, Capricorn, it has particular importance.

Vitamin C aids in all forms of gum disease, such as bleeding gums, soft and receding gums, pyorrhea, and tooth cavities—all common Capricorn complaints. (Most Capricorns spend a good deal of time and money at the periodontist.) Vitamin C has been proven to lessen most allergy, hay fever, and asthma problems, and, of course, your usual yearly bout of bacterial and/or viral upper-respiratory infections.

This marvelous vitamin also helps to heal wounds and bone fractures, and it decreases swelling in painful joints. It also helps the body to form collagen, which if retained in insufficient supply, may cause the cells in your bones to lose their supportive strength. Because Capricorns are prone to back and knee problems, you should be certain that you always have an adequate supply of vitamin C, as included in your Capricorn Reducing Diet.

FOODS RICH IN VITAMIN C

Almonds	Grapefruit
Apples	Green peppers
Asparagus	Lemons
Bananas	Oranges
Beets	Orange juice
Blueberries	Parsley
Broccoli	Pineapple
Brussels sprouts	Skim milk
Cantaloupe	Strawberries
Carrots	Tomatoes
Celery	Watercress
Currants	

Vitamin D

Without adequate vitamin D, the body could not properly assimilate calcium. The result would be soft bones. Your back and spine are sensitive areas for all Capricorns and so you must be sure to have an adequate intake of vitamin D.

Vitamin D improves absorption and utilization of the calcium and phosphorus required for bone formation. It also helps regulate the nervous system and your heart's rhythmic action. In addition, recent research indicates that vitamin D may play an important role in alleviating arthritic pain, so often a Capricorn complaint.

FOODS RICH IN VITAMIN D

Bass	Oysters
Butter	Salmon
Cheese	Sardines
Herring	Shrimp
Liver	Sunflower seeds
Mackerel	Tuna
Milk	Watercress
Mushrooms	Yogurt

Bioflavonoids

Bioflavonoids act with vitamin C to prevent cholesterol build up, which can cause clotting of the arteries, veins, and capillaries. Bioflavonoids act with vitamin C to maintain "clean blood." Because of the anticlotting effect, bioflavonoids can also be quite effective in preventing varicose veins.

FOODS RICH IN BIOFLAVONOIDS

(Bioflavonoids are nutrients mainly found in the rinds of citrus fruits.)

Apples	Parsley
Apricots	Peanut butter
Blackberries	Prunes
Black currants	Salmon
Buckwheat	Sardines
Cherries	Shrimp
Grapes	Sunflower seeds
Grapefruit	Sweet potato
Green pepper	Turkey
Lemons	Wheat germ
Oranges	

Vitamin E

Vitamin E's most important function is to serve as an antioxidant and anti-aging vitamin. It prevents red blood cells from combining with toxic peroxide and instead promotes their combining with oxygen. Vitamin E also helps to dissolve blood clots and dilates the blood vessels so that oxygen-rich blood is freely carried to all parts of the body.

Many specific health problems, Capricorn, result from impaired circulation—varicose veins, for example. Because of vitamin E's positive effect on circulation, it both prevents and relieves varicose veins.

FOODS RICH IN VITAMIN E

Apples	Chicken
Asparagus	Eggs
Avocados	Halibut
Broccoli	Liver
Cabbage	Milk
Carrots	Mushrooms
Cheese	Parsley

Lecithin

Lecithin is an emulsifying agent: It breaks down large fat globules into microscopic bits, which helps prevent cholesterol plaque from forming on the walls of your arteries. Lecithin, one of the ingredients in bile, acts to break down fats aiding the function of the gallbladder. Capricorn's do have a sensitivity to gallbladder problems and for this reason it is a good idea to have adequate lecithin in your diet.

FOODS RICH IN LECITHIN

Avocados	Rice
Barley	Sesame seeds
Beef	Sunflower seeds
Chicken	Tuna
Liver	Turkey
Milk	Veal

Capricorn Sample Maintenance Menu

When you reach your desired goal, please follow the maintenance eating hints found in the "General Diet and Maintenance Guidelines for All Sun Signs" at the beginning of this book for proper calculations of caloric intake.

I'm including a sample maintenance menu based on your sun sign for optimal Capricorn maintenance. Try to choose many of the foods you eat from your Capricorn Maintenance Food lists.

2,000 Calories Per Day

BREAKFAST	CALORIES
2-inch wedge honeydew melon	50
2-egg omelette with 1 oz. Swiss cheese,	
made with 1 Tbsp. diet butter	300
1 toasted English muffin	145
coffee or tea	0
	495

LUNCH

4 oz. dry white wine (optional)	75
½ avocado stuffed with ½ cup crabmeat and endive on a bed of lettuce	298
1 dinner roll with 1 tsp. diet butter	130
coffee, tea, or no-sodium diet soda	0
	503

MIDAFTERNOON SNACK

1 cup fresh strawberries	45

DINNER

4 oz. dry red wine (optional)	75
5–6 oz. roast beef	575
1 cup braised celery and mushrooms	50
1 baked potato with 1 Tbsp. sour cream and chives	120
green leafy salad with alfalfa sprouts, watercress, parsley, seasoned with lemon juice, garlic, and dill	100
	920

SNACK

1 cup any flavor ice milk	160

TOTAL DAILY CALORIES   2,123

Remember, drink 8 glasses of water every day.

Restaurant Eating the Capricorn Way

Perhaps you have seen the following dishes on restaurant menus. Maybe you have ordered them, and maybe not. Included here are dishes chosen to specifically appeal to the Capricorn palate. Note that all of the recommended dishes contain the nutrients especially important for you and which are included in your Capricorn Maintenance Foods lists. All the foods listed are prepared lightly and are good restaurant choices for low-calorie eating. Note the high level of calcium foods and vitamin D, especially found in the salmon and sweetbreads. Note the incorporation of pasta and cheese dishes, especially akin to Capricorn. And of course, to complement your very earthy nature, the American bill of fare is especially suited to your taste, Capricorn. In all cases, one appetizer plus one entrée equals approximately 500–600 calories.

French Restaurant

APPETIZERS

Eggplant with caviar

Salad of crabmeat and lemon

ENTRÉE

Seafood baked in a light wine sauce

Loin of lamb with fresh mint

Braised sweetbreads with mushrooms

Chicken in wine sauce

Italian Restaurant

APPETIZERS

Thinly sliced beef with herb sauce

Roasted fresh peppers and anchovies

ENTRÉES

Fettucine and ricotta cheese with sage

Veal in a green basil sauce

Striped bass in wine, capers, and anchovies

Veal cutlet stuffed with ricotta cheese and spinach

Chinese Restaurant

APPETIZERS

Wonton soup

Chicken egg drop soup

ENTRÉES

Diced chicken with broccoli

Sliced beef with watercress and snow peas

Moo Shu pork with 1 cup white rice

Baby shrimp with steamed water chestnuts in garlic sauce

American Restaurant

APPETIZERS

Fresh fruit cup

Jumbo shrimps or clams on the half shell

ENTRÉES

Broiled chicken and ribs

Hamburger every way under the sun

Shrimp and salad bar

Prime ribs au jus

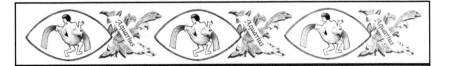

AQUARIUS

January 21–February 19

The Aquarius
Personality

"Let me try that."

Naturally, Aquarius, you would be the first one to start your own Sun Sign Diet. Visionary, open to new ideas, independent, original, experimental, and intuitive, you always dare to test new waters even before others have discovered them. Indeed, you seek them out.

Not that you have an inborn weight problem, at least not compared to other zodiac signs. Quite the contrary, Aquarians tend to be tall and lean. Ruled by the distant planet Uranus, symbol of sudden change, inventiveness, and inspiration, you are so forward-thinking, you sometimes seem to be just a little out of this world. You are so engrossed in your mental pursuits—be it planning your next career move, pursuing yet another cause, or conversing with the waif you lately befriended in the park—you often just forget to eat.

And your hands are usually too busy creating to find their way to your mouth. You might be photographing, painting, or sculpting. Or fine-tuning your newest invention. If your fingers are not actually occupied, the rest of you, body and soul, is probably given over to the experience of airplane flying or to hot-air ballooning or your daily practice of transcendental meditation, yoga, or kung fu.

Humanitarian, individualistic, and unpredictable, you are leaps and bounds ahead of other people—in food, facts, and the future. Many of you February people become vegetarians because you oppose the inhumane treatment and slaughtering of animals, and, of course, you have explored the benefits of a meat-free diet. Intrigued by its philosophy, or just the fact it is something new and different, you might eat according to zen macro-biotics. Generally you believe there is something spiritual about living basically on fruits, grains, vegetables, nuts, and unprocessed foods. On the other end of the spectrum, there are those of you unusual, opinionated, and rebellious Aquarians who are strictly meat-and-potatoes types and swear you will waste away to a feather without a daily quota of animal protein.

But you may also be interested in futuristic foods. You are fascinated by anything to do with space travel, and have probably tried the foods astro-nauts eat. On the other hand, you consume your share of good old Ameri-can junk food, usually the salty variety, like potato chips, corn chips, pretzels, and peanuts. You are mad for anything salty and salt most of your food. No wonder: Your ruling cell salt is sodium chloride, better known as common table salt.

As children, you Aquarians tend to distinguish yourselves with your weird eating habits. Peanut butter and banana sandwiches for breakfast. And lunch. And dinner. Fifty-two weeks out of the year. As adults, your tastes are no less unusual, although they are more prone to change. You love caviar on bagels, applesauce over mashed potatoes, stone-ground whole pumpernickel bread with chili. You will go miles out of your way for a taste of the foods you crave—spinach tortellini, cheesecake, and tart desserts like lemon meringue. You have a special fondness for cucumbers, yogurt, eggplant, and potato salad. Fruits and cold cuts are high on your food list, and you can make a meal of a good salad, especially a Caesar salad with a dash of Worcestershire and Tabasco sauce. You can live on sardines or boursin cheese for days, or go on runs of root beer and brown rice, and you will survive. The truth is, you have only a passing interest in food, for the most part. It is one of life's necessities, and you don't pay much more attention to it than you do to your clothing and shelter—and that isn't much. Your mind tends to be preoccupied with grander things. You prefer foods with a reputation for providing energy. You eat as little as you need to get by and still keep going on your tireless pursuit of the Aquarian.

Friendship is the true consuming passion of the Aquarian. Brotherly—and sisterly—love is perhaps a more accurate term. It is far easier for you to give of yourself to humanity than it is for you to give yourself to a single individual. One representative of the species will serve as well as the next for your investigations into the human condition. Not that your interest at the time is not genuine; it is. It's just generally not sustained, that's all. Inquisitive and restless, you are like the honey bee that alights on a flower, extracts its nectar, and goes on to the next beautiful bloom.

Others may lose themselves in a crowd, but not the humanitarian Aquar-ian. That is where you find yourself. In a peace march, a political conven-tion, an encounter group, any place where people congregate. Everyone is your friend, at least potentially. But to really get close to one person, to sustain an intimate relationship, that is your most difficult challenge. To love some one, first you must be friends, and then you must fall in love with the person's mind. To love you is to love your causes. For you to commit yourself to one relationship, you must feel that the two of you together are a whole truly greater than one. When you do fall in love, you are apt to communicate it in the most novel ways. You may tell your loved one you care by carrier pigeon, walkie-talkie, or satellite transmission, though skywriting is your passion, and it does seem like such a logical way to communicate your thoughts.

You do seem to be at home in the upper reaches of the stratosphere, airy Aquarius. Anyway your mind often seems to be somewhere else besides here on this planet. Sometimes you seem not to be listening, or to be listening in space. You have a way of going off that can be disconcerting to those around you, but you can't help yourself. You need space, and when you find yourself feeling confined or claustrophobic—especially in intimate relationships—off you go into the wild blue yonder. But when you are here, engaged in a passionate discussion about the application of holography to the development of computer technology or exuberantly expounding upon the Russians' fascinating research into the field of parapsychology, you are so present and charming, who can resist?

You live on the wave of the future, scientific Aquarius, and perhaps you like to think the rest of us will catch up with you someday. You love things technological the way a child loves toys. Even your kitchen looks like a stainless-steel monument to space-age cookery. While you do not consider yourself to be the gourmet of the zodiac, you do believe if one must cook, it should be done, in ultramodern convenience. You probably have every imaginable gadget, from a computerized blender to an electronic garlic press—and perhaps you have made them all yourself. Undoubtedly you are the first in the neighborhood to have a domestic robot that cooks, bakes, and cleans up. You believe every household should have one. Not in the future, but *now.* Probably you have track lights and shelves lined with lucite, glass, and chrome utensils and objects. And, last but not least, on your counter is your cordless telephone, an absolute must in the Aquarian home for that unexpected, fast "takeoff" away from it all and into another room. You know how you hunger for freedom and space.

Yes, Aquarius, you even like foods that contain space—airy, puffy, flaky things like whipped cream, meringue, cotton candy, croissants.

Unfortunately, they are not as light as they seem. When you have had a bit too much of these goodies, or the dairy foods, cheeses, and pastas you like to binge on, or one too many exotic meals, you begin to feel weighed down, and then it's time to reduce. Always drawn to the offbeat and unconventional, you are no different when it comes to choosing a diet. Beware, rash Aquarius, this is the one time you should not get caught up in the fly-by-night. You are a fixed sign, so when you do gain weight it is harder for you to lose it. You may go on a fad diet, take off a pound or two, then put it right back on. Well, no more watermelon fasts or grapefruit diets for you, flighty Aquarius. For permanent weight loss, you need something down-to-earth and sensible. Believe it or not, that is the only way to keep that high Aquarian energy flying.

Well, seek no more, wandering one. Your Sun Sign Diet is as unique as you are. It has original recipes for you and you alone, designed to satisfy your exotic cravings at the same time it provides high-energy nutrition. Share your new-found discovery with friends, of course. Start a low-calorie gourmet club. You know how well you feel when you have the comrade-ship and support of a group, and your typical enthusiasm will be inspiration for everyone.

You are about to embark upon the most futuristic diet of your lifetime, Aquarius. It is the breakthrough you've been looking for.

Sexual Appetite

In the mid-1960s, in the iconoclastic rock musical *Hair,* the chorus sang about the "the dawning of the age of Aquarius," while the entire ensemble took off their clothing for the first time in Broadway history. Sexual libera-tion, open marriage, separate vacations—we can probably thank you, Aquarius—or blame you—for all of it. You are not one to abide by custom when there are new horizons to be explored, and that goes as well for sex and marriage as it does for anything else in your life. Your inventiveness can make for a very exciting sex life—as long as it lasts. And if you finally settle down, it will probably be forever. But your need for space and change can make marriage a very difficult proposition for anyone daring enough to try it with you. Or very dynamic for anyone who succeeds.

First of all, you have an irresistible charisma, beautiful Aquarius. Your captivating smile and presence make others want to know you. You know you are unique and sought-after, both for your physical charms and your remarkable intelligence; yet you usually prefer to remain emotionally de-tached. You can be seduced, aloof Aquarius, but your clever lover will have to carve a very intriguing path to your bed—and heart—via the mind. For you, sexual intimacy is always and only an expression of intellectual inti-macy. Your partner must be your friend and companion first, and lover second.

Even then, once you have been lured, your interest in sexual expression may be as erratic as your interest in food. Your need to be unfettered and free usually far surpasses your need for personal intimacy. Eventually, the solitary mood overtakes you, and off you go to cloister yourself in your study or your studio, or maybe to take a space ship to the moon. Or you may simply stay in bed, lost in some impenetrable dreamland right beside your lover. Your total refusal at these times to acknowledge your involvement can be a devastating experience, as anyone knows who has ever had a hot Aquarian lover turn suddenly distant and cold. I know, eccentric Aquarius, that given a little space, you'll be back and hotter than ever. However, your partner may not understand this and may cling in desperation just when you most want to be left alone.

Think about this, Aquarius, the next time you find yourself at your refrigerator door at 2 A.M., feeling dissatisfied and asking the bottom of the container of eggnog you just finished off, "How come no one understands me? When I tell someone I just need some space, it doesn't mean I'm not interested, it just means I need space!" Well, you do have this way of putting yourself on another planet and radioing back to earth, you are not to be bothered. "Understand me or leave me" is a pretty tough assignment even for the most dedicated partner. Understanding usually requires communication, and not everyone in the zodiac is blessed with your extrasensory perception, Aquarius. Many of us still need to resort to old-fashioned methods, like the personal conversation.

So, if you have been overeating lately and feeling sexually ungratified, let me make a suggestion. Start right now to try for a little more intimacy in your life—emotional intimacy. Scare you? All Aquarians have an unconscious fear that true, mutual love will clip their wings and put them forever in locks and chains. Your kind prefer detachment. You may even have just cause for your feelings. After all, how can you devote yourself to a single person when humanity needs you? Well, there is an old saying that "charity begins at home." If you want to help the needy masses, Aquarius, there is probably one of their number in your kitchen right now who is overeating and starved for your attention. It is unfortunate but true that your mate is more likely than you to have a serious weight problem. Do a good deed and share this book with your lover. Just reading this chapter on Aquarius may help ease the frustration by adding to his or her understanding.

You do your part, too. Don't run in fear from intimacy, but take it as a challenge. Share and care for your mate like your best friend—because he or she really is. *Communicate.* You of all the signs of the zodiac, Aquarius, are capable of giving a person the freedom necessary to grow. And that is what relationship is all about. Let your partner know how desperately you want to share yourself, but that you sometimes feel that you must discover other parts of yourself first; then you will share them (you might even tell the world.) But until then, you need private time to be alone.

Your partner will quickly realize the benefits of giving you all the independence you need. After all, it's not as if you go off philandering, loyal Aquarius. You are just recharging your psychic batteries on some cosmic journey. When you do return to the nest, your lovemaking is likely to produce some pretty celestial fireworks. And that is something worth waiting for.

Your innovative, experimental mind is quite creative about sex, and you should take advantage of it to keep boredom out of the bedroom. You may not hang from chandeliers or be the first to buy X-rated videos, but exotic situations do arouse your desire. Love in an igloo in Alaska or a tent in Tangiers is stimulating to your imagination. You have a delicious rebellious streak that loves to make love where no one can tell on you, where you can act out your fantasies with complete abandon. Some of your fantasies do remain daydreams, of course. But Aquarian daydreams feed the psyche and satisfy the soul. And that is much better than eating. Besides, Aquarius, your body says make love only on an empty stomach.

Eating/Entertaining at Home

When guests come to your home, Aquarius, they should expect the unexpected. The type of food, the combinations, the table service, the decor, and even the company—all promise to be unusual when Aquarius entertains.

Your home may be chaotic, especially at mealtimes, due to your unpredictable life. A guest may arrive prepared for an intimate dinner for two only to find a third party at your table, probably some wayfarer you met at a bar and took home to share your meal. You may send out advance invitations to a dinner party, then serve your company food you picked up at a takeout place. Or you will call your friends at the last minute and then treat the spontaneous company to a three-course meal of your favorite foods.

This repast might start with a soup, like cold cucumber soup or watercress and parsley soup, definitely something different. Then will come the sandwich—halvah and peanut butter on pumpernickel bread, or some other strange variation on the peanut butter theme. Dessert might be a selection of exotic fruits—papaya from Bangkok, mango from Mexico, kiwi from New Zealand, pomegranate from Israel—and each one will have a story. You will point to the photographs of foreign lands on your wall to illustrate each tale.

Whatever you serve, it is likely to evoke questions from your company. "What is this?" or "What is in this?" are typical ones. Not that you serve foods mysteriously blended. Actually, you prefer things served discreetly. Peas and corn will have their own separate bowls and meat will have its own serving platter. But you will offer a menu of the most unusual foreign fare, from kosher Japanese food to dishes from a Tibetan kitchen. You have a penchant for sour rather than sweet foods, and you really like a smorgasbord or buffet style of serving, so your guests can help themselves to the variety of interesting foods you set out. By the way, "interesting" is a commonly heard adjective around the Aquarian table.

Your place settings may be extraordinary, also. A handwoven cloth from Peru, plates thrown by a Japanese ceramist, and forks, knives, and spoons collected from flea markets across the nation. That is, if there are utensils at all. You might prefer eating with chopsticks, or Indian-style, with the hands. You might use carved tableware from the century before the Babylonian empire, and glasses—rather, goblets—from some other fallen civilization. You love music to accompany any meal, but what kind of music will be dictated strictly by your mood at the moment. You may play heavy metal with the Beef Wellington and Brahms with the hot dogs. In any case, it will be played on equipment imported from the twenty-first century and piped into every room in the house.

Ambiance, appearance, and taste are more important to you than nutrition, and everything you serve will be light and delicious, if a little offbeat.

For example, I once attended a beautiful dinner party hosted by two Aquarians. I was told to wear something blue, which I did. And when I arrived I found twenty other people also dressed in blue. We sat down at a table set with royal blue cloth, and above us from the ceiling hung blue helium balloons. We were served luscious blueberries on blue plates followed by blue and white delft china plates heaped with white and blue macaroni (that's right, it was dyed blue). We were offered blueberry muffins in white baskets and corn muffins in blue baskets. Then came a lovely salad with blue cheese dressing, and last but not least, coffee with blueberry liqueur served with blueberry crepes suzettes. Maybe my Aquarian friends were having their blue period or maybe it was blueberry season. I never learned the reason for the event—not that Aquarians need such earthly reasons—but it was a most memorable, charming, and special evening, as dining in an Aquarian home always is.

Food Shopping

Gifted, intelligent Aquarius, there are many things you do well in life, but shopping isn't one of them. In fact, you are probably the world's worst food shopper. You are not very interested in food per se, and your motivation for buying where, what, and how you do would baffle the most adept market researcher. You like to shop quickly, but you invariably shop without a list. (Not to be easily categorized, of course, one typically eccentric

Aquarian I know does make out a shopping list. However, she puts it in her pocket until checkout time, then reads it over to see if she remembered everything. It is a game that absolutely delights her Uranian mind.) You tend to buy on impulse, which would be disastrous to the diet of anyone who cared more about food than you. Basically, grocery shopping is something you just like to get over with as quickly and painlessly as possible.

Generally speaking, you tend to go through the supermarket as though you are in a trance. Perhaps you just tune out all the brand names on the shelves as you go by. At any rate, you look as though a person could run naked down the aisle and you wouldn't notice.

When you are not buying out of impulse, you buy out of habit. You tend to stock up on staples, which may include anything that you usually want around the house, like salty junk foods and all kinds of Mexican-style things. Although you are not given to sweets, you are crazy about cheeses and cannot resist cheesecake in any form. Pickles are a particular Aquarian passion, and you will buy jars at a time—sour pickles, new pickles, little ones, big ones.

You do not really pay attention to prices, but you can sort of intuitively tell when a store is not giving its customers value. Then you will avoid it on principle, even though it is the most convenient market in your area. You will not spend time reading labels, either. But you have your clairvoyant Aquarian ways of seeing past inflated claims about the natural and healthful contents of various products. Animal-loving Aquarius, you probably know more about the pet foods in the store than you do about the human varieties. You will succumb to items marked "new" and "improved," however, because you cannot resist trying the unknown.

You prefer to patronize the small neighborhood groceries, which you feel are more homey and human in scale than the sprawling food shopping centers (although the latest computerized supermarket checkouts that scan your groceries, announce the price, and do everything but pack your bags for you may temporarily appeal to your futuristic eye). On the other hand, a supermarket chain that advertised that all its profits for a certain week would go to aid the hungry in Africa would surely attract Aquarian customers, and you wouldn't think twice about the inconvenience or increased price. Your own stomach, philanthropic Aquarius, is rarely your primary concern.

Social Dining

When you think of social dining, friendly Aquarius, the emphasis is on *social.* The society you keep is more important than the food you eat, and the thought of dining out conjures up images primarily of company and conversation in the Aquarian mind. Long after the meal is over, you will forget the name of the place you had dinner, what you ate, or when it was, but you will always remember who was there and what was said. Dull people bore you quick-minded Uranians. However, you like people who are smart, not smart-asses.

You love to try different types of foods, and the more strange and exotic, the better. A Scandinavian smorgasbord, an Indonesian rijstafel, soul food, Moroccan food—if someone names it, you'll try it. An unusual eating arrangement might also interest you—sitting on a floor of a Japanese restaurant, or viewing an open tandoori oven in an Indian one. You enjoy English pubs and honky-tonks, if the music is lively, and Mexican restaurants where a strolling guitarist serenades. You love any sort of buffet, especially the Sunday-morning-brunch type that features a vast array of foods around a magnificently carved ice statue. (You Aquarians are often fabulous sculptors, and you may have attempted one of these yourself.) You may draw the line at the price of a restaurant. With so many starving children in the world, it's difficult for the liberal Aquarian to justify spending one hundred dollars on a meal for two. If it is a $1,000-a-plate dinner to raise money for refugees, however, I am sure we can count you in.

European-style cafés where you can linger over a cup of espresso for hours and talk, talk, talk with friends, are especially appealing to the brainstorming Aquarian. You love to surround yourself with writers, artists, and intellectuals, people with whom you can tackle metaphysical questions and share your profound insights. If there is a palm reader or astrologer making the rounds of tables, all the better. Then your friends can glimpse the future you have spent entire conversations telling them about.

Because the conversation is far more titillating to you than the food, Aquarius, restaurant eating does not present so much of a threat to your diet. You are usually so busy talking, you do not have much time for chewing, and it is not unusual for a waiter to come to clear your table to find most of your food still on your plate.

Special-Occasion Dining

There is no such thing as dieting on a special occasion for you, Aquarius. You are a crowd pleaser, and would not want to hurt the feelings of your hosts and their guests by bringing up your diet, a topic of conversation you consider boring in the first place. The problem is, social Aquarius, you have a way of making all your life into a special occasion. Paddling down the river, sipping a bottle of beer? Who could think of dieting? Who can think of dieting when you're going on a champagne brunch—on horseback, that is. Unusual? Of course, Aquarius: You planned it. And then there's the hot toddy and hot chocolate at the end of a day of ice skating (a favorite Aquarian pastime). Too much of a special occasion to give that up.

Whenever you are attending some social gathering, you will be as gracious as if you were the host. You will go out of your way to introduce people to one another and to make sure everyone is well fed and watered. Of course, as a guest, you will never arrive empty-handed. You always seem to know the proper house gift, although it will never be anything so common as cocktail napkins, candy, or a cheese board.

On the other hand, you cannot be pushed or coerced into making an appearance at some special function just because everyone else is doing it. In fact, that is one of the best reasons you have not to go, nonconforming Aquarius. Just because all the family goes to Grandma's the third Sunday of every month is no reason you should.

Well, you can be stubborn when you want to be, Aquarius. So just decide you won't eat on the next occasion, no matter how special, and you know what? You won't.

Your Health

Aquarius, you are one of the signs least given to excess weight, partly due to your nature at time of birth and partly to the strong influences of your personality. Sometimes, you just get too involved in projects to even think of food, and there aren't too many people who can say that, lucky Aquarius. You also are perfectly happy at times to eat a dinner of Korean egg rolls, Greek salad, Spanish chicken and rice, and some Italian gelato to round off the meal. The more unusual the fare, the more your taste buds salivate. Well, you must have a charmed star in your constellation because generally you are able to keep your weight under control and you are able to maintain your good health throughout your life.

In typical Aquarian fashion, you also have a way of coming up with some clever, if bizarre—and sometimes none too healthy—means of losing weight, when and if you see the pounds creeping on.

You active February people do have to beware not to overdo things. Your desire for constant change and ever new vistas often leads to an erratic life-style, which can create stress that you may not even be aware of—but that is damaging to the body just the same. It is not easy to turn off that always inquisitive mind of yours at night, and you may suffer bouts of insomnia. You may not feel you require more sleep (and many Aquarians do require little), but beware that you do not push too hard.

Aquarius rules the lower legs, ankles, and blood circulation in general. Diseases to which Aquarians are subject include:

Anemia	Nervous diseases
Cramps in the legs	Oxygenation problems
Hardening of the arteries	Ruptures
Muscle spasms	Sprained or broken ankles
Myelitis	Swollen ankles

Sodium chloride is the Aquarius cell salt. Cell salts are naturally occurring minerals that are normal constituents of the body cells. They are found in trace amounts in foods, and plants, animals, and human beings require these compounds for proper nutrition. And, like vitamins, cell salts get used up. Sodium chloride is commonly known as table salt; however, adding table salt to your meals will not satisfy your sodium chloride needs. This is because ordinary table salt is too coarse to enter the bloodstream where it can be utilized by the body. Sodium chloride regulates the water level within the cells in the body; it controls how much water enters and leaves each cell. Water, which makes up 70 percent of the human organism, must be properly distributed. Unhealthy distribution, due to a sodium chloride deficiency, can cause several problems, including catarrh, dropsy, diarrhea, and weight gain. Sodium chloride also regulates the amount of hydrochloric acid that enters the stomach during food digestion. If the amount of hydro-chloric acid is not properly regulated, digestive problems may ensue.

FOODS RICH IN SODIUM CHLORIDE

Apples	Figs
Asparagus	Lentils
Cabbage	Radishes
Carrots	Shellfish
Celery	Spinach
Corn	Strawberries

You should maintain a diet that keeps your blood clean and well oxygenated. And that means eating a lot of oxygen-rich, detoxifying natural, raw foods like fresh fruits and vegetables, as well as limiting your consumption of carbohydrate foods like starches and sugar, which rob the body of oxygen. You should also avoid high-cholesterol, fat-laden foods, because Aquarians are prone to hardening of the arteries later in life. Incorporating foods rich in vitamin C, bioflavonoids, and vitamin E will help purify your blood as well as strengthen the veins, reducing the risk of varicose veins and phlebitis. Finally, remember to include many of the B-vitamin foods and to avoid anemia by following the regimen based on your sun sign requirements.

Supercharged Aquarius, you are so busy helping others and your mind is so filled with ideas the rest of us won't have for maybe another century, eating takes up quite a small part of your thoughts. Don't forget that you do need healthy nourishment in the here and now, however. Perhaps you are already dining on some natural, predigested, packaged space-age fare. If it is the wave of the future, I can count on you to track it down.

Aquarius Daily Nutritional Supplements

- One general multivitamin with minerals
- 400 mg vitamin E
- 2,000 mg vitamin C with bioflavonoids
- Fiber foods

Remember, Aquarius...

This diet is uniquely prepared to address your sun sign and *should not be interchanged with any other Sun Sign Diet.* It is important that you follow the diet exactly as it appears, for optimum weight loss and assimilation. Before starting your Aquarius diet, carefully read "General Diet and Maintenance Guidelines for All Sun Signs," found at the beginning of this book. Remember, drink 8 glasses of water daily.

I know, Aquarius, that you have always tried the latest diet available, the most unusual you could find. You are now about to embark on a sensible reducing diet that has been prepared to meet your nutritional needs.

Good luck, and *go for it.*

The Aquarius Seven-Day Reducing Diet

Aquarius, here is a diet designed specifically for your constitution. It incorporates the foods you need to keep your blood pure and well oxygenated and your cholesterol and fat levels low, and to give you the nutritional components you need while maintaining a low calorie count.

I have included a Substitution Day, which gives guidelines to use other diet days for variety or additional choice.

For the first time you have a diet that has been prepared for your own specific needs and likes. When the combinations are followed a specific dynamic action takes place, and for that reason no substitutions are permitted. If you do not like a particular food, just omit it. At anytime, if you wish to exchange lunch with dinner, or vice versa, you may do so as long as you do not use a lunch or dinner from another day's menu.

And of course, a binge day has been included for those crazy days when you feel that you cannot go on any longer. You will find instructions for the Aquarius Total Binge Day at the end of your Seven-Day Reducing Diet.

Food is easily prepared and can be ordered in most restaurants. Plan to do your weekly shopping for all the items so that you have no excuses.

You will note that some items have an asterisk (*). I have indicated the importance of each of these specific foods that has been included in your diet and the vitamin and/or mineral content in the section "Notes to Aquarius Seven-Day Reducing Diet."

One last word, Aquarius: Do not salt your food. You will find that the inclusion of so many natural sources of sodium chloride foods in your Sun

Sign Diet will make the use of that salt shaker unnecessary. And much more healthful.

You may repeat this diet week after week until you have reached your goal weight. Go for success, Aquarius.

DAY ONE

This day has been designed to cleanse your system Aquarius, while giving you a dieting boost. You have been overtaxing your system on salty foods and many toxic foods. So get started with an alkaline fruit day.

BREAKFAST
>   4 oz. unsweetened grapefruit juice
>
>   tea or herbal tea—sugar substitute if desired

MIDMORNING SNACK
>   1 medium-sized banana

LUNCH
>   1 orange*
>
>   1 apple
>
>   1 oz. sunflower seeds
>
>   tea or herbal tea—sugar substitute if desired

MIDAFTERNOON SNACK
>   1 orange*

DINNER
>   papaya—up to 3 whole papayas
>
>   herbal tea or regular tea
>
>   water
>
>   *Absolutely nothing else.*

This is a high-enzyme fruit day. You will feel energetic and will be happy when you see the scale tomorrow.

Remember, drink 8 glasses of water every day.

DAY TWO

BREAKFAST

1 slice whole grain or stone-ground bread*

1 small apple

1 oz. Camembert cheese*

coffee or tea

LUNCH

fresh fruit salad*—up to 3 cups absolutely fresh fruit of your choice

black coffee, tea, or no-sodium Perrier or no-sodium club soda.

Nothing else.

MIDAFTERNOON SNACK

1 tangerine or 4 oz. unsweetened apple juice

DINNER

¼–½ chicken breast* (baked or broiled without skin) prepared with ginger and dry sherry; mix with 2 tsp. raisins

½ cup brown or wild rice

1 cup salad of watercress, parsley, cauliflower, broccoli, and spinach,* served with dressing of lemon juice and garlic pepper

no-sodium seltzer with lime

Remember, drink 8 glasses of water every day.

DAY THREE

BREAKFAST

1 cup assorted honeydew and cantaloupe balls (fresh or frozen)

1 oz. sunflower seeds*

black coffee, tea, or herbal tea

LUNCH

3½ oz. Chinook salmon*

4–5 artichoke hearts canned in water, seasoned with 2 Tbsp. horse-radish*

no-sodium seltzer with lime, iced tea, or no-sodium diet soda

water, water, water

DINNER

4 oz. dry white wine (optional)

6 oz. broiled or baked filet of sole of flounder baked with ¼ cup Mexican salsa*

1 baked potato or ½ cup linguine with 2 Tbsp. Parmesan cheese

½ sliced cucumber

no-sodium seltzer with lime

EVENING SNACK

1 cup fresh strawberries*

Remember, drink 8 glasses of water every day.

DAY FOUR

BREAKFAST

½ cup cottage cheese mixed with ½ cup unsweetened applesauce

2 Tbsp. wheat germ and 5 almonds*

tea or coffee

LUNCH

2-egg mushroom omelette with basil, chervil, and parsley, topped with 3 anchovy filets*

1 whole sliced tomato

1 glass iced tea, no-sodium seltzer, or no-sodium diet soda

water, water, water

DINNER

4 oz. dry white wine (optional)

4–6 oz. veal scallopine* stir-fried in low-sodium soy sauce

1 cup fresh mushrooms* and ½ cup steamed broccoli,* served with 2 Tbsp. Parmesan cheese

1 cup fresh strawberries

1 cup iced black coffee, tea, or no-sodium seltzer with lime

Remember, drink 8 glasses of water every day.

DAY FIVE

BREAKFAST

½ cup water-pack mandarin or tangerine sections

1 slice pumpernickel bread with ¼ cup skim-milk ricotta cheese

black coffee, tea, herbal tea, café au lait (2 oz. skim milk)

LUNCH

3½ oz. Pacific sardines* with dill sauce (drain oil from can)

salad of watercress, alfalfa sprouts, and black olives mixed with ¼ cup plain yogurt and dill

iced tea, no-sodium Perrier, or no-sodium seltzer

MIDAFTERNOON SNACK

10 pistachio nuts

DINNER

¼–½ broiled or baked chicken prepared in tomato juice or ¼ cup Mexican salsa sauce

1 cup lightly steamed fresh mushrooms

1 cup salad of watercress,* fresh string beans, and black olives seasoned with lemon juice and garlic pepper

iced tea, water, or no-sodium seltzer

Remember, drink 8 glasses of water every day.

DAY SIX

BREAKFAST

> ½ cup granola cereal
>
> ¾ cup skim milk
>
> café au lait (2 oz. regular milk)

LUNCH

> fresh fruit salad (Repeat lunch from Day Two; up to 3 cups of any fresh fruit.)
>
> black coffee, tea, or water
>
> *Nothing else.*

DINNER

> 4 oz. dry red or white wine (optional)
>
> 1 cup long-grain brown rice or 1 cup vegetable pasta steamed and served with 3 tablespoons grated Parmesan cheese

and

> 1 box frozen broccoli spears served with 2 Tbsp. Mexican jalapeño sauce
>
> ½ medium sized baked eggplant with 1 oz. hard cheese and herbs
>
> iced tea, no-sodium Perrier with a twist of lime, or espresso
>
> What a delight!
>
> *Remember, drink 8 glasses of water every day.*

DAY SEVEN

BREAKFAST

4 oz. orange juice

1 thick slice pumpernickel bread

2 oz. smoked salmon

1 Tbsp. cream cheese

café au lait (2 oz. skim milk)

MIDMORNING SNACK

1 bunch of grapes (20–30)

DINNER

turkey and avocado* salad (4 oz. turkey, ½ avocado) with large tossed salad of mixed greens, green pepper, cucumber, lettuce, and 2 tsp. blue cheese dressing

1 oz. Camembert cheese on rye cracker

espresso coffee

or

1–2 lb. boiled or broiled lobster (no butter, use lemon juice)

large tossed green salad with 2 tsp. blue cheese dressing

1 oz. Camembert cheese on rye cracker

espresso coffee or 4 oz. white wine

Remember, drink 8 glasses of water every day.

SUBSTITUTE DAY

If you are unable to keep to any day's menu, or wish to change for any reason, you may at any time substitute the following days from your reducing diet as many times as you wish: Day Two, Day Three, Four, Six.

Notes to Aquarius Seven-Day Reducing Diet

You will have found most of your food explanations on your daily reducing diet sheet. I am quite aware that Aquarians like to see the "whole picture" at once.

Aquarius Diet Notes—Day One
* Oranges are rich in vitamin P (bioflavonoids).
A good day for internal cleansing and weight loss

Aquarius Diet Notes—Day Two
* Whole grain bread is high in fiber and excellent for the digestive tract.
* Camembert cheese, is actually lower in fat than most cheeses. It is therefore, perfectly fine, wary Aquarians, to eat this delicious dairy product in the amount given above.
* The enzyme action of the fresh fruit is most beneficial for cleansing the system of toxic wastes.
* Chicken is high in vitamin E, phosphorus, and B-6.
* Spinach is rich in bioflavinoids.

Aquarius Diet Notes—Day Three
* Sunflower seeds are an excellent source of calcium.
* Salmon is an excellent source of low-cholesterol, high-protein food that is extremely rich in vitamins A, B, and E.
* Horseradish is an excellent blood cleanser.
* Mexican salsa is made from red peppers, chili, onions, and parsley. It is rich in vitamins A, B, and C.
* Strawberries act as a blood purifier.

Aquarius Diet Notes—Day Four
* Almonds are rich in protein, potassium, manganese, and phosphorus.
* Anchovy is an excellent source of protein that will keep your taste buds

nourished for your desire of salty food. A low-calorie, power-packed protein lunch.

* The veal is rich in B vitamins and a low-cholesterol choice of first-quality protein.

* The mushrooms and broccoli are a rich source of vitamin B-12.

Aquarius Diet Notes—Day Five

* Sardines are a major source of low-cholesterol protein, with excellent satiating power. It will keep your energy level high—rich in B-12.

* Watercress is an excellent source of calcium.

Aquarius Diet Notes—Days Six and Seven

* Grapes are a good source of vitamin P (bioflavonoids).

* The avocado is an excellent vegetable protein, high in vitamins A, C, B-1, potassium, sodium, and magnesium.

The balance of your reducing diet is designed to combine the proper amount of proteins, complex carbohydrates, fats, and enzyme-rich food. Your Aquarius Reducing Diet is programmed for high energy and easy digestion, but is nutritiously abundant in vitamins B, B-12, C, E, and the bioflavonoids.

Your calcium needs are met by the various green vegetables, but most important, *watercress* and *parsley*. Make sure you include these two foods when indicated.

Do not drink any milk or milk products when you have fruit meals. The milk lactose will stop the enzyme action of the fruit.

Make a habit of using no-sodium diet soda whenever possible. The more salt you have, the more your body will demand.

AQUARIUS TOTAL BINGE DAY

Aquarius, when you feel internal cravings and must deviate from your diet or die, follow the rules below.

Before You Binge

1. Drink water.
2. Drink water.
3. Drink water.
4. Rest.
5. Brush your teeth and rinse with your favorite mouthwash.
6. Chew sugarless gum for 20 minutes.

You may find that the desire to binge has passed. However, if you are still suffering from intense food frustration, follow these basic binge rules:

Rule One

Under no circumstances should you ever binge before completing Day Five of your reducing diet. This will ensure a maximum weight loss with a minimum of food frustration.

Rule Two

If, for example, you binge on the sixth day of your diet, resume your diet the following day (Day Seven) with the menu for Day Six. If you binge for just one meal, such as lunch on Day Six, resume your reducing diet with dinner on Day Six of your reducing diet.

Rule Three

Bingeing is for when you get that creepy, anxious feeling, when you feel like pulling out your hair—strand by strand—and you cannot endure dieting for even one more moment. Before you climb the walls, give yourself a binge day. It is hoped that this will not be necessary more than four times a month.

Rule Four

After you have lost your first 10 pounds, you may vary your binge day with the binge day of the sun sign opposite yours, which is Leo.

Remember, an occasional binge day—when necessary—will still allow you to lose weight (without guilt). Here, Aquarius, is your binge day menu.

Binge Day Menu

BREAKFAST

bagel or blueberry muffin with 1 Tbsp. peanut butter 1 Tbsp. diet jam and/or diet margarine

café au lait or tea

MIDMORNING SNACK

1 oz. bag Dorito chips

LUNCH

1 slice pizza

½ cup Tofutti frozen dessert or ½ cup ice cream

no-sodium diet soda or light beer

MIDAFTERNOON SNACK

20 pistachio nuts or 1 small bag of M&M's

DINNER

1 cup Wonton soup with about 20 Chinese noodles steamed shrimp and vegetables in soy sauce

½ cup white rice

2 Chinese fortune cookies

tea

Maintaining Your Ideal Weight

Aquarius Maintenance Foods for Optimum Health

When you have achieved your desired weight goal, you should follow a maintenance diet rich in the specific nutrients that you, Aquarius, need each and every day.

Vitamin E

Vitamin E is an antioxidant. It prevents red blood cells from forming with toxic peroxide and promotes oxygen filtration of the blood; ensures proper flow of blood to all parts of the body by dissolving blood clots and dilating blood vessels. Since most of Aquarius' health problems involve the circulatory system (everything from shivering to varicose veins), vitamin E is a necessity, for it is crucial to the maintenance of healthy circulation.

FOODS RICH IN VITAMIN E

Apples	Eggs
Asparagus	Halibut
Avocados	Hazel nuts
Broccoli	Leeks
Cabbage	Liver
Carrots	Milk
Cheese	Mushrooms
Chicken	Peas

Parsley
Peanut butter
Salmon
Shrimp

Sunflower seeds
Sweet potatoes
Turkey
Wheat germ

Vitamin C

One of the many jobs of vitamin C is aiding in the maintenance of blood-vessel elasticity and preventing hemorrhaging of blood vessels. Thus vitamin C will help Aquarius in avoiding circulatory problems. Vitamin C also aids in the production of collagen, which constitutes about 40 percent of the body's protein. If insufficient amounts of collagen are produced, cells in the bones lose their supportive strength. Prone to broken ankles, Aquarians cannot afford to lose any supportive strength in the bones. The body cannot manufacture its own vitamin C, so vitamin C must be supplied in your daily diet.

FOODS RICH IN VITAMIN C

Alfalfa sprouts
Almonds
Apples
Asparagus
Bananas
Beets
Blueberries
Broccoli
Brussels sprouts
Cantaloupe
Carrots
Celery
Chicken liver
Cranberries

Currants
Grapefruit
Green peppers
Lemons
Oranges
Orange juice
Paprika
Parsley
Pineapple
Skim milk
Strawberries
Tomatoes
Watercress

Vitamin B-12

Vitamin B-12 is necessary for proper metabolism of protein, carbohydrates, and fats. Also, without vitamin B-12, red blood cells cannot be manufactured effectively within the bone marrow, and anemia results. Because, Aquarius is susceptible to anemia, it is important for you to include foods rich in vitamin B-12 in your diet.

FOODS RICH IN VITAMIN B-12

Alfalfa

Beef

Bran and wheat flakes

Chicken

Chicken liver

Cottage cheese

Eggs

Green peas

Herring

Muscle meats

Pickled foods

Prunes

Raw oysters

Sardines

Shellfish

Skim milk

Soy bean products

Swiss cheese

Trout

Yogurt

Bioflavonoids

Bioflavonoids act with vitamin C to prevent cholesterol buildup, which can cause clotting of the arteries, veins, and capillaries; to maintain the elasticity of the blood vessels and to help prevent and alleviate many of the other circulatory problems to which Aquarius is susceptible.

FOODS RICH IN BIOFLAVONOIDS

Apples

Apricots

Blackberries

Black currants

Buckwheat

Cherries

Grapes

Grapefruit

Green peppers

Lemons

Oranges

Parsley

Prunes

Rose hips

Spinach

Aquarius Sample Maintenance Menu

When you reach your desired goal, please follow the maintenance eating hints found in "General Diet and Maintenance Guidelines for All Sun Signs" at the beginning of this book for proper calculations of caloric intake.

I'm including a sample maintenance menu based on your sun sign for optimal Aquarius maintenance. When you create your own menus for yourself, try to choose many of the foods you eat from your Aquarius Maintenance Foods lists.

2,000 Calories Per Day

BREAKFAST	CALORIES
½ grapefruit	39
1 bagel	163
2 Tbsp. cream cheese	99
2 oz. smoked salmon	100
coffee	0
	401

MIDMORNING SNACK	
1 banana	105
1 Tbsp. peanut butter	95
	200

LUNCH	
Super Tuna Pita:	
½ cup tuna salad	175
3 slices tomato	10
2 leaves lettuce	5
1 slice Swiss cheese	50
½ Tbsp. diet mayonnaise	20
1 whole wheat pita	150
8 oz. milk	100
	510

MIDAFTERNOON SNACK	
¼ cup sunflower seeds	201

DINNER	
4 oz. white wine (optional)	85
4 oz. lean roast beef	266
1 baked potato with 1 Tbsp. diet margarine	135
mixed green salad with 1 Tbsp. low-calorie dressing	160
	646

EVENING SNACK

1 oatmeal raisin cookie   69

TOTAL DAILY CALORIES   2,027

Remember, drink 8 glasses of water every day.

Restaurant Eating the Aquarius Way

Perhaps you have seen the following dishes on restaurant menus. Both the dishes and the types of restaurants chosen will appeal to your Aquarius palate and satisfy your nutritional needs. Your penchant for exotic, unusual foreign food will be satisfied by the intriguing Indian, Thai, and Danish menus. And who knows, maybe you will be lucky enough to find your favorite—a buffet-type restaurant that lets you choose one dish from every nation. Options, choices—that's the Aquarius way.

In all menus, one appetizer plus one entrée equals approximately 600–700 calories.

Chinese Gourmet Restaurant

APPETIZERS

Shark's fin soup

Sliced jellyfish

ENTRÉES

Sesame beef, sautéed in spicy sauce, on a bed of bean sprouts, sprinkled with sesame seeds

Blue crabs in Hunan wine sauce

Baby shrimp and bits of chicken cooked over high flame, then sautéed with fresh vegetables

Chicken chunks in a tingling hot sauce

Indian Restaurant

APPETIZERS

Chicken chunks in a sharp mint sauce

Yogurt shake, served mildly salted

ENTRÉES

Minced chicken flavored with fresh herbs and spices

Fish marinated in special spices and grilled in clay oven

Tandoori mixed grill

Lamb or beef cooked with spinach and fresh Indian spices

Thai Restaurant

APPETIZERS

Shrimp curry

Beef salad

ENTRÉES

Squid sautéed with onion and hot pepper

Chicken curry

Beef sautéed with onion and chili pepper

Chicken sautéed with basil leaves and chili

Danish Restaurant

APPETIZERS

Fresh salmon, cured in old-style Danish dill sauce

Imported Danish shrimp

ENTRÉES

Boiled chicken in creamed asparagus garnished with parsley

Copenhagen omelette, with Danish shrimp and mushrooms

Chopped prime beef mixed with chopped onion, red beets, capers, parsley, and potatoes

Danish roast beef hash with fried egg

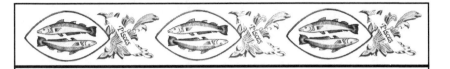

PISCES

February 20–March 20

The Pisces
Personality

"I'm on a seafood diet. When I see food, I eat it."

Pisces, you are creative, imaginative, intuitive, and intelligent. Not bad credentials for a fish confused about his—or her—ability and self-image. I know it has been hard for you to find a diet that works. The one you began at nine o'clock in the morning is usually overboard by three in the afternoon, cast off when some leviathan mood reared its ugly but familiar head in the sea of your psyche.

Emotional eating is your foremost diet problem. Inner turmoil makes you nervous, and you often try to swallow your anxiety away with food. The smallest slight to your sensitive ego sends you bingeing on sweets, chocolates, ice cream, or anything creamy. Inevitably the pounds pile up, and the vicious cycle of depression and overeating is set in motion. You also have an unfortunate propensity to retain fluids in your body because you are a water sign. You frequently feel bloated, which only exacerbates any weight problem.

Next time you reach for that piece of cheesecake, ask yourself if it really helps assuage your hurt feelings. I think that is just one of your self-indulgent illusions, Pisces. You have as many moods as the sea has currents, and they are as capable as the most powerful undertows of drowning you —but only if you let them. The truth is you do have willpower. Just dive within that oceanic consciousness of yours, and you will find it.

Once you commit to a diet, I know you will follow it to a tee. You are very good at taking advice and guidance, and actually like to be told what to eat. (Then you cannot blame yourself for failure.) Decision-making is not your forte, even when it comes to something as basic as choosing what you will have for lunch. When you go to a restaurant, you tend to order whatever your companion is having. If someone asks what you like to eat, you will simply answer "everything." And you mean it. This can be exasperating to your host or partner, as I personally discovered the first year of marriage to my own lovable Pisces spouse. You really are one easy-to-please fish, Pisces, and happy to eat whatever we feed you. You have a few staples in your diet, like seafood, salad, martinis, and lots of orange juice. There are also certain strong aromas, like ripe Brie or cooking broccoli, that offend your sensitive nose. But except when you are depressed, you rarely have a craving for any one kind of taste and almost never decline to eat a particular food.

Left to your own devices you have a tendency to eat at random. Each new day brings something different. Usually, whatever is in the refrigerator will do. Leftovers are fine; so is a five-course gourmet meal. You probably won't cook anything fancy for yourself, but if you can feed somebody else, your creativity in the kitchen knows no bounds.

Some members of your school, Pisces, do cultivate an interest in nutrition, following a keen instinct that it would benefit their own constitution. Even then, you health-conscious fish manage to eat in a way that defies logic. You will dine on junk food one week, then organic food the next, and convince yourself you have an excellent pattern of nutritious eating. Or you will eat an instant breakfast of powdered chemicals (with two tablespoons of wheat germ added for good measure), call it your "vitamix," and feel totally justified in consuming two cupcakes for your lunch.

How long have you been dreaming about losing weight, Pisces? You are a grand master of deception and seem particularly adept at fooling yourself. Some of you pretend you are not really heavy; others exist under the illusion that you are. Sometimes you pretend to put yourself down in front of others while holding yourself in good esteem. Your fantastic, subtle mind is capable of weaving such complex webs of avoidance, evasion, and denial that it is sometimes hard even for you to discern the truth in your life anymore.

You are known to be the great actors and actresses of the zodiac, Pisces, and you do have a penchant for exaggeration and drama. However, you sometimes hide behind your guises as insulation from what seems to you like a cold, hard world. And you are not without good reason. Pisces sensitivity and compassion are unmatched by any other sign. Psychic and impressionable, you are easily affected by forces outside yourself and by what others think of you. You have a deep desire to be loved by all, and you tend to put everyone else's needs above your own. On the other hand, your exceptional warmth, gentleness, and humor are immediately endearing and you exude an ethereal charm and grace others find irresistible. You have a deeply giving nature, and people sense this in you instantaneously. And yes, beware, unselfish Pisces, they often take advantage of your wonderful nurturing soul.

Do you really have to be the one to eat the leftovers? And when someone asks you what type of restaurant you prefer to go to, do you always have to say, "Oh, it doesn't matter. Where would you like to go?" Do you have to say, "I'm sorry," when you have nothing really to be sorry about?

I know you can see the pattern, my perceptive friend. Also know you have the choice to change it. Start thinking about what you really like. No false modesty; no self-deprecating waves of the hand. The "I don't deserve it syndrome" has to go. Guilt only increases your stress levels. Learn to say "no" without justifying yourself or giving explanations. You cannot be best friend to the world without being your own worst enemy, Pisces.

I know you think you are being judged all the time, as though you are onstage, but I want you to start to participate in your life rather than perform. Don't blame circumstances on someone else. Take responsibility for your life, and it will manifest into a positive attitude toward dieting. Start asking for the emotional support you want from others, and you will no longer need to eat to feel nurtured. Learn the lessons of self-worth and assertiveness, and you will cease sabotaging your efforts to lose weight.

I know you are ready for a big breakthrough in your eating patterns, because you have taken the first step of commitment by purchasing *The Sun Sign Diet.* So, no more excuses, elusive Pisces. I have heard every one in the book from you:

"My biorhythms are off this week."
"It's not my fault. My mom [spouse, child, etc.] won't let me stay on my diet."
"My friends say I look haggard."
"I had to postpone the diet because I was visiting friends for the weekend and didn't want to be a stick-in-the-mud."
"I was doing great on this new diet. Then my boss [teacher, classmate, brother] told me that hers [his] is easier, simpler, better."
"My astrology chart has so many rough aspects this month."
"A little taste couldn't hurt."

Have I left any out?

If it seems as though I am being tough on you, Pisces, it is just because I know how much you want to get control of your eating habits. And I am on your side. Successful dieting will come to you once you learn to put yourself first. It will take some mastery over your emotions to start saying "no," but *discipline will ultimately give you the freedom you seek.* Put your extraordinary consciousness to work for yourself in a positive way. Imagine how you will look when you have lost weight and keep the picture clear in your mind. Start your diet with a friend who can support you as much as he or she will benefit from your ever-present, good-natured support. And take comfort in the fact that the Pisces Sun Sign Diet will not only address all your nutritional needs, but also your emotional makeup and personality characteristics. I guarantee you will take to it . . . like a fish to water.

Sexual Appetite

Dreamy Pisces, you have been accused more than once of being in love with love. You don't mind. You like the world through your rose-colored glasses. If you are not in love, your world falls apart.

Admittedly, you are one easy fish to fall in love with. You are seductive, alluring, charming—and don't pretend you don't know it, my adorable, theatrical friend. Even your eyes have a look that says, "I love you. Let me take care of you." Male or female, you have one of the tenderest hearts in the zodiac. You are accepting, trusting, and giving almost to a fault, and you have a keen sense of touch, which you express with armloads of physical affection. You are extremely vulnerable and intense. And deep as the waters your sign rules.

You Pisces females are the epitome of womanhood. You know how to use your attributes to the hilt—and you do, with the most calculated subtlety. Your mate will hardly know what hit him. But when the fish bites the hook, the question is: Who has been caught, the fisherman or the fish?

You Pisces men cast your own sort of spell. Poetic, inspired by art and beauty, you carve the classic romantic figure. Who says the age of chivalry is dead? No woman who has ever been courted by a Pisces man. You bring flowers to your lovers, open doors, walk them home, even make sure they are tucked into bed at night—and that, after the honeymoon is technically over. You are typically described by females as "a man I can really talk to," and there is nothing more appealing than that.

One reason you fish are so good at romance is that you have studied it so carefully. All you Pisces are looking for storybook passion. You have cried at all the greatest love stories in literature and on the silver screen, and have been seduced by torrid tales of romance on the soaps and in dimestore novels.

The problems arise when you begin to judge your own happiness in life by Hollywood standards. If you believe you must have drama, passion, and romance to sustain the spirit, Pisces, your unrealistic expectations of love will be a source of extreme frustration to you, emotionally and sexually. You know it is time to reevaluate your dreams and fantasies when you find yourself seeking solace at the refrigerator door.

There are a few other typically Piscean pitfalls to look out for in relationships if you are ever to get your emotional eating—and weight—under
control. First of all, you have a tendency not to feel good about your love
life unless you surrender completely. However, it really isn't necessary—
or even good for you—to relinquish all your power to your mate. Save
some for you, Pisces. Ask yourself if your libidinal and emotional needs are
being met, and if not, work to change this. Were you disappointed the night
you dimmed the lights, played soft music, made yourself enchanting and
available—but your partner failed to sweep you off your feet? Well, if it is
passionate lovemaking you want, don't wait for someone else to make it
happen. Speak up for what you desire, and take an active role in creating it.
And you don't have to play sick or weak to get the attention you crave. If
your relationship is ridden with pressure and emotional upset, get professional counseling if you cannot work it out between you. Trying to "make
believe" the problems do not exist will surely have an outlet—and usually
it is food.

Also, beware that you do not play victim or martyr. I know, you feel that
sacrifice is part of all true love. Just make sure that when you put the wishes
and desires of your lover above yourself that you are not setting yourself
up to feel as though you have been taken for granted. Resentment uncom-
municated often is swallowed away by food. Your capacity for devotion
and sacrifice sometimes borders on the unhealthy.

You want love so badly, you have been known to take it in whatever
form you can get it. Be wary of hot-tempered, domineering types who will
take pleasure in how easily you fish can be intimidated. And don't be so
willing to slave over a hot stove for the adoration of your family or run
yourself ragged catering to their needs at the cost of your own self-esteem.

The fact that many fish fall prey to this dangerous trap is confirmed by
the high number of Pisces who do well losing weight at health spas. What
accounts for this success? In questioning hundreds of Pisces reducing at
various spas, I have heard one answer almost consistently: "Well, my family
is not here, so I do not have to take care of them. Here I get to look after
myself first."

A lot of rage is often suppressed in that response. Let some of the anger
and bitterness surface. You are everybody's favorite sounding board, sym-
pathetic Pisces. Now take your turn. You deserve to have your feelings
heard, too. Stop stuffing down your emotions with food. Just getting them
off your chest will make you feel lighter immediately.

Do maintain some sense of proportion about love. You get so caught up
in the drama, the end of an affair can leave you wondering if life is really
worth living. Well, you know perfectly well it is. No single event can ruin
your life. Emotions cannot kill you, even though the pain of a breakup may

hurt you a lot. And you don't have to eat to kill your emotions, either. Tell your loved one what displeases you, write a beautiful poem. Above all, call upon your wonderful sense of humor, and transcend the sorrow with laughter.

Remember, food cannot satisfy the voracious Pisces appetite for love. More than anything, your own poor body image is what stands between you and the fulfillment you seek. When you lose the weight you desire, your sexuality will let loose like a tidal wave. And no one is more tantalizing and irresistible than Pisces when you feel sexy.

Eating/Entertaining at Home

An open door and a well-stocked refrigerator are two unmistakable signs of the Pisces home. You love to entertain guests almost as much as they love to be entertained by you, and it is not uncommon for your friends to drop by unannounced, help themselves to whatever is in the icebox, and settle comfortably in front of your television, just as though they were at home. And that is just the way you like it to be. You probably keep a store of assorted cocktail foods and dessert goodies in the freezer for just such occasions. Your home is a haven for anyone seeking sustenance, warmth, compassion, and an attentive ear. And the simple, aesthetic, and gracious style of the surroundings are a reflection of the soft presence of the Pisces hostess or host.

When your friends receive a formal invitation to dine at your home, they know they are in for very special treatment.

Planning a menu is the hardest part of home entertaining for the indecisive fish, but you usually keep a library of cookbooks or file of recipes on hand so you are ready and able to go when the mood strikes. If your guests have any special diet requirements, they can be assured you will take their needs into consideration to the best of your ability. You never mind making lots of food, because leftovers are things you like to eat anyway. Once you finally decide what to prepare, the rest comes rather easily—not unlike the way you plan finally to start a diet.

Presentation is very important to your artistic sensibilities, Pisces. Your table is sure to be beautiful, with color-coordinated china and linens. You will create just the right ambiance with soft lights and music—very cozy and a bit dramatic. The various savory spreads and dainty canapés with fluted edges which will probably precede the meal are a dead giveaway of the thought and care you put into the evening's preparation. You like to serve a full-course meal which will be complemented from hors d'oeuvres to after-dinner mints with a fine selection of alcohol, wines, and liqueurs from your bar. Undoubtedly, the entrée will be fish, which you have grown up to believe is "brain food," that is, the kind that develops analytical skills, to compensate for the feeling Pisces always has that you came into this world with more gray matter on the creative, intuitive side of your brain.

You look upon entertaining as a time to catch up on news and with the lives of your friends. You love to watch others enjoy the foods you serve, and don't have much patience with people who pick at their food indifferently. You tend to spend your evening being the charming host or hostess and as a result, you probably do very little eating—as long as guests are there. It is when the company goes home and you are left to clean up the leftovers that trouble strikes. Take my advice, Pisces. Save the wrapping-up for your mate. It really is your dieting downfall, and forewarned is forearmed.

Your real gratification comes not from the food, anyway, but from the compliments you receive from your guests. Of course, you will *pretend* "it was absolutely nothing." But the truth is nothing could please you more than to know your company has gone home feeling that they love you and care about you and that your love and conversation is important in their lives. Your guests will also go home carrying hefty CARE packages, if I know you, my giving friend. Just as well, too. It means less left over for Pisces to consume.

Food Shopping

Pisces has no special day or time to go food shopping. You go when you are in the mood, and *only* when in the mood. It is not an activity you find to be exciting, and you regard it basically as a chore.

The one sure thing that can be said about your shopping habits is that you will always take home a big load of groceries. You prefer the convenience of one-stop shopping at a supermarket offering everything your heart could desire. Indeed, you buy according to whim; consumer logic has little to do with Pisces' choice of foods or brands. You frequently cut out coupons but rarely use them. You don't mind a bargain but won't shop to find one. You will try a new or improved product because you saw it advertised in a magazine, heard it touted on radio or TV, or simply have a hunch that you might like it. You will buy gourmet or specialty foods if company is expected but probably not for yourself alone.

You do have certain limitations. You do not like to buy generic products or "no-name" brands because your superior intuition says, "There might be something hidden," or, "The FDA probably doesn't control it"—just a feeling that something isn't right for you. Your tastes do tend to be rather simple. You will bypass the fresh bakery counter and head straight to the packaged cookie section, probably to pick out the same brand you have been eating since you were a kid.

Crafty Pisces, you will probably sneak some other junk food snacks into your shopping cart, too. Don't deny it. Probably something in the chocolate family, right? An economy pack of candy bars, six for the price of five? Do you really expect me to believe your excuses—suddenly you are a consumer maven? Chocolate relaxes you? What an imagination.

Well, for someone who doesn't like to shop, you manage to spend more time than necessary doing it. Your impulsive and psychic methods of food selection tend to be somewhat inefficient, and you do have a habit of spacing out while trying to make decisions. Also you are always letting people cut ahead of you on the checkout line. Your generous, adaptable nature just doesn't allow you to say no to someone whose basket has only ten items when yours is filled to overflowing.

As cursory as your interest is in buying food at the supermarket, you often develop a sudden, insatiable curiosity to taste it on the drive home. If you must eat while driving, Pisces, try to choose a piece of fresh fruit and not some chocolate unmentionable. Better still, eat something satisfying on the ride *to* the food store, so you will not be swayed by a growling stomach to purchase tempting goodies in the first place.

Social Dining

When selecting a restaurant, the fish looks for friendly waters. You like gracious service, good companionship, and distinctive but unpretentious atmosphere. If the maitre d' knows you and the waiters sing as they serve your meal, so much the better. You will be back. But you look for quality in the food, too, and a long-stemmed rose in a crystal vase on your table will not compensate for an appetizer consisting of two artichoke leaves or an entrée of overcooked fettucine.

Chinese, Italian, Japanese restaurants are perennial Pisces favorites. And any establishment with a good oyster bar or specializing in seafoods will always fit your bill. If it overlooks the seashore, you cannot ask for more—except perhaps to be afloat in an old ship turned into a restaurant. You also like eateries that evoke a sense of distant times or places—ones that serve foods prepared from almost-forgotten recipes or that display turn-of-the-century splendor—dark and handsome, with original gaslight fixtures. Even a simple mural of a Parisian street scene will please you.

You are not one for heavily spiced foods, but rather prefer dishes that are light and flavorful made with delicate sauces. Your well-developed senses can detect the slightest scent, and you are bound to experience ecstasy in an establishment where ever so subtle aromas waft from the kitchen and finely flavored foods arouse your taste buds. Do you smell the faint scent of chocolate from the pastry case? If you decide you deserve a treat, you will probably order the thickest, deepest chocolate cake you can find, laced perhaps with a Grand Marnier.

Of course, no meal would be complete without the opening martini, the toast of champagne, and the bottle of wine. To the wine, add good food and lingering conversation among old friends, and Pisces has found a restaurant experience of poetic perfection. You are not unwilling to pay for such an evening. You often tip more than other signs (you don't want the waiters to think of you unfavorably), and you will always tip generously when you have occupied a table many hours.

A final word on social dining, Pisces. You may want to spare yourself some torture and opt like many of your dieting comrades to eat at home during this period. The sign of two fishes swimming in opposite directions, you are bound to be torn between your higher and lower selves when faced with a twenty-six-item dessert menu. If you must dine out, you will ultimately feel more secure in your diet resolve if *you* choose the restaurant—no small order for someone who usually defers this responsibility. Pick a place where you are familiar with the menu, or better still, where you know the management will prepare your order to specifications, and you will be in safe waters.

Special-Occasion Dining

Special-occasion dining can present you fish with exceptional dieting difficulties. New and different settings affect Pisces moods, and moods arouse your appetite. You might think it is your appetite for food, but look deeply into the clear waters of your psyche and you will probably discover what you hunger for is really something less concrete—yet more substantial: companionship, love, perhaps spiritual fullness. Know this about yourself, and you will be better equipped to enjoy any special occasion without sabotaging your reducing efforts.

Boating, sailing, or a day by the seashore is especially dangerous to watery Pisces. Relaxed by the motion of the water and mesmerized by the sight of billowy sails, you are likely to "throw caution to the wind," as the expression goes. Salt air does have a way of making a person hungry and thirsty, so even if your hosts have told you "don't bring anything," I suggest you do. Pack your own special food supply for these kinds of journeys, and you will be proud of your own tenacity afterward.

Unless you are very close with the people, it is not like you, unassuming

Pisces, to mention to your hosts that you are dieting, or to ask them to prepare for your needs. If the occasions do not come too frequently, you might consider eating less during the day, "saving" the calories for the big bash. While I am not an advocate of this type of eating, I also know from working with hundreds of Pisces clients that this strategy, more than most, seems to suit your psychological and emotional makeup. If you *do* decide to blow your diet for some celebration, don't abandon ship the rest of the week just because you went overboard once. Some of you tricky little fish have been known to use that one wedding or holiday meal as an excuse to bail out. Now, can you *imagine* that.

And watch your liquor consumption, too. You tend to forget what you are eating when you have had too many drinks.

By now, you might be asking yourself, 'What chance do I have anyway? I always am the one to make the parties, invite people to my home, keep up the Cousins Club meetings, and host the Thanksgiving, Christmas, and Groundhog Day celebrations.' It is true that your nurturing instincts and charm make you a natural for the host or hostess position. But you also get plenty of invitations yourself from friends and relations, endearing one. Be sure that during your dieting weeks you defer all burdensome entertaining responsibilities to everyone else. You may be gratified to learn you are loved despite the fact you weren't the one who cooked the meal.

Your Health

Physically, Pisces is a generally healthy sign, although your intense emotional life can cause you to suffer stress-related illnesses. We all have bad days, but the trick is not to let your feelings have such an overshadowing effect on you, Pisces, that they manifest in the body as disease. Even Western medicine now recognizes the relationship between mental and physical health. And in Pisces, which according to astrology rules the superconscious and subconscious minds, that relationship is particularly powerful. Your tendency to become pessimistic when you feel under the weather only delays recuperation. Rather than dwell on your problems and ailments, think about how soon you will be out of the sickbed. The more you think about recovery, the quicker it will come.

Your general dieting pattern is that you pile up the pounds rather than gain weight suddenly. That is because you are emotional eaters. You do not overeat at one meal but snack in between or grab some milk and cookies late at night—whenever you are in the mood for some "mothering."

You would do well to learn some stress-management techniques, Pisces, if you want to control your weight and retain your healthy constitution. Learn to find constructive outlets for your feelings. Write or keep a journal.

Realize that you can help your friends work out their problems without taking on their worries and emotional turmoil. Most Pisces are highly developed spiritually, and you may be drawn to various forms of yoga or meditation. These techniques have been shown to be effective in reducing stress and increasing relaxation—and are far better means of releasing tension than the use of mind-altering drugs. Besides, Pisces forms addictions far too easily. Self-hypnosis, visualization, and other mental techniques have also produced some successful results for dieters and might be particularly effective when practiced by Pisces' powerful mind. Remember, the key to maintaining your good health is a healthy emotional state. An optimistic Pisces is a healthy Pisces.

Pisces rules the feet, toes, and their muscles and bones (particularly, those of the heels and ankles). Pisces rules, as well, the pineal gland and circulation of the body's fluids to its extremities.

Problems and diseases to which Pisces are predisposed include:

Alcoholism	Fungus
Allergies	Gout
Bowel disorders	Muscular dystrophy
Bunions	Swollen glands
Duodenitis	Tender feet
Excessive mucus discharge	Water retention
Foot ailments	

The Pisces diet should be rich in vitamins C, B-12, and B-6, iron, folic acid, and pantothenic acid. The Pisces who frequently suffers from allergic reactions will find that the inclusion of plenty of foods containing vitamin C and pantothenic acid will help relieve symptoms. Most Pisces have slow metabolisms; vitamin B-12 should help strengthen it. Lack of the B vitamins can be detrimental to the health of your nervous system.

Iron phosphate is the Pisces cell salt. Cell salts are naturally occurring minerals that are normal constituents of the body cells. They are found in trace amounts in foods, and plants, animals, and human beings require these compounds for proper nutrition. Like vitamins, cell salts get used up. Of the twelve cell salts, iron phosphate is the only metal. It is found in the body mainly in the hemoglobin. Iron phosphate is necessary for healthy red blood cells. A deficiency causes red corpuscles to become weak and unable to fight off infection. It can also cause anemia. Iron phosphate aids oxygen distribution to all body tissue, too. All body cells and tissues need ample oxygen to function normally. Without enough oxygen, bodily processes slow down, causing a lethargic feeling. By increasing the amount of oxygen flowing to tissues, iron phosphate helps speed up recovery and promote rapid healing.

FOODS RICH IN IRON PHOSPHATE

Almonds	Lettuce
Barley	Lima beans
Beef	Onions
Beef liver	Radishes
Cabbage	Spinach
Cucumbers	Strawberries
Lentils	Walnuts

Up to now, one of your biggest reducing problems has been that most diets have left you feeling tired and listless. You probably have felt the diets you tried were not "balanced" for you, and you have been right. Pisces are susceptible to iron phosphate deficiency, which leads to feelings of fatigue, headache, and depression. Note that many of the foods listed above, which are rich in iron phosphate, have been included in your Pisces Reducing Diet. Also be sure to note the various foods on your maintenance foods lists. After you lose your desired weight, design your menus around these foods, which are so important for your unique chemical and physical makeup.

Pisces Daily Nutritional Supplements

- One general multivitamin with minerals
- Time-release B-complex B-100
- 2,000 mg vitamin C with bioflavonoids

Remember, Pisces . . .

This diet is uniquely prepared to address your sun sign and *should not be interchanged with any other Sun Sign Diet.* It is important that you follow the diet exactly as it appears, for optimum weight loss and assimilation. Before starting your Pisces diet, carefully read "General Diet and Mainte-nance Guidelines for All Sun Signs," found at the beginning of this book. Remember, drink 8 glasses of water daily.

I know, Pisces, that you have been confused with all the diets on the market, wondering which one is the best choice for you. There are no more decisions to be made, because you have just found the Pisces Reducing Diet, designed specifically to meet your nutritional, chemical, and behav-ioral needs. No more wishing for the perfect diet . . . your dreams have been answered.

Good luck, and *go for it.*

The Pisces
Seven-Day
Reducing Diet

The Pisces Seven-Day Reducing Diet has been designed to meet all your nutritional needs and to incorporate foods that will help you deal with stress. It is important that you try not to eat processed or refined foods (white bread, white sugar) and that you eat natural, unadulterated foods as much as possible. Your diet also includes foods with high concentrations of vitamin B-1 to protect your sensitive digestive system, vitamin B-6 for regulating your protein metabolism, vitamin B-12 for the production of red blood cells, pantothenic acid, and folic acid. Vitamin C foods have been included to work with the pantothenic acid foods to keep your body producing antibodies that battle viruses. In addition you will note that the Pisces Seven-Day Reducing Diet is rich in potassium foods, which will act as a diuretic to your water-retentive body. Potassium will also be very beneficial to you for your leg cramps and fatigue. If your sodium/potassium level is not balanced, the result is a toxic buildup of sodium that is locked in as "water weight."

Your Pisces Reducing Diet, enriched with extraordinary amounts of the B vitamins, will allow you to lose weight without the feeling of lethargy or depression. In fact, I guarantee you will have more energy than you have ever had before.

You may choose to try a diet aid known in the United States as Glucomannan. It can be purchased in any health food store. It is extracted from the Japanese konjac root, a tuber that is very high in fiber. A final monograph on its effectiveness has not yet been established by the FDA, as it has no history of use in the United States before 1958; however, the konjac root has been cultivated and eaten in Asia for over a thousand years.

Glucomannan contributes to a decrease in cholesterol and triglyceride levels, and aids in maintaining low-density lipoprotein levels. It acts as a dietary fiber to increase viscosity and moisture content of food as it is digested, so that it forms a smooth, soft mass that moves easily through the intestinal tract. Digestion is slowed, so normal blood sugar levels are maintained after a meal.

In addition I would like to recommend the use of 2 tablespoons of apple-cider vinegar in an 8-ounce glass of water or no-sodium club soda. Stir and sip slowly with your food. Like wine (but with few calories) it is a fermented product rich in potassium and phosphorus. It also helps reduce cravings for alcohol.

You will note, as you look at the Pisces Reducing Diet, that some foods are marked by an asterisk (*). It indicates that the explanation of the food value, and its importance, appears in the pages following the diet, in the section "Notes to Pisces Seven-Day Reducing Diet."

At the end of the chapter you will find a binge day menu. The Pisces Total Binge Day has been designed so that if you must "blow your diet" you will not feel guilty. The calories and combination will not allow you to lose weight, but you should not gain weight either. It has been included so that you do not tear your hair out if you feel that you cannot go on any further. Try to keep your binge days down to four a month and never use a binge day until you have completed Day Five of your diet.

You may continue on the reducing diet as long as you wish. It is highly nutritious, available, and easy. Just make sure to take yourself into consideration as a number one priority, and do your shopping at the beginning of the week so that you have everything you need to ensure your success.

One final hint: Pisces, when you feel you are overcome with an emotional problem and wish to grab something, remember your comfort foods:

- A hot cup of herbal or regular tea. I think you will find the tea satisfies that Piscean urge for warmth and solace. If you wish the uplift of caffeine, choose one of the many flavorful varieties on the market. Darjeeling, orange pekoe, mint, Japanese, Chinese Formosa oolong, jasmine, Ceylon breakfast, and English breakfast are most pleasant. Add a little sugar substitute or drink it with a dash of lemon and/or cinnamon, and you have a tasty, low-calorie drink that will assuage your hunger, fill your hands, and keep your body warm.
- A cup of Lipton Trim Soup or any low-sodium chicken soup. Chicken soup is also wonderfully calming and satisfying.
- Water, water, water. Two glasses will calm your nerves. Try it.

You, Pisces, wished upon a star, and your dream has come true. Your very own Pisces Sun Sign Diet is your way to a "heavenly body."

DAY ONE

Pisces is a water sign. And oh, how you retain water. Especially around the ankles. It is important that you start your diet with a combination of food that will rid the body of water, which appears to give you that bloated look and of course registers on the scales.

BREAKFAST

½ cantaloupe*, or ½ fresh pineapple*, or 1 whole papaya

black coffee, tea, or water

MIDMORNING SNACK

½ cantaloupe

LUNCH

1 lb. fresh or frozen steamed asparagus* seasoned with lemon juice and garlic pepper.

black coffee, tea, or water

MIDAFTERNOON SNACK

fresh or frozen steamed asparagus (as much as you want) and 1 sliced cucumber

DINNER

2 large baked potatoes,* seasoned with garlic pepper, chervil, and poppyseeds

water, water; herbal tea, or regular tea

Remember, drink 8 glasses of water every day.

All of the above foods are excellent diuretics when eaten exactly as specified. In addition, the cantaloupe and baked potatoes are a rich source of potassium, which will force the sodium out of your system. You will urinate a great deal today. Do not use lemon juice on your cantaloupe. Do not drink any beverage but water, herbal tea, regular tea, or black coffee. Do not put milk in your coffee—it will stop enzyme action.

DAY TWO

BREAKFAST

3–4 kiwis,* sliced, with 1 heaping Tbsp. peanut butter*

black coffee, tea, or water

MIDMORNING SNACK

2 cups tea, with sugar substitute and lemon if desired

LUNCH

1 cup gazpacho*

2-egg mushroom, artichoke, or broccoli omelette* prepared with very little margarine

diet no-sodium soda, black coffee, or tea

MIDAFTERNOON SNACK

1 cup Lipton Trim Soup

or

1 can Yoo-Hoo diet chocolate drink

10 pistachio nuts*

DINNER

1 cup Lipton Trim Soup

¼–½ baked or broiled chicken,* seasoned with lots of ginger*

1 cup lightly steamed mushrooms

1 medium cucumber on a bed of lettuce, seasoned with dill

no-sodium diet soda, tea, or no-sodium Perrier with a twist of lime

Remember, drink 8 glasses of water every day.

DAY THREE

BREAKFAST

> 1 apple,* sliced, with 1 oz. Edam, Swiss, or Gouda cheese

> *or*

> 1 Tbsp. peanut butter

> tea

LUNCH

> ½ cantaloupe or 1 large apple, with ½ cup cottage cheese

> 2 sesame breadsticks

> 2 cups tea

MIDAFTERNOON SNACK

> 10 pistachio nuts

> 1 cup Lipton Trim Soup

DINNER

> ***Veal Scallopine* in Marsala, with Artichokes and Apricots***
> 4 oz. veal scallopine, sautéed in ¼ cup Marsala wine with 1 cup water-pack or frozen artichokes, and 5 dried apricots; simmer until veal is brown.

> salad of watercress,* parsley,* endive,* and sliced tomato with basil, seasoned with lemon juice and garlic pepper

> 1 35-calorie Jell-O frozen pudding pop

> 1 can Yoo-Hoo diet chocolate drink

> *Remember, drink 8 glasses of water every day.*

DAY FOUR

BREAKFAST

Pineapple Cheese Delight*

Blend ¼ fresh pineapple with ¼ cup skim-milk ricotta cheese or ½ cup plain yogurt* in blender. Use sugar substitute and 2 ice cubes and blend until frothy. Absolutely delicious.

LUNCH

1 cup natural instant miso soup* (Edwards & Sons is an excellent brand.)

⅔ cup brown rice* served with just a scant hint of butter seasoned with herbs of your choice

or

½ avocado* with ½ cup diced chicken and 2 olives with 2 tsp. reduced-calorie dressing (eliminate miso soup with this choice)

DINNER

1 cup gazpacho

4–6 oz. baked or broiled salmon,* filet of sole, flounder, halibut, trout, or cod prepared with lemon juice and garlic pepper

1 small green pepper

all the D-Zerta diet gelatin you want

tea or no-sodium Perrier with a twist of lime

Remember, drink 8 glasses of water every day.

DAY FIVE

BREAKFAST

½ cantaloupe*

or

1 cup fresh strawberries*

or

1 small banana*

5 almonds*

LUNCH

3½ oz. canned tomato herring*

1 Tbsp. horseradish and 1 whole tomato with ½ bunch watercress*

or

up to 3 cups fresh fruit salad of your choice

tea or coffee

Nothing else.

DINNER

1 cup Lipton Trim Soup

¼–½ baked chicken* seasoned with lots of ginger and 1 cup lightly steamed mushrooms* and parsley*

sliced cucumber seasoned with dill on a bed of lettuce

no-sodium Perrier with a twist of lime

tea, herb tea, or Yoo-Hoo diet chocolate drink

Remember, drink 8 glasses of water every day.

DAY SIX

BREAKFAST

½ cantaloupe

or

1 cup fresh strawberries

or

1 small banana

¼ cup skim-milk ricotta cheese or cottage cheese

MIDMORNING SNACK

1 cup hot tea

LUNCH

1 large cucumber sliced in half spread with ¼ cup farmer cheese, 4 green olives, and 4 anchovy filets

tea or no-sodium diet soda

or

up to 3 cups fresh fruit* salad of your choice

tea or black coffee

Nothing else.

DINNER

4 oz. chicken livers* sautéed in dry sherry, seasoned with garlic and ½ medium-sized onion

2 cups fresh salad of watercress, parsley, and cucumber, with low-calorie dressing of your choice (not more than total 70 calories)

iced tea, hot tea, or apple-cider vinegar and water

or

Flounder* Wrapped with Broccoli* in Wine

Sauté 4–5 oz. flounder wrapped with broccoli until done in ½ cup dry white wine.

watercress and spinach salad (as much as you want), seasoned with lemon juice and garlic pepper

no-sodium Perrier with a twist of line

EVENING SNACK

1 35-calorie Jell-O frozen pudding pop, strawberry

Remember, drink 8 glasses of water every day.

DAY SEVEN

BRUNCH

4 oz. orange juice

Pita Bread Tuna Sandwich*
Combine the following and toss in whole wheat pita bread: alfalfa sprouts, ½ cup lettuce, ¼ cup red cabbage, 1 scallion, ¼ cup chopped green pepper, ½ tomato, 1 cup Monterey Jack cheese, and 2 Tbsp. Pritikin no-oil salad dressing.

iced or hot tea, or no-sodium diet soda

or

4 oz. orange juice

2 scrambled eggs (use little margarine)

1 toasted bagel with 1 Tbsp. cream cheese

coffee with ½ cup milk

DINNER

*Papaya Pineapple Shrimp**
Sauté 4–6 oz. shrimp in 2 Tbsp. orange juice concentrate mixed with whole cubed papaya and ¼ cup fresh pineapple.

1 cup cauliflower with endive

or

1–2 lb. whole broiled or steamed lobster* (no butter, use lemon juice)

1 baked potato seasoned with lemon juice and garlic pepper

iced or hot tea, or espresso

D-Zerta diet gelatin—as much as you want

Remember, drink 8 glasses of water every day.

Notes to Pisces Seven-Day Reducing Diet

Pisces Diet Notes—Day One
* Both cantaloupe and pineapple are rich in your needed vitamin C and have excellent diuretic properties. No milk is allowed on this day because it will stop the enzyme production and you will not have a good weight loss.

* Asparagus is an excellent diuretic vegetable. It is a good source of vitamins C and B-1, and folic acid. In addition, it is rich in the enzyme asparagine, which helps to break up accumulated fats in the cells.

* Potatoes are rich in potassium and will be most filling. They act as nature's diuretic and rid the body of excess water. When combined with the rest of your day's menu you will notice excellent results when you step on the scale tomorrow morning.

Pisces Diet Notes—Day Two

* The kiwi and peanut butter are excellent examples of readily absorbed fructose and protein.

* Gazpacho is an alkaline vegetable soup that helps to rid the body of toxins, makes you feel more energized, and has all of the necessary nutrients from your maintenance lists. Prepare in the following manner:

Pisces Gazpacho
2 cups tomato juice
¼ cup diced cucumber
¼ cup diced celery
¼ cup diced green pepper
1 tsp. Worcestershire sauce
1 tsp. fresh parsley
2 Tbsp. Pritikin no-oil salad dressing

Combine all ingredients and chill overnight. Makes two servings.

* Egg omelette is high in protein, low in carbohydrates
* Pistachio nuts —remember, only 10. They are rich in phosphorus, iron, potassium, and magnesium, a quick pick-me-up when you feel tired.
* Chicken is naturally high in your needed vitamin B-6. It is low in calories, high in protein. The ginger nourishes the nervous system, and helps fight fatigue and digestive problems.

Pisces Diet Notes—Day Three

* Apple is a good source of sodium, potassium, magnesium, and vitamins B and C; coupled with peanut butter or cheese, it provides additional protein and appetite satiation. Helpful combination for those Pisces nerves.

* Watercress, parsley, and endive should be used as often as possible. They are an excellent source of calcium and vitamin C. They're rich enzyme power aids in the removal of toxins from the body. And if that is not enough reason for including them in your diet, note that they are also rich in folic acid. Endive is another excellent source of folic acid.

* Veal is a low-calorie, easily digested quality protein.

Pisces Diet Notes—Day Four

* Pineapple is rich in bromelin and chlorine, two properties that stimulate urination. Water-retentive Pisces, take heed.

* The yogurt will make your breakfast vitamin B-12 inclusive and will cleanse the intestinal tract of unwanted bacteria.

* Miso soup is an excellent source of soy bean–rich protein, containing vitamin B-12, iron, phosphorus, and calcium. This is a particularly calming soup for Pisces and should be used often in your maintenance program. Similarly, the brown rice and avocado are both excellent sources of the B vitamins.

* Salmon is an excellent low-cholesterol, high-protein food that is extremely rich in vitamins A, B, and E.

Pisces Diet Notes—Day Five

* The almonds are a good source of iron. If you choose them you will have an extra boost of energy to get you through to lunch.

* Fruits are all high in vitamin C, potassium, and folic acid, a good energy source and a positive diuretic aid for Pisces.

* Herring is rich in protein and vitamin B-12, which is so very important for your nervous system.

* Chicken is rich in vitamin B-6, which aids in protein metabolism and minimizes water retention.

* Mushrooms are an excellent source of pantothenic acid, which helps in the production of antibodies, thus building resistance to disease.

* Parsley and watercress supply a good amount of vitamin C.

Pisces Diet Notes—Day Six

* Fresh fruit salad has the most dynamic enzyme action of any food. It gets your fires burning and stimulates metabolic action, which helps oxidize your food more quickly. No milk is to be combined with fruit. Not even one swallow. It will stop enzyme action.

* Chicken livers are a source of iron, pantothenic acid, folic acid, and B-12, all of which are Pisces' nutritional requirements.

* Similarly, you will find the combination of flounder and broccoli meets your chemical nutritional requirements. The choice is yours.

Pisces Diet Notes—Day Seven

This is an excellent protein-packed day.

* Tuna is rich in vitamin B-6, and when combined with vegetables is a rich satisfying balance of protein and carbohydrates.

* Both the shrimp and lobster are good sources of vitamin B-12 and iodine. The cauliflower and lobster are chock full of pantothenic acid.

PISCES TOTAL BINGE DAY

Pisces, with all the extreme pressures and responsibilities you undertake, there are times you just must let go. However, this time your digression will not lead to guilt because it has been programmed into your Pisces Reducing Diet. When you reach the point where you "can't go on," choose a binge day. Enjoy the day. The following day you must return to your Pisces Seven-Day Reducing Diet.

Before You Binge

1. Drink water.
2. Drink water.
3. Drink water.
4. Rest.
5. Brush your teeth and rinse with your favorite mouthwash.
6. Chew sugarless gum for 20 minutes.

You may find that the desire to binge has passed. However, if you are still suffering from intense food frustration, follow these basic rules:

Rule One

Under no circumstances should you ever binge before completing Day Four of your reducing diet. This will ensure a maximum weight loss with a minimum of food frustration.

Rule Two

If, for example, you binge on the sixth day of your diet, resume your diet the following day (Day Seven) with the menu for Day Six. If you binge for just one meal, such as lunch on Day Six, resume your reducing diet with dinner on Day Six of your reducing diet.

Rule Three

Bingeing is for when you get that creepy, anxious feeling, when you feel like pulling out your hair—strand by strand—and you cannot endure dieting for even one more moment. Before you climb the walls, give yourself a binge day. It's hoped that this will not be necessary more than four times a month.

Rule Four

After you have lost your first 10 pounds, you may vary your binge day with the binge day of the sun sign opposite yours, which is Virgo.

Remember, an occasional binge day—when necessary—will still allow you to lose weight (without guilt). Here, Pisces, is your binge day menu.

Binge Day Menu

BREAKFAST

4 oz. orange juice

1 thick bagel (any type)
1 Tbsp. cream cheese
2 oz. lox with sliced onion

LUNCH

1 all-beef frankfurter with roll, smothered in sauerkraut

or

1 slice pizza

4 oz. vanilla, chocolate, strawberry, or coffee ice cream or ice cream cone

Yoo-Hoo diet chocolate drink or light beer

DINNER

2 glasses wine or champagne, or 1 martini or Bloody Mary (optional)

Parmesan Fettucine Broccoli

8 oz. cup fettucine served with 1 cup broccoli spears, Parmesan cheese, chopped chives and basil prepared with 1 tsp. butter or margarine.

2-inch-wide slice garlic bread

½ cup sherbet

Remember, drink 8 glasses of water every day.

Maintaining Your Ideal Weight

Pisces Maintenance Foods for Optimum Health

When you have achieved your desired weight goal you should follow a maintenance diet rich in the specific nutrients that you, Pisces, need each and every day.

Vitamin C

Two of vitamin C's more important jobs are concerned with the body's ability to resist dangerous bacteria and infection. Vitamin C aids in the formation of collagen. Collagen is a substance that constitutes about 35 to 40 percent of the body's protein. It fortifies cells, keeping them in their natural formations and allowing them to resist any invading infections. Vitamin C is also extremely important in the production of white blood cells, which protect the body from invading bacteria. The proper intake of vitamin C will reduce Pisces' susceptibility to allergies, too.

FOODS RICH IN VITAMIN C

Alfalfa	Blueberries
Almonds	Broccoli
Apples	Brussels sprouts
Asparagus	Cantaloupe
Bananas	Carrots
Beets	Celery

Chicken
Cranberries
Currants
Grapefruit
Green peppers
Lemons
Oranges
Orange juice

Paprika
Parsley
Pineapple
Skim milk
Strawberries
Tomatoes
Watercress

Vitamin B-12

Vitamin B-12 is essential for healthy metabolism of proteins, fats, nerve tissue, and carbohydrates. Pisces have the slowest and least dynamic metabolism of the twelve signs. A diet rich in vitamin B-12 should help strengthen your metabolism. (Remember, Pisces, a healthy metabolism is crucial to a reducing diet's success.) It is also important for the maintenance of a healthy nervous system, and can be helpful in alleviating insomnia. The Pisces hectic schedule is likely to wear your nerves thin and at times can cause sleeplessness. Keep this list of foods in mind on your next late evening date; you'll appreciate it when you finally fall into bed and are ready to relax.

FOODS RICH IN VITAMIN B-12

Alfalfa sprouts
American cheese
Beef
Bran
Chicken
Chicken liver
Cottage cheese
Dairy products
Eggs
Green peas
Herring
Liver

Milk
Muscle meats
Pickled foods
Prunes
Raw oysters
Sardines
Shellfish
Skim milk
Soy bean products
Swiss cheese
Trout
Yogurt

Folic Acid

Folic acid is a member of the B-complex vitamins, and is most effective when taken with vitamin B-12. Folic acid also works well with vitamin C and pantothenic acid. One of folic acid's functions is carrying carbon, which is necessary for the production of red blood cells. A deficiency of folic acid can cause anemia or atherosclerosis. Folic acid is also important for the proper function of glands. Pisces rules the thymus gland, thus this area could prove to be a sensitive one.

FOODS RICH IN FOLIC ACID

Asparagus	Kale
Avocado	Lamb
Beet greens	Lima beans
Brewer's yeast	Liver
Broccoli	Peanuts
Brown rice	Potatoes
Chard	Smoked ham
Cottage cheese	Spinach
Endive	Turnips
Green leafy vegetables	Wheat bran
Kidney	

Pantothenic Acid

Pantothenic acid is a member of the vitamin B complex and is most effective when taken with B-12 and B-6. Pantothenic acid primarily helps fortify the body's defense against disease by aiding in the production of antibodies. Pisces rules the lymphatic system, where these antibodies battle bacteria and viruses. Foods rich in pantothenic acid will maintain a healthy lymphatic system.

FOODS RICH IN PANTOTHENIC ACID

Avocados	Eggs
Beef kidney	Lobster
Beef liver	Mushrooms
Broccoli	Orange juice
Cauliflower	Pineapple juice
Chicken heart	Skim milk
Chicken liver	Watermelon
Chick peas	

Vitamin B-6

Vitamin B-6 has numerous functions, ranging from preventing tooth decay to relieving acne. It is "nature's antihistamine," as it is crucial to the body's production of antibodies. Vitamin B-6 is also quite effective in alleviating water retention, a typical problem for the water sign Pisces. Recent research has indicated that asthma, to which Pisces are prone, can be greatly relieved by extra vitamin B-6 intake. It also seems to alleviate painful burning feet, another common Pisces ailment.

FOODS RICH IN VITAMIN B-6

Alfalfa sprouts	Lentils
Avocados	Mackerel
Bananas	Peanuts
Beef liver	Prunes
Brewer's yeast	Salmon
Cabbage	Skim milk
Chicken liver	Sunflower seeds
Egg yolk	Tuna
Fish	Wheat germ
Green peppers	White meat chicken
Honey	Whole milk
Lamb	

Iron

Iron is one of the more important minerals in the body. It works in the red blood cells, uniting copper with protein to produce hemoglobin. Iron also assists in the production of globulin, which transports oxygen to the muscles, giving them the ability to contract. Lack of iron can lead to anemia. A diet sufficient in iron will ensure proper oxygenation and a good supply of energy—important to Pisces, who tends to overestimate the body's endurance, and as a result, gets run down keeping up a hectic, romantic schedule.

FOODS RICH IN IRON

Alfalfa sprouts	Broccoli
Almonds	Chicken
Avocados	Dried beans
Beef	Egg yolk
Beets	Green beans

Green peas	Mushrooms
Kidney	Olives
Lamb	Onions
Liver	Red wines

Pisces Sample Maintenance Menu

When you reach your desired goal, please follow the maintenance eating hints found in "General Diet and Maintenance Guidelines for All Sun Signs" at the beginning of this book for proper calculations of caloric intake.

I'm including a sample maintenance menu based on your sun sign for optimal Pisces maintenance. When you create your own menus for yourself, try to choose many of the foods you eat from your Pisces Maintenance Foods lists.

2,000 Calories Per Day

BREAKFAST	CALORIES
6 oz. orange juice	83
2-egg tomato and onion omelette (1 tomato, ¼ chopped onion, 1 tsp. diet margarine)	275
1 slice whole wheat toast	58
1 Tbsp. apple butter	37
coffee with milk	25
	478

LUNCH	
1 juicy cheeseburger	324
1 American roll	114
10 french fries	137
½ cup coleslaw	86
1 light beer	95
	756

MIDAFTERNOON SNACK	
12 pecans	50

DINNER

4 oz. dry white wine (optional)	83
6 clams on the half shell	120
6 oz. shrimp with green peppers and 1 oz. peanuts	372
1 cup salad of alfalfa sprouts, cabbage, endive, and raw broccoli	100
	675

EVENING SNACK

1 cup fresh strawberries	45

TOTAL DAILY CALORIES   2,004

Remember, drink 8 glasses of water every day.

Restaurant Eating the Pisces Way

Perhaps you have seen the following dishes on restaurant menus. Both the dishes and the types of restaurants chosen will appeal to your Pisces palate and satisfy your nutritional needs. Note that all of the recommended dishes contain the nutrients specified in your Pisces Maintenance Foods lists.

I know, Pisces, that often you leave the choice of a restaurant to others, saying, "Oh, it doesn't matter where we go . . . I like everything," even when you secretly hope their choice will be Japanese, Italian, Chinese, or Continental seafood fare. I've tried to cover all these bases.

In all menus, one appetizer plus one entrée equals approximately 600–700 calories.

Italian Restaurant

APPETIZERS

2 glasses dry white wine (Pisces, you may opt to skip an appetizer and instead enjoy wine with your meal.)

Prosciutto with fresh fruit

ENTRÉES

Assorted fresh fish in red wine sauce

Angel hair pasta with fresh vegetables (ask for no oil)

Stuffed veal chop

Breast of chicken in garlic

Japanese Restaurant

APPETIZERS

Fresh clams with ginger sauce

Boiled vegetables, served with vinegar and sesame seeds

ENTRÉES

Sushi

Sukiyaki

Casserole of fish and vegetables

Prime rib broiled with green onion

Chinese Restaurant

APPETIZERS

Egg with crabmeat or shrimp

Fish soup

ENTRÉES

Beef with scallions

Braised fish with sweet and sour sauce

Diced chicken with almonds

Eggplant with garlic sauce

Seafood/Continental Restaurant

APPETIZERS

Sliced tomato and red onion salad

Watercress soup with dill

ENTRÉES

Boiled or broiled lobster dipped in lemon juice—not butter

Avocado and shrimp salad

Brook trout stuffed with crabmeat

Broiled swordfish steak, in a lemon/wine sauce

Bibliography

Adams, Catherine, *Nutritive Value of American Foods*. Pamphlet prepared by Agricultural Research Service, U.S. Department of Agriculture, Washington, D.C., 1975.

Adams, Rex. *Miracle Medicine Foods*. West Nyack, N.Y.: Parker, 1977.

Adams, Ruth. *The Complete Home Guide to All the Vitamins*. New York: Larchmont Books, 1972.

Anderson, Jefferson. *Sun Signs, Moon Signs*. New York: Dell, 1978.

Arroyo, Stephen. *Astrology, Psychology, and the Four Elements*. Vancouver, WA: CRCS, 1975.

Bartlett, John. *Bartlett's Familiar Quotations*. 13th ed. Boston: Little, Brown, 1955.

Beilier, Henry G. *Food Is Your Best Medicine*. New York: Random House, 1965.

Bircher-Brenner, M. *Eating Your Way to Health*. New York: Penguin Books, 1973.

Bragg, Paul C. *The Miracle of Fasting*. Burbank, CA: Health Science, 1969.

Brewster, Letitia, and Michael F. Jacobson. *The Changing American Diet*. Pamphlet prepared by Center for Science in the Public Interest, Washington, D.C., 1978.

Bricklin, Mark. *The Practical Encyclopedia of Natural Healing*. Emmaus, PA. Rodale Press, 1976.

Bruch, Hilde. *Eating Disorders*. New York: Basic Books, 1973.

Buscaglia, Leo. *Living, Loving, and Learning*. New York: Ballantine Books, 1982.

———. *Loving Each Other*. Thorofare, N.J.: Slack, 1984.

———. *Love*. New York: Fawcett, 1972.

Carrington, Hereward. *Fasting for Health and Long Life*. Mokelumne Hill, CA: Health Research, 1953.

Carter, C. E. O. *An Encyclopedia of Psychological Astrology*. London: Theosophical Society, 1963.

Clark, Linda. *Know Your Nutrition*. New Canaan, CT: Keats, 1973.

———. *Rejuvenation*. Old Greenwich, CT: Devin-Adair, 1979.

Corbin, Cheryl. *Nutrition*. New York: Holt, Rinehart and Winston, 1980.

Cornell, Howard Leslie. *Encyclopedia of Medical Astrology*. 3rd ed. New York: Weiser, 1972.

Cunningham, Donna. *An Astrological Guide to Self-Awareness*. Vancouver, WA: CRCS, 1978.

Davidson, William M. *Davidson's Medical Astrology*. Monroe, N.Y.: Astrological Bureau, 1979.

Davison, Ronald. *Mundane Astrology*. New York: National Astrological Society, 1975.

DeRosis, Helen A. *Women and Anxiety*. New York: Delacorte Press, 1979.

Dietary Goals for the U.S. 2nd ed. U.S. Senate, Select Committee on Nutrition and Human Needs. Washington, D.C.: Government Printing Office, 1978.

Dobin, Joel C. *The Astrological Secrets of the Hebrew Sages*. New York: Inner Traditions International, 1983.

Duff, Howard M. *Astrological Types*. Duff, 1948.

Duz, M. *A Practical Treatise of Astral Medicine and Therapeutics*. London: W. Foulsham, 1966.

Ebertin, Rheinhold. *Psychological Interpretation of the Chart*. New York: National Astrological Society, 1973.

Ehret, Arnold. *Mucusless Diet Healing System.* New York: Benedict Lust, 1976.

Epstein, Alan. *Psychodynamics of Injunctions.* York Beach, ME: Weiser, 1984.

Evans, Jane A. *Twelve Doors to the Soul: Astrology of the Inner Self.* London: Theosophical Society, 1979.

Fredericks, Carlton. *High-Fiber Way to Total Health.* New York: Pocket Books, 1976.

Garten, M.O. *The Natural and Drugless Way for Better Health.* New York: Arc Books, 1969.

Gauquelin, Michael. *How Cosmic and Atmospheric Energies Influence Your Health.* New York: Aurora, 1971.

Geddes, Sheila. *Astrology and Health.* Northamptonshire, England: Aquarian, 1981.

George, Llewellyn. *A to Z Horoscope and Delineator.* 29th ed. St. Paul, MN: Llewellyn, 1973.

Gerras, Charles (ed). *The Encyclopedia of Common Diseases.* Emmaus, PA: Rodale Press, 1976.

Goodman, Linda. *Sun Signs.* New York: Taplinger, 1968.

Gray, Henry. *Gray's Anatomy.* New York: Bounty Books, 1977.

Hand, Robert. *Horoscope Symbols.* Gloucester, MA: Para Research, 1981.

————. *Planets in Transit: Life Cycles for Living.* Gloucester, MA: Para Research, 1976.

————. *Planets in Youth.* Rockport, MA: Para Research, 1977.

Jacobson, Roger. *Calculation of the True Nodes.* New York: National Astrological Society, 1972.

Johnson, Robert A. *We: Understanding the Psychology of Romantic Love.* San Francisco: Harper and Row, 1983.

Keane, Jerryl L. *Practical Astrology: How to Make It Work For You.* West Nyack, N.Y.: Parker, 1967.

Kundalini Research Institute. *Foods for Health and Healing.* Berkeley/Pomona, CA: Spiritual Community/ K.R.I., 1983.

Landscheidt, Theodore. *Structures of Prime Numbers and Distances Between Planets.* New York: National Astrological Society, 1973.

Lappé, Frances Moore. *Diet for a Small Planet.* New York: Ballantine Books, 1974.

Lundsted, Betty. *Transits: The Time of Your Life.* York Beach, ME: Weiser, 1980.

Marks, Tracy. *How to Handle Your T-Square.* Arlington, MA: Sagittarius Rising, 1979.

Marsh, Edward E. *How to be Healthy with Natural Foods.* New York: Gramercy, n.d.

Marshall, Mel. *Real Living with Real Foods.* New York: Fawcett, 1974.

Martine. *Sexual Astrology.* New York: Dell, 1976.

Meyer, Michael R. *A Handbook for the Humanistic Astrologer.* Garden City, N.Y.: Anchor Books, 1974.

Michaels, Marjorie. *Stay Healthy With Wine.* New York: New American Library, 1981.

Newman, Laura. *Make Your Juicer Your Drugstore.* Simi Valley, CA: Benedict Lust, 1972.

Pearson, Durk, and Sandy Shaw. *The Life Extension Companion.* New York: Warner Books, 1983.

Pennington, Jean A. T., and Helen Nichols Church. *Food Values of Portions Commonly Used.* 14th ed. New York: Harper and Row, 1985.

Raman, B. V. *The Spiritual Value of Astrology.* New York: National Astrological Society, 1972.

Raphael. *Raphael's Medical Astrology.* Ontario, Canada: Provoker, 1978.

Recommended Dietary Allowances. Washington, D.C.: National Academy of Sciences, 1979.

Reuben, David. *Everything You Always Wanted to Know About Nutrition.* New York: Avon Books, 1972.

Rosenblum, Bernard. *The Astrologer's Guide to Counseling.* Reno, NV: CRCS, 1983.

Rudhyar, Danr. *The Sun Is Also a Star.* New York: E. P. Dutton, 1975.

Sakokian, Frances, and Louis S. Acker. *The Astrologer's Handbook.* New York: Harper and Row, 1973.

Scott, Cyril. *Cider Vinegar.* Northamptonshire, England: Aquarian 1968.

Schull, Martin. *Celestial Harmony.* York Beach, ME: Weiser, 1980.

Shelton, Herbert M. *Fasting Can Save Your Life.* San Antonio, TX: Natural Hygiene Press, 1981.

———. *Food Combining Made Easy.* San Antonio, TX: Dr. Shelton's Health School, 1951.

———. *Superior Nutrition.* San Antonio, TX: Dr. Shelton's Health School, 1951.

Simonson, Maria, and Joan Rattner Heilman. *The Complete University Medical Diet.* New York: Warner Books, 1983.

Starck, Marcia. *Astrology Key to Holistic Health.* Birmingham, MI: Seek It Publications, 1982.

Sutton, Nancy. *Adventures in Cooking with Health Foods.* New York: Pyramid Press, 1972.

Tarnower, Herman. *The Complete Scarsdale Medical Diet.* New York: Rawson Wade, 1978.

Townley, John. *Planets in Love: Exploring Your Sexual Needs.* Gloucester, MA: Para Research, 1978.

Verrett, Jacqueline, and Jean Carper. *Eating May Be Hazardous to Your Health.* New York: Simon and Schuster, 1974.

Viscott, David. *How to Live With Another Person.* New York: Pocket Books, 1974.

Wangemann, Edith. *The Birthplace Houses.* New York: National Astrological Society, 1972.

Wanson, George. *Nutrition and Your Mind.* New York: Harper and Row, 1972.

Wassmer, Arthur C. *Making Contact.* New York: Fawcett, 1978.

Weingarten, Henry. *The Study of Astrology.* New York: ASI, 1977.

Weiss, Clara A. *Astrological Keys to Self-Actualization and Self-Realization.* New York: Weiser, 1980.

Wentzler, Rich. *The Vitamin Book.* New York: Gramercy, 1978.

Zerof, Herbert G. *Finding Intimacy.* New York: Random House, 1978.

Zolar. *It's All in the Stars.* New York: Fawcett, 1962.

INDEX

BIOGRAPHY

Gayle Black, B.A., M.P.H., majored in psychology at Adelphi University, Long Island, New York, and received a master's degree in health care and hospital administration from C. W. Post Graduate School, Greenvale, New York. She is licensed by the State of New York and has taught both yoga and astrology in the Nassau County School System. She has studied nutrition and diet therapy for the past fourteen years, both in Europe and the United States, and has served as a consultant to physicians. She presently lives in New York City, where she maintains a private practice.

Ms. Black was assistant administrator of Bennett Community Hospital, Fort Lauderdale, Florida, and was elected U.S. Representative in Health Care for one year at St. Thomas's Hospital, London, England. For five years she held the position of assistant professor and deputy chairperson of the Health Care Management Department at St. Francis College, Brooklyn, New York.

She is a member of the American Public Health Association, American Association of University Professors, American Hospital Association of America, Eta Sigma Phi Health Honor Society, the Royal Society of Health, and the American Federation of Astrologers.